Culture, Madness and Wellbeing

Jason Lee

Culture, Madness and Wellbeing

Beyond the Sociology of Insanity

Springer

Jason Lee
Leicester Media School
De Montfort University
Leicester, UK

ISBN 978-3-031-37529-3   ISBN 978-3-031-37530-9 (eBook)
https://doi.org/10.1007/978-3-031-37530-9

This Springer imprint is published by the registered company Springer Nature Switzerland AG
The registered company address is: Gewerbestrasse 11, 6330 Cham, Switzerland

If I had feelings, I'd have a nervous breakdown.
Andy Warhol.
Blessed are the cracked, for they shall let in the light.
Groucho Marx.
The madman is not the man who has lost his reason. The madman is the man who has lost everything except his reason.
G.K. Chesterton.

Acknowledgements

This book was completed while I was the recipient of a British Academy Innovation Fellowship 2022–2024, IF\220089. My thanks to the British Academy and to my innovation partner Jones Bamber Productions.

Many thanks to Professor Brian Brown, Dr Nishi Yarger, Professor Rusi Jaspal, Professor Justin Smith, and Professor Stuart Price for reading versions of this manuscript and research support.

I would especially like to thank all those who contributed to the interviews in Chap. 5, offering their invaluable insight and precious time.

Thanks to my family during the writing process, especially to Rebecca Griffith for her input.

Many thanks to Springer for their patience.

Elements of Chap. 2 on post-traumatic stress disorder appeared as—Jason Lee, 'Post-traumatic stress disorder in the films *Taxi Driver* and *You Were Never Really Here*: A comparative progressive approach', in *Normalizing Mental Illness and Neurodiversity in Entertainment Media—Quieting the Madness*, ed. Malynnda Johnson and Christopher J. Olson (London: Routledge, 2021).

Aspects of Chap. 3 on sexuality were published in *Film International* as—Jason Lee, 'Are You Kidding? Re-assessing morality, sexuality, and desire in *Kids*', *Film International*, Vol 16 Issue 3, 2018.

A version of Chap. 6 was presented as the following conference paper—Inside Voice: Shamanism, Ventriloquism and Radars in Search of Transcendent Originality. Imperial College, Great Writing Conference, June 2012.

Contents

About the Author

Jason Lee (https://cjplee.com) is Professor of Film, Media, and Culture at De Montfort University, Leicester, and a Chartered Psychologist with the British Psychological Society. Lee is the author of numerous books, including *Nazism and Neo-Nazism in Film and Media* (Amsterdam University Press, 2018) and *Sex Robots—The Future of Desire* (Palgrave, 2018).

List of Abbreviations

AAW	Amherst Artists & Writers
ADHD	attention deficit hyperactivity disorder
BBC	British Broadcasting Company
BPD	borderline personality disorder
CBT	cognitive behavioural therapy
CEO	chief executive officer
DID	dissociative identity disorder
DSM	Diagnosis and Statistical Manual of Mental Disorders
ECT	electroconvulsive therapy
FGM	female genital mutilation
IMDB	Internet Movie Database
MIT	Massachusetts Institute of Technology
LSD	lysergic acid diethylamide
NHS	National Health Service
PRN	pro re nata (in the circumstances or as required)
PTSD	post-traumatic stress disorder
SRA	satanic ritual abuse
UK	United Kingdom
VR	virtual reality

Part I
History and Happiness

Chapter 1
The Unhappiness Industry

1.1 Introduction: Why the Transrational?

The media reports daily of a mental health crisis. In this volume I shall argue that overemphasizing the rational and ignoring the transrational has influenced an upsurge in mental health problems.[1] Unlike the transrational most people know what rational means. In this introduction I explain what the transrational is. Part of the problem includes the long history of the prioritisation of thinking over feeling. The philosopher Plato positioned reason as the higher part of the human that needs to be prioritised. The majority of academic Western philosophy of the last 500 years has been situated within rational discourse and has promoted reason as a higher realm. Descartes' 'I think therefore I am' is probably the most popular and commonly known phrase from philosophy.

Our personality type dictates how we view the world.[2] Some would agree with the view that our thoughts make up who we are, they construct our world. Others believe experience is, 'Only real in the way/That I feel from day to day', to quote Canadian singer song writer Neil Young.[3] Social scientists, psychiatrists, psychologists, anthropologists, historians, and philosophers applied here all assert the importance of the transrational.[4] Some are known as anti-philosophers, recognizing reason does not tell us everything.[5] While being primarily cultural studies engaging with an intersectional approach this book utilizes creative practice studies along with film and media studies, communication studies, history, psychology, and sociology.

---

[1] Unfortunately, the dominate discourse is to contain discourse, that is restricted it in a binary fashion. This text argues against this process. Being able to hold two opposing views is a sign of maturity and being healthy.

[2] Jason Lee, *The Psychology of Screenwriting* (London: Bloomsbury, 2014), pp. 85–103.

[3] Neil Young, World on a String.

[4] Including Bataille, Laing, Foucault, Irigaray, and Deleuze.

[5] Terry Eagleton, *The Meaning of Life* (Oxford: Oxford University Press, 2007).

J. Lee, *Culture, Madness and Wellbeing*, https://doi.org/10.1007/978-3-031-37530-9_1

This interdisciplinarity affirms the transrational imagination. Before we get any further into explaining what the transrational is and explicating the history of 'madness', a summary of each chapter will be beneficial.

This chapter examines the histories and theories of 'madness', including psychological, historical, and sociological approaches. Post-institutionalization of the 'mad', society became institutionalized, maximizing surveillance and control. Chapter 2 assesses the culture of 'madness', including film, television, and theatre. We find culture, especially film, can be a transrational mechanism for healing and wellbeing, given the heightened 'affective volume'.[6] There is an analysis of subgenres of films on 'madness', fictional television shows, plus reality television is examined. Film is shown to be a primary medium for the transrational and a way of explaining the impact of post-traumatic stress disorder and depression.

Gender, sexuality, and racism addressed in Chaps. 3 and 4 have are often prioritized in cultural studies, but the stigma of mental illness is one of our deepest.[7] Given, 'popular culture and the mass media come to serve as the only frames of reference available for the construction of collective and personal identities',[8] the focus here on media and culture is pertinent. Chapter 3 evaluates 'madness', gender, sexuality, and adolescence, investigating influential female writers and contemporary film. How women have been demonized in literature, film, and celebrity culture is expounded upon. We learn how engaging with fiction is important for wellbeing.

Chapter 4 interrogates 'madness' and race through a focus on colonialism, postcolonialism, and psychiatry, delineating the development of black 'madness' and white 'madness'. Insanity was viewed as a breakdown of the higher functions and not thought possible in non-white populations. Those outside the West were believed to be non-thinking and suffering from none of the sense of fear, loss, anticipation, alienation, and regret of 'civilized' countries. Michel Foucault's work became a colonising movement fortifying the individual in the containing system appealing to the individualism of the West.[9] Postcolonial theory is utilized, including the work of psychiatrist and activist Frantz Fanon, 'the purveyor of the transgressive and transitional truth'.[10]

Ethnographic interviews with those impacted by 'madness' personally and professionally are employed in Chap. 5. Real-life experiences of 'madness' are personal frameworks within mediated and remediated narratives, part of a double hermeneutic, or triple if we include the reader's interpretation. Narration is all: people tell a story about their past at a certain point in time and space then this is remembered and

[6]Norbert Wiley, 'Emotion and Film Theory', *Studies in Symbolic Interaction*, Vol. 26, 2003, pp. 169–187, p. 179.

[7]Nassir Ghaemi, *A First-Rate Madness: Uncovering the Links Between Leadership and Mental Illness* (London: Penguin, 2011), p. 256.

[8]Dominic Strinati, *An Introduction to Theories of Popular Culture* (London: Routledge, 1995), p. 239.

[9]Ibid.

[10]Homi Bhabha, *The Location of Culture* (London: Routledge, 2009), p. 57.

interpreted later, the reader reinterpreting this. These powerful narratives show the real impact of 'madness', how it has been treated, and what we can learn from personal experiences.

Chapter 6 examines 'madness' and creative practice, including fictional and personal experiences, dissecting 'madness' and its relationship with voice, creativity, and the transrational. Philosopher Emmanuel Levinas, theologian Karen Armstrong, and psychologist Stephen Pinker are utilised, among others. Previously, psychology primarily focused on the limiting aspects of mental health problems.[11] There has been a shift towards wellbeing and positive aspects of psychology which could be problematic. There is evidence that what is often thought of as mental ill-health, like hearing voices, leads to greater creativity and Chap. 6 confirms this.

Chapter 7 analyses 'madness', leaders and gurus explaining how great leaders possess a 'madness' so they can function well in a crisis.[12] This counteracts one definition of 'madness', that it means the inability to function.[13] Most gurus go through a process of psychic re-awakening, what could be termed constructive 'madness'. From ancient religious myths to modern films, the role of the hero and guru proves that only by resisting the apparent sanity of the system and status quo can a protagonist and the world encounter a deeper reality and awake.[14] There is also an analysis of group psychosis and the Witch Craze, a form of group psychosis explained by economics. Female healers were a threat socially and economically to the patriarchy so were destroyed. Other forms of popular group psychosis are examined, including celebrity culture.

Chapter 8 concludes by furthering an understanding of the creative value of transrationality, and through examining the politics of self and its adaptivity with regards to 'madness'. Social media, video games, and popular music are explored, along with the concept of authenticity. 'Madness', free will, and choice in the context of the fatalism of economic markets are expounded on. An alternative way of discerning ontology (the nature of being) is confirmed. This moves us away from a priori reason towards the openness of the transrational which is beneficial for wellbeing, contesting an accepted definition of normality concerning the functional utility of the human. There is a challenge to the 'mad' activity and over-production and consumption of capitalism which functions as a desperate attempt to overcome anxiety.[15] What was thought to be the cure is part of the illness.

Let us return to the fact that the transrational is not a commonly used, known, or understood term. This supports my initial argument that it is overlooked. So, what is it? One thing to point out immediately is that it is not the opposite of reason or the

---

[11] Sarah Andrews, 'Creativity and Mental Health', Media Discourse Centre seminar presentation, De Montfort University, 10 March, 2019.

[12] Ghaemi, op. cit.

[13] Anthony Storr, *Feet of Clay – Saints, Sinners, and Madmen: A Study of Gurus* (London: HarperCollins, 1996).

[14] Joseph Campbell illustrates this in *The Hero with a Thousand Faces* (London: Fontana, 1993).

[15] Erich Fromm, *The Fear of Freedom* (London: Routledge, 1989), p. 79.

rational. It is reasonable to assume it might be, because most of us have been programmed to think and feel in this either-or fashion, but as this book will show such a stance is limiting. The varied definitions of the transrational concern those experiences that do not conform to cause-and-effect structure. Definitions vary from the work of philosopher Ken Wilbur (1995) to analytical psychologist Jerome Bernstein (2000) to Franciscan theologian Richard Rohr (2011) who is my main source.[16] Significantly, the transrational is not the opposite of reason or the rational but includes the rational. The rational tries to exclude feelings and instinct which, as we shall see, is not possible. A rational approach is one side and denies part of the human, the feeling part, leading to mental health problems. This book continually returns to film, because in film feeling is paramount. So, we can see that film prioritises an aspect of the transrational and then can lead to wellbeing overcoming mental health problems. Editing provides the DNA of a film and the ideal cut satisfies six criteria with the number one criterion emotion rated at 51%.[17]

Analytical psychology is useful when it comes to incorporating the transrational and moving from binary one-side knowledge for wellbeing, so this shall be used throughout this book.[18] To paraphrase its founder, C.G. Jung, the conscious attitude of the neurotic is one-side, coming from the conscious which is unnatural. This must be balanced by the unconscious which includes integrating instinctive forces, including dreams, which can be thought of as part of the transrational. We shall understand in this book how films relate to dreams, plus the nuances concerning emotion and film. The unconscious can contain elements that should be conscious, if not then instinct can be full of prejudice and the natural symbol-producing function becomes distorted.[19] In a healthy sense, there is a dialectic between the inner and outer, between the hypothetical (the imaginal) and the experimental (the embodied), and through this analytical psychology can elaborate on how films 'create the feeling of meaning'.[20] Creating the feeling of meaning is an innovative way of explaining the affective experience of film and how the transrational works.

Most of us have experienced what could be described as 'mad' events, met someone we believed was 'mad, or behaved in ways others perceived as 'mad'. Sometimes 'madness' is seen as the opposite of meaning. 'Mad' is one of those

---

[16] Ken Wilbur, *Sex, Ecology, Spirituality – The Spirit of Evolution* (Boulder, Colarado: Shambhala, 1995); Jerome Bernstein, 'Listening in the Borderlines', *The Salt Journal*, Issue 2.2, January/February, 2000, pp. 13–21; Richard Rohr, *Falling Upward* (London: SPCK, 2011).

[17] Walter Murch, *In the Blink of an Eye. A Perspective on Film Editing* (Los Angeles: Silman-James Press), p. 18.

[18] Jung used alchemy as a symbol of this. The alchemic process was one that was both physical and psychic and extended through the whole of nature. The symbol for this was both empirical and transcendental. See C.G. Jung, *Mysterium Conjunctionis: An Inquiry into the Separation and Synthesis of Psychic Opposite in Alchemy* (Princeton: Princeton University Press, 1970), p. 554.

[19] See C.G. Jung, *The Practice of Psychotherapy* (Princeton, NJ: Princeton University Press, 1966), and *Psychological Types* (London: Routledge, 2006).

[20] Angela M Connolly, review of Greg Singh's *Film after Jung: Post-Jungian Approaches to Film Theory* (London: Routledge, 2009) in *Journal of Analytical Psychology*, 2011, 56, 134–147, p. 140.

sensitive words full of ambiguity, which is sometimes used as an adjective, more specifically as a superlative. A colloquial way of using the term 'madness', as in something is sheer 'madness', is that it is folly, stemming from the twelfth-century French folie which means 'madness'. The sequel to *Joker* (Todd Philipps, 2018), the highest grossing R-rated movie ever made, is *Joker: Folie à Deux* (Todd Phillips, 2014), 'madness' of two or folly of two. Often this concerns a romantic relationship where 'madness' can spread by association.[21] This suggests 'madness' is not purely biological, but one aim of this book is to move away from a binary either/or approach to the subject of 'madness'. Someone experiencing 'madness' can behave in a way that is abnormal and unacceptable, but we will see that accepted behaviour can also be 'mad'. What is the agreed normality, what is normal, and who defines this?

This book explains how 'madness' shapes culture, just as culture shapes 'madness', and how denying the transrational has caused 'madness'. One definition of 'madness' is the inability to tell a convincing story. Written and visual stories are dominated by tales of 'madness'. Good stories offer something that is just out of reach, a 'mad' occurrence that cannot be completely explained away rationally. In this sense, they step into the transrational, and this is how we make sense of the world. Attempts to grasp 'madness' have been intrinsic to human culture. In a cultural sense 'madness' is normal. One example is that of King Nebuchadnezzar in the book of *Daniel* c. 603 BC where living as an animal apart from God in the wilderness the king loses his mind which is only restored when he acknowledges God.[22] Nebuchadnezzar's, 'body was drenched with the dew of heaven until his hair grew like the feathers of an eagle and his nails like the claws of a bird'.[23] After seven years the king then looks to heaven and declares, 'my sanity was restored'.[24] In the following century, Hippocrates separated medical science from philosophical, religious, and magical beliefs; the environment was considered a component of insanity, but the brain was found to be paramount.[25] Plato's dialogue *Timaeus* c. 360 BC comments on the, 'soul's accession of wisdom in a condition of divine madness allied to prophecy', and Shakespeare frequently employs the 'conventional association' of dream with madness in several plays, especially *Hamlet* and *King Lear*.[26]

Written and visual culture has endeavoured to incorporate 'madness', but it remains dangerous for it challenges established rational methods of comprehension. The work of 'mad geniuses' in the nineteenth century, including philosopher Friedrich Nietzsche and painter Vincent van Gogh, was considered the height of creativity encapsulating the 'triumph of madness'.[27] For paediatrician and

[21] Also known as shared delusional disorder.

[22] Daniel, 4.1-34. *The Bible*, Revised Standard Version (London: Collins, 1977), p. 714–715.

[23] Daniel, 4.33. Ibid.

[24] Ibid.

[25] Anthony Masters, *Bedlam* (New York: Michael Joseph, 1977), pp. 23–24.

[26] Marjorie Garber, *Dream in Shakespeare. From Metaphor to Metamorphosis* (New Haven: Yale University Press, 2013), p. 5.

[27] Michel Foucault, *The Archaeology of Knowledge* (London: Routledge, 1989), p. 288.

psychoanalyst Donald Winnicott 'little madnesses' are our most deeply felt enthusiasms, investments, and attachments in the sphere of culture.[28] Winnicott worked with the BBC framing the U.K.'s national narrative on what constitutes mental health. Here he equates 'madness' with a joy, part of the leap of faith we all need to make life meaningful. Overall, in these terms we can see then the necessity of 'madness', historically, culturally, and personally.

Technological progress has been thought of as 'madness'. Warnings against the problems of social media exacerbating mental health problems can be viewed as part of this discourse. Virtual reality (VR) has been used to successfully treat areas such as psychosis. One major reason for the promotion of VR is cost, given automated delivery offers greater access. Interestingly, social media contagion spreads certain forms of 'madness'. Dissociative identity disorder (DID) has become popularised, like Tourette's syndrome, through platforms such as TikTok. People who may not have a disorder or syndrome can believe they have disorders and syndromes such as these through using popular media. For Heidegger technology is detrimental to the human, but it is possible to have a freeing relationship with it if we are questioning.[29]

As the narrator of Evelyn Waugh's 1945 novel *Brideshead Revisited—the sacred and profane memories of Captain Charles Ryder* put it between World War 1 and 2:

> We could watch the madmen, on clement days, sauntering and skipping among the trim gravel walks and pleasantly planted lawns; happy collaborationists who had given up the unequal struggle, all doubts resolved, all duty done, the undisputed heirs-at-law of a century of progress, enjoying the heritage at their ease.[30]

Ryder sees 'madness' here as absolute certainty and in a religious sense if we are totally certain then there is no need for faith making religion redundant. People who are certain they own the truth are blinkered and we can recognize doubt then is part of sanity.

During the 1950s 'madness' began to be celebrated by youth culture and intellectuals, especially the Beat generation led by poet Allen Ginsberg. The opening line of Ginsberg's most famous poem *Howl*, dedicated to his friend Carl Solomon who he met in a mental hospital, begins, 'I saw the best minds of my generation destroyed by madness'.[31] *Howl* attacks capitalism and the bomb, then ecstatically celebrates the 'Mad generation!'. By the 1960s novelist and Merry Prankster founder Ken Kesey and Harvard psychologist and acid-tripper Dr. Timothy Leary, used 'madness' as a metaphor in a multitude of ways, including protesting against American imperialistic wars.[32] The late 1970s and 1980s witnessed London band Madness, the

---

[28] Annette Kuhn, ed., *Little Madnesses: Winnicott, Transitional Phenomena, & Cultural Experience* (London: I.B. Tauris, 2013).

[29] Martin Heidegger, in *The Question Concerning Technology and Other Essays,* trans. William Lovitt (New York: Harper and Row, 1977), pp. 3–4.

[30] Evelyn Waugh, *Brideshead Revisited – the sacred and profane memories of Captain Charles Ryder* (London: Penguin, 1945), p. 10.

[31] Allen Ginsberg, *Howl and Other Poems* (San Francisco: City Lights, 1955).

[32] See Timothy Leary, *The Politics of Ecstasy* (Berkeley: Ronin Publishing, 1968).

Nutty Boys, triumphing in the UK hit parade and at this time calling someone a 'nutter' was sometimes a term of affection, but more commonly it is a term of abuse. Cadbury's chocolate 1992 advertisement confirmed, tongue in cheek, 'everyone's a fruit and nut case'.

'Madness' has been understood and misunderstood, and interpreted in a plethora of ways, including: the supernatural with 'madness' as evil, sin, and possession; the biological; psychological; sociological; as well as the historical and cultural. There is no agreement on, 'what mental illness is, what causes it, what will cure it'.[33] 'Madness' is a slippery term relating to the out of the ordinary functioning as a foil to the status quo which could itself be 'mad'. Despite 'mad' or crazy meaning quirkily attractive, and its celebratory nutty side, it remains taboo, considered antithetical to wellbeing, dangerous, and frightening. 'Madness' is so popular, but this is one way our fears surrounding 'madness' are not faced, given 'madness' points to an agreed normality, annihilating difference.

Psychopathology is a medical term from the Greek pathology which means suffering. The term was also used, 'to connote passions or feelings more generally'.[34] Mental health is currently in vogue, often framed as wellbeing. A focus on wellbeing in the workplace can be a cheap way of offering something to employees, rather than better hours and wages.

> The NHS is obsessed with the "wellbeing" of its staff. In theory, this makes sense: when you can't manage to recruit any more staff, it figures you'd try to hang on to those that you have. In practice, this is the kind of wellbeing that takes the fact that you're struggling with, say, regularly watching people die and then lying awake at night with your heart pounding wondering whether you could have done anything more to save them, and asks if maybe *you could just be a bit more cheerful*?[35]

The transrational, while including the rational, also includes the imagination and feeling, and so is a good concept when examining culture. We want culture, such as movies and theatre and novels, to move us. Unlike the transrational, the rational mind finds it impossible to fathom and process the major areas of life, including love, suffering and death.[36] The emotional world is part of the transrational. Difficulties in dealing with emotions lead to mental unwellness.

The transrational does not divide it incorporates. The greater our understanding of the transrational, which contains the imagination, emotions and the rational, the more wellbeing will result. We tend to think in binaries, but transnationality does not contradict reason, or the rational. The transrational concerns emotions, experiencing, and witnessing, allowing for an 'open system', leading to a deeper understanding, healing, and better mental health and wellbeing.[37] The transrational emphasises

---

[33] Roy Porter, *A Social History of Madness – Stories of the Insane* (London: Phoenix, 1996), p. 8.

[34] M. Guy Thompson, *The Death of Desire. An existential study of sanity and madness* (London: Routledge, 1993), p. 3.

[35] Anonymous, 'Confessions of a Junior Doctor', *The Times Magazine*, 13 August, 2022, p. 21.

[36] Rohr, op. cit.

[37] Ibid., p. xxxi

experiential knowledge. Sometimes transrational experiences are put down as 'mad' because they may not fit normal descriptions of an agreed-on reality, so we can see there is a relationship between the transrational and conceptions of 'madness'. According to Einstein it is emotion, not reason or the rational, which is at the heart of art and science.[38] 'On balance, a creature who lacked emotions would not just be less *intelligent* than we are; it would be less *rational* too.'[39]

Virginia Woolf's essay *On Being Ill* (1926) and her novel *Mrs. Dalloway* (1925) function as a defence of 'madness' as interiority, an interiorized space of psychic freedom, a privacy resisting the interpretive authority of patriarchal experts.[40] As the meme puts it, reversing Warhol, in the future everyone we will be private for 15 min. In a social media dominated world, it is hard to resist the pressure to always share, to constantly make oneself public to gain the gaze, although sharing if balanced is a healthy activity. With identity normally carved through external measures via the ego reflecting Freud's performance principle especially in a selfie-obsessed culture, an alternative internality such as that proposed by Woolf is required to re-address the balance. This is where transrational knowledge and experiencing the transrational is vital, because it requires engaging with the complex world of the interior life and emotions which many try to avoid through various external behaviours and addictions.[41] Michelle Obama makes a similar point when she explains that during the pandemic lockdown, she realised her over-activity which was now curtailed had a neurotic element.[42]

The transrational is associated with the imagination, attempting to unite the individual with the whole, 'of desire with realization, of happiness with reason'; this is not in the Aristotelian sense of recalling the repressed, only to repress it again—'purified'.[43] The transrational reinvigorates human emotions, and this is where healing and wellbeing arise.[44] What I am saying with regards to the transrational is simple and obvious, but the hegemonic power dynamics that seek to control societies often obfuscate this truth.[45] As the world's foremost authority on post-traumatic stress disorder puts it, from drug addiction to self-injurious behaviours, mental health issues commence as a way of trying to cope with the pain of

---

[38] Todd Macalister, *Einstein's God – A Way of Being Spiritual Without the Supernatural* (Berkeley: Apocryphal Press, 2008).

[39] Dylan Evans, *Emotions* (Oxford: Oxford University Press, 2003), p. 123.

[40] Jennifer Spitzer, Article Abstract, unpublished, *Transgressive Culture*, 2012.

[41] Jason Lee, ed., *Cultures of Addiction* (New York: Cambria, 2010).

[42] Michelle Obama, *The Light We Carry – Overcoming in Uncertain Times* (New York: Viking, 2022).

[43] Herbert Marcuse, *Eros & Civilization* (London: Abacus, 1973), p. 110.

[44] For C.G. Jung there is a middle path between external and internal which draws on the symbol. This contains both the rational and irrational, drawing together the world of external perception and sensory stimuli, and perception of the unconscious which he relates to the spiritual.

[45] These are economic, but often cultural.

emotions.[46] To paraphrase Dr. Johnson, people become beasts through activities, like excessive drinking, to get rid of the pain of being human. Through emotions we are human, but emotions are denied and then our humanity is lost. Emotions form part of the transrational and successful films concern the emotions and the transrational, but emotions inside the cinema are different to those outside given inside they are more controlled.[47] What I am saying is not justifying the approach that claims everything is offensive, everything is triggering; we do not have the right to not be offended.

In a world that prioritizes inhuman data over the emotions the transrational has been relegated, leading to dehumanization and to mental illness.[48] Robots take on attributes that are more human than those of humans with stories about robots functioning to remind us of our humanity.[49] Paradoxically, 'madness' involves not blindly accepting what C.G. Jung called the shadow self. The shadow enables us to keep searching and not just settle into quelling our anxieties.[50] To not acknowledge this shadow, part of our deeper transrational knowledge and understanding, would be at best live a half-life, at worst a living death, as we numb our shadow and feelings with drugs, alcohol, or any other addiction.

Divisions between reason and 'madness' are porous. The 'mad' can believe they are experiencing the height of reason. Tony Blair's belief in the 2003 Iraq War could be an example of this, although this is more hubris syndrome than 'madness'.[51] Psychiatrist Nassir Ghaemi makes a strong argument for the benefits of 'madness', that is mental health problems for leadership in a crisis situation which is discussed further in Chap. 7.[52] As interviewee A.6 in Chap. 5 points out, 'madness' is only known after the event, in recovery, when the 'mad' absolute truth of what went before is seen as false. During the event, the 'mad' believe they are experiencing the height of reason. 'The madman is not the man who has lost his reason. The madman is the man who has lost everything except his reason.'[53] Regardless of whether someone is 'mad', to believe in the totality of reason is a form of 'madness' hence the need for transrational knowledge.

---

[46] Bessel van der Kolk, *The Body Keeps the Score: Mind, Brain and Body in the Transformation of Trauma* (London: Penguin, 2014), p. 76.

[47] Norbert Wiley, 'Emotion and Film Theory', *Studies in Symbolic Interaction*, Vol. 26, 2003, pp. 169–187.

[48] James Brindle, *New Dark Age: Technology and the End of the Future* (London: Verso, 2019).

[49] Jason Lee, *Sex Robots – The Future of Desire* (London: Palgrave, 2018).

[50] Rohr, op. cit., p. 55.

[51] Ghaemi, op. cit., p. 248.

[52] Ghaemi, op. cit.

[53] G.K. Chesterton in M.J. Cohen, *The Penguin Dictionary of Epigrams* (London: Penguin, 2001), p. 239.

1.2 Freedom and Control

During the classical period 'madness' was linked to vice, then later to social failure, and then to degeneracy when it was assumed that 'madness' of the most violent kind was only common in 'the lower depth of society'.[54] 'Madness' was seen as the result of a fall from grace, asylums the embodiment of hell. In *The New Testament* Jesus and his disciples heal people seen as possessed by evil demons, as if 'madness' is a curse for transgressions. Some of these demoniacs we might think have an illness like epilepsy. Even today illness of any kind, but especially mental illness, can be thought of as a punishment from God. When things go wrong it is natural to believe God or the gods are against us, that there is something endemically wrong with us, but belief goes deeper than this and Chap. 2 examines the relationship between 'madness' and evil further.[55] In Innuit communities when an individual possesses their spirits, they become a shaman; when the spirits possess the individual, they are sick and unworthy of becoming a shaman.[56] This is a revelatory point similar to the idea that we are not our diagnosis. Someone is not a schizophrenic; they have symptoms that have been bundled up under this diagnosis.

Since the Enlightenment's insistence on prioritizing the rational world, transrational knowledge has been relegated to the realms of the imaginary.[57] This we will learn here has been problematic for a deeper understanding of the human condition. The Enlightenment's other name, the Age of Reason, is telling. I am not dismissing reason or the Enlightenment. This period was when human equality was asserted. What I am arguing is that because an over-emphasis on the rational took hold an imbalance has led to mental health problems. Despite the myths surrounding the rational as akin to objective, any rational judgement is always partial and prejudicial.[58] The transrational includes the rational, but the rational is mistakenly believed to be superior. During the Age of Reason even in matters of faith reason took hold. Christian reformers, such as Calvin and Luther, believed that through reason they could advance faith. For others their approach epitomized 'madness'.[59] The 1789 French revolution made the Church subordinate to the state, but this desire to replace religion with the 'cult of reason' for its enemies was 'a cult of insanity'.[60]

---

[54] Michel Foucault, *Madness and Civilisation. A History of Insanity in the Age of Reason*, trans. Richard Howard (London: Tavistock/Routledge, 1989), p. 260.

[55] There is the alternative view that having a sick person in your household draws you to God; in this sense illness is a blessing rather than a curse.

[56] Robert Moss. *Dreaming the Soul Back Home: Shamanic Dreaming for Healing and Becoming Whole* (New York: New World, 2012), p. 250.

[57] Karen Armstrong, *The Battle for God* (London: Ballantine Books, 2001), p. 69.

[58] Michael Vannoy Adams, *The Fantasy Principle. Psychoanalysis of the Imagination* (New York: Brunner-Routledge, 2004).

[59] John Dickie, *The Craft – How the Freemasons Made the Modern World* (London: Hodder & Stoughton, 2020).

[60] Armstrong, op. cit., pp. 111–112.

This eighteenth-century movement desired liberty, egality, and fraternity, but for 'mad' subversives in the nineteenth century this meant liberty's antithesis—being caged.

Enlightenment thinkers attempted to replace religion by faith in humanity. Schopenhauer's sound criticism of Kant was that the Enlightenment was a 'secular version of Christianity'.[61] Those who tried to step beyond belief and faith through reason established the church of reason which had its own blind faith. Drawing on Eastern ideas, for Schopenhauer personal identity, free will, and moral autonomy are false notions. He attempted to undermine the belief in the human subject that underpins Christianity and humanism.[62] In the nineteenth century belief in transrational knowledge bubbled under the surface, condemned as part of the occult. Traditional knowledge keepers within the academy found such activity treacherous.

'Mad' has a maddeningly wide 'lexical range', including anger and the slang synonymous with 'too or really', although what was slang now appears standard dictionary definitions.[63] We shall return to group psychosis in the context of celebrity worship and the Witch Craze in Chap. 7, but in postcolonial terms there is group, 'psychosis of patriotic fervour'.[64] A shift from negative psychology, focusing on symptoms, to positive psychology focusing on wellbeing, is benign but can be superficial. The well-adapted person is not evidence of proof of mental health.[65] With their own politicization, 'madness', mental illness, wellbeing, are interrelated and contested terms. In 2016 the United Arab Emirates appointed H.E. Ohood Al Roumi as the minister of state for happiness. In 2019 New Zealand made wellbeing their focus, rather than gross domestic product. Concerns around wellbeing are central to human existence, but to prioritize wellbeing over economic growth makes headline news, as if it is 'mad' to sacrifice the economy for wellbeing. The concentration on endless economic growth targets is part of the limitations of the colonial rational mindset discussed in Chap. 4 that has ignored transrational knowledge. 'Waste is the highest virtue one can achieve in advanced capitalist societies'.[66]

A synonym of rational is sane but despite the ideological myths that fused Nazism and fascism it was the blind rational will of the twentieth century led to the 'mad' machinery of Auschwitz and the bombs on Hiroshima and Nagasaki. The war with Japan was essentially over, but America was compelled to test its technology for scientifical rational purposes, regardless of the horrific consequences.

---

[61] John Gray, *Black Mass – Apocalyptic Religion and the Death of Utopia* (London: Farrar, Straus, and Giroux, 2007), p. 41.

[62] Ibid, p. 44.

[63] Therí Alyce Pickens, *Black Madness:: Mad Blackness* (Durham, NC: Duke University Press, 2019), p. 4.

[64] Bhabha, op. cit., p. 7.

[65] Daniel Burston, *The Wing of Madness. The Life and Work of R.D. Laing* (London: Harvard University Press, 1996), p. 155. They may be adapted to a society that is not healthy, such as Nazi Germany.

[66] Haruki Murakami, *Sputnik Sweetheart* (2003), p. 19.

Notwithstanding the openness of the Beat generation in the 1950s and postmodernism's rise wrongheaded dualism dominates today. This is true in constructions of the rational versus the irrational, but the transrational overcomes this. This bifurcation is less pronounced in the East where Taoism, Buddhism and Hinduism prevail.[67] Ideas concerning authenticity and meaning are not universal, especially in a psychological and psychotherapeutic context.[68] Without engagement with the transrational we cannot be fully human, and this is at the core of creative narratives globally and transhistorically.[69]

The classical period's unchained animality view of 'madness' was restrained by discipline in the nineteenth century. This was followed by reformers such as those of the York Retreat.[70] Established in 1820, the Lincoln Asylum was the UK's first total-asylum. Here in 1837 it dawned that the 'mad' could be handled without mechanical restraints which at the time was a revelation.[71] The building of British asylums was believed to help cure insanity, but with an increase in professions to treat the 'mad' there was, 'a startling and continuing rise in the proportion of the population officially recognized as insane'.[72] On 5 April 1877 *The Times* reported that given the rise in lunacy the insane would soon be in the majority in the country and they would then free themselves and lock up the sane.[73] Explanations were sort at the time, but two of the assumptions of the era have been more recently identified.[74] Firstly, it was assumed during this period that there was a finite number of 'mad' people so there must be a finite number of sane people. In *The Quantity Theory of Insanity* (1993) Will Self satirizes this notion, a higher level of insanity in one part of the country leading mathematically to a lower level elsewhere.[75] Self is also mocking the dangerous deification of data. The second assumption was the mistaken identification of the 'mad' as objective and unchanging.[76] This was an error in the nineteenth century and is a common belief today.

If patients are permanently branded with a particular diagnosis and label they may act only within that framework. What labels me negates me is a popular phrase attributed to Kierkegaard. Having a diagnosis could alleviate some angst but in an existentialist sense it is inauthentic and in a Jungian sense the only 'madness' is an

---

[67] A binary division of the world into East and West is erroneous, but to a degree this point is still valid.

[68] Ruthellen Josselson, *Narrative and Cultural Humility: Reflections from "The Good Witch" Teaching Psychotherapy in China* (Oxford: Oxford Scholarship Online, 2020).

[69] Joseph Campbell, op. cit.

[70] Andrew Scull, *Museums of Madness: The Social Organization of Insanity in Nineteen-Century England* (London: Allen Lane, 1979) p. 70.

[71] Ibid.

[72] Ibid., p. 222.

[73] Ibid., p. 225.

[74] Ibid.

[75] Will Self, *The Quantity Theory of Insanity* (London: Penguin, 1991).

[76] Scull, op. cit., p. 234.

identification with the diagnosis. A definition of insanity at this period included, 'one whose intellect has been perverted', from a text by Thomas Mayo, *Medical Testimony and Evidence in Cases of Lunacy* (1854).[77] When we position everyone not deemed appropriate for society as 'mad' the asylums begin to fill up.[78] What is 'perverted' and 'appropriate' became key to the developments of English psychiatry in the nineteenth century. Chapter 4 shows how English psychiatry had a global influence and how morality and 'madness' have always been entwined. This continues to this day.[79]

First published in 1952, *The Diagnostic and Statistical Manual of Mental Disorders* (DSM) had its fifth edition in 2013. This is used globally to diagnose versions of 'madness' and if followed to the letter everyone would have a mental disorder.[80] In the 1960s a number of identity scandals occurred in American mental asylums with researchers posing as patients, leading to the view that maintaining the drama of differentiation between staff and patients was problematic.[81] We can see how power dynamics might be problematic for healing, but it is not always the therapist that has the power. Joseph Heller's 1961 novel *Catch-22*, adapted for cinema in 1970 and directed by Mike Nichols, and turned into a mini-TV series in 2019, shows the absurdity of how definitions of 'madness' are used. World War 2 pilot Captain John Yossarian claims insanity to free himself from future missions. This proves his sanity. Clinically, a denial of diagnosis can be seen as further evidence of 'madness'. More accurately this interpretation can be reversed—a complex becomes pathological when we delude ourselves that we have got it.[82] People can cling to the boundaries of a diagnosis which limits them.

Psychiatrist Thomas Szasz, in works such as *Ideology and Insanity—Essays on the Psychiatric Dehumanization of Man* (1970), revealed how control became justified by the prevailing mental health ideology.[83] Szasz's work has been simplistically attacked for dismissing mental illness as a myth, but this is an inaccurate view.[84] What he was getting at was the performative nature of the patient who takes on the diagnosis which is verified in mental patient wards. This removes an existential crisis—who am I—and offers a twistedly optimistic answer for an identity—a mental patient with a diagnosis. Such a framework offers the fragmented psyche a position to operate within initially, a personal narrative and personality paradigm but

---

[77] Ibid.

[78] Ibid., p. 253.

[79] One interviewee for this book was sectioned after 'immorally' showing her breasts to the police.

[80] Leader, op. cit., p. 108.

[81] Erving Goffman, *Asylums – Essays on the Social Situation of Mental Patients and Other Inmates* (London: Routledge, 1991), p. 105.

[82] See C.G. Jung, *Psychological Reflections: A New Anthology of His Writings, 1905-1961* (London: Routledge and Keegan Paul, 1971).

[83] Thomas Szasz, *Ideology and Insanity – Essays on the Psychiatric Dehumanization of Man* (London: Marion Boyars, 1973).

[84] B. Lawrence, Social Work and Mental Health, Unpublished PhD, University of York, 1998, p. 128.

has its dangers. You are not your illness, disorder, or condition, even if this is a personality disorder which according to psychiatry is not something that changes.[85]

The Reality of Mental Illness was a popular reply to the anti-psychiatry movement.[86] American psychologist Paula Caplan made a significant impact in the anti-psychiatric diagnosis field.[87] For Robert Youngson, terms like 'mental pathology' or 'mental disease' are thought to be, 'metaphors, but have been used so often that the metaphors have acquired solidity'.[88] In certain circumstances this view is correct, but not all. Psychiatrist and broadcaster Anthony Clare made it clear that Szasz's division between physical diseases and mental disorders was inaccurate using phobic anxiety state as an example.[89]

For historian Eric Hobsbawm the late twentieth century was the age of 'madness' and he also used 'schizoid', 'insane' and 'lunacy' to describe the era.[90] Philosopher Zlavoj Žižek claimed US policy in the first decade of the twenty-first century was, 'definitively approaching a stage of madness'.[91] Chapter 7 examines how US president 2016 to 2021 Donald Trump was often considered 'mad' by mental health professionals and the media. In this historical and political context 'madness' means instability and incoherency. Hobsbawm's focus was on the Cold War period from 1947 to 1991 finishing with the disbanding of the Soviet Union. This was also the era that produced the DSM, now developed in collusion with the pharmaceutical industry.[92] This level of complicity is disappointing given the DSM was originally created for benign purposes and intended for much more flexible use; for example, in the 1980 edition it was noted that it was so imprecise it should never be used for forensic or insurance purposes.[93]

Unfortunately, the DSM has since become the main mental health bible for legal and insurance purposes. Scientific culture, driven by capitalism and financial interests, became much more literal and there was a rise of religious fundamentalism across many religions. During this period mental health became dictated to by data, which became a higher truth divorced from humanity, the rational prioritized over the transrational. Data is a commodity and capital and it is easy to forget it is never a

[85] Ibid.

[86] Martin Roth and Jerome Kroll, *The Reality of Mental Illness* (Cambridge: Cambridge University Press, 1986).

[87] Paula Caplan, *They Say You're Crazy – How The World's Most Powerful Psychiatrists Decide Who Is Normal* (London: Hachette Books, 1996).

[88] Robert Youngson, *The Madness of Prince Hamlet and Other Delusions* (London: Robinson Publishing, 1999), p. 29.

[89] Anthony Clare, *Psychiatry in Dissent – Controversial Issues in Thought and Practice* (London: Routledge, 1989), pp. 28–30.

[90] Eric Hobsbawm, *Age of Extremes. The Short Twentieth Century 1914-1991* (London: Abacus, 1991).

[91] Slavoj Žižek, *Living in the End Times* (London: Verso, 2011), p. 56.

[92] Darian Leader, *What is Madness?* (London: Penguin, 2011).

[93] Kolk, op. cit., p. 29.

neutral artefact.[94] Data was the new holy scripture. Decisions were made once data flows had been maximised, but counter-intuitively this led to worse decision making. This was found to be overt in behavioural psychology where more was found to be less. An experiment on MIT business students found that greater knowledge concerning investments led to poorer decision making, an excess in information and data flows creating a deprivation of awareness.[95]

From the 1950s to the 2000 the rate of use of mental health services tripled in America, suggesting a lowering of stigma attached to mental health, and a broader definition of what it is.[96] Despite those with mental illness suffering more violence than those without, from 1950 to 1996 the assumed 'dangerousness' of those with more serious mental illnesses like psychosis (often perceived as actual 'madness') increased two and a half fold; evidence shows this was, in part, through the effects of the media, with de-institutionalization also playing a role.[97]

The supernatural and paranormal have strong affinities with conceptualizations of 'madness'. This has been impacted by the media with currently 320 television shows on the subject available in the UK. The correlation between evil and 'madness' has not dissipated, but this is where the boundaries between the rational and irrational breakdown. The contemporary blind-belief in apparently rational data as always teleologically insightful can be interpreted as irrationally 'mad'. Data became framed as a paranormal pure intelligence. The belief in the purity of data is the worship of the untouched rational which is then irrational, aligning reality in the past, present, and future. Technological systems have collapsed time and space; 'computation conflates past and future'; while erroneously, 'data is modelled as the way things are, and then projected forward'.[98] This promotes a dangerous a priori predetermination from one tool that humans think will enable total control over the outer world. Computation does not simply direct our actions in the present but constructs an 'immanence' that best fits its parameters.[99]

The 1973 book *Sybil* by Flora Rheta Schreiber concerns a woman with multiple personality disorder, today more accurately termed dissociative identity disorder (DID). The book was adapted into the made-for-television film *Sybil* (Daniel Petrie 1976) and is promoted on the back-cover blurb as, 'the true story of a woman possessed by sixteen separate personalities'. The supernatural and paranormal correlate here with mental ill-health to tempt potential readers—evil sells. *Lie To Me* Season Two Episode 1 (2011) also hints at a connection between a diagnosis of DID

---

[94] Natalie Fenton, et al., *The Media Manifesto* (Cambridge: Polity Press, 2020), pp. 51–57.

[95] Jonah Lehrer, *The Decisive Moment. How the Brain Makes Up its Mind* (Edinburgh: Canongate, 2009), p. 155.

[96] Jo C. Phelan, Bruce G. Link, Anne Stueve and Bernice A. Pescosolido, 'Public Conceptions of Mental Illness 1950 to 1956: What Is Mental Illness and Is It to be Feared?' In *Journal of Health and Social Behaviour*, Vol. 41, No. 2, June 200, pp. 188–207.

[97] Ibid., p. 202.

[98] Bridle, op. cit., p. 44.

[99] Ibid.

and the paranormal, using the iconography of the devil. Despite awareness campaigns by celebrities and the demystifying by philosophers, mental ill health and 'madness' are still viewed as caused by evil and leading to violence. Mental illness is feared, viewed as a threat, not just to the individual but the entire group.

Psychiatry developed as a lucrative science of observation, classification, and containment. This classification stems from the industrial revolution and nineteenth-century rationalism, but a binary logic today will not suffice. A scientific binary approach to knowledge, ignoring the transrational, has led to more mental illness, but a wholeness is required, what St. Bonaventure called the 'coincidence of opposites'.[100] Nothing is true that compels us to exclude.[101] Scientific discourse in this field of mental health is led by a medical paradigm that often excludes the transrational, so this needs questioning.

Popular culture has continually played with this mistaken identity theme, especially the horror film genre such as *Unsane* (Steven Soderbergh, 2018), a feature shot on an iPhone. Seeking to capitalize, when the medical industry finally caught up with these private retreat 'madhouses' treatment did not lead to better results.[102] The question over what is healthy with regards to functioning is of key significance when we address 'madness', and we examine this in Chap. 8 from a legal perspective. In *What is Madness?* (2011) psychoanalyst Darian Leader explains that one of Britain's most prolific serial killers Dr. Harold Shipman, who murdered possibly 700 patients, would be termed normal and sane because he was functioning.[103]

Definitions of mental illness, 'madness', and normality fail us, especially when we label normal behaviour as that which consists of the ability to function. To be sure, 'madness' is the rule rather than the exception.[104] The medical profession continued to reinvent paradigms for divisions of 'madness' in collusion with the pharmaceutical industry.[105] A plethora of studies have revealed how mental distress has risen, especially depression and anxiety, between the 1930s and 1990s.[106] New diagnoses meant new treatments, new drugs gaining more profit, but levels of unhappiness and mental illness rose. The complexities of 'madness', race, and colonialism are addressed in Chap. 4. The origins of American psychiatry were in the treatment and classification of immigrants.[107] Sociologically, accounts of mental health frameworks and negotiations with power include the neo-Durkheimian,

---

[100] Rohr, p. 83.

[101] Albert Camus, *Summer* (Penguin: London, 1995), p. 68.

[102] Ibid., p. 253.

[103] Leader, op. cit.

[104] Leader, op. cit.

[105] Kolk, op. cit.

[106] Jean Twenge, 'Are Mental Health Issues On the Rise?', in *Psychology Today*, October 12 2015, Are Mental Health Issues On the Rise? | Psychology Today (accessed October 07, 2021)

[107] Thomas Szasz, *Ideology and Insanity – Essays on the Psychiatric Dehumanization of Man* (Syracuse University Press: New York, 1970), p. 214.

neo-Weberian, and neo-Marxian and poststructuralist.[108] The neo-Weberian is the most applicable here in consideration of the medical model and the development of the history of treatments of insanity. Psychiatric medicine creates a technical and exclusive language which then maintains its social status excluding others. This means there is power over clients, new recruits, and other occupational groups, creating a hierarchy.[109] This is confirmed in interview responses in Chap. 5. Sociologists Rogers and Pilgrim inaccurately claim a difference between sociologist Andrew Scull and historian of ideas Michel Foucault over the period when mass incarceration began.[110] Incarceration in Britain and Europe was different. With war being rampant in mainland Europe subversives were more likely to be locked up.

When the metaphorical is always replaced by the literal this creates difficulties because then anything can be viewed as a disorder. While not wanting to downplay trauma and its impact, it needs noting there has been a rise of people self-identifying as victims of trauma which might mean those suffering deep trauma do not get the services they need. Similarly, 'anything anyone might do in the company of another may now be defined as psychotherapeutic'.[111] A decline in the popular belief in the need for a cure of sick souls was replaced by the need for the cure of sick minds.[112] There is a problem when the pressure to regard mental illness as an unchanging fact rather than a judgement is acquiesced to. In, 'psychiatry the classificatory act functions as a definition of social reality'.[113] This definition of social reality becomes a means for control and a way of defining morality.[114]

Another definition of 'madness' is an inability to conceive of the other. Through relationships with another our subjectivity and freedom are called into question paradoxically creating a more meaningful self. 'Madness' by its alterity can deny alterity, bringing about a certain freedom from others. But this then can form the trap of mental and possibly physical isolation through incarceration. If homogenization prevails through mental health treatment ideology, individuality is over-ridden. Cults have taken this approach to ironing out difference, as Chap. 7 shows. The happiness industry frequently does the same.

What are taken to be the defining features of 'madness'—delusions, hallucinations, and so on—are secondary symptoms; they are less the constitutive nature of 'madness', but responses to it.[115] The ever-increasing size of the DSM is a stark example: 'Wearing ink-stained clothes' according to the DSM is part of a schizoid

---

[108] A. Rogers and D. Pilgrim, *A Sociology of Mental Health and Illness* (Open University Press: Maidenhead, 2010), pp. 135–137.

[109] Ibid., pp. 134–135.

[110] Ibid., p. 141.

[111] Szasz, op. cit., p. xii.

[112] Ibid.

[113] Ibid., p. 207.

[114] Ibid., p. 219.

[115] Leader, op. cit., p. 17.

personality disorder.[116] Those who ignore the transrational tend to emphasise the literal, because it is easier than a more nuanced transrational metaphorical approach. Mental disorders are defined on political whims and aesthetic tastes and with the emphasis on surface over depth the DSM naturally increases categorizes.[117] The number of those diagnosed with psychosis has increased five-fold, the drug industry working hand-in-glove with mental health researchers creating diagnostic categories; 'with each new category came a new medication, creating market niches'.[118]

Epicurus (341-270 BC) wrote that it is never too late to 'secure the well-being of one's mind'; we must study philosophy and meditate on happiness, because if we have that we have everything.[119] This behaviour is akin to contemporary paths to wellbeing via bibliotherapy and meditation. Given the dominance of the medicalization model today it is hard to recognize that 'madness' is not necessarily an illness. There is an assumption it relates to a neuro-chemical imbalance, but this takes personal responsibility. According to Anthony Clare 'madness' is 'lack of adjustment to the world'.[120] This forms part of how the happiness industry takes over. Behind this outlook is the problematic New Age mantra, change your thoughts and you change your world.[121] If this was all people did then what would happen to social action. While philosophically it is easy to understand the potential benefits of such a belief, it has filtered into cognitive behavioural therapy and become equated with fact.

For popular spirituality guru Eckhart Tolle, 'there is no other, and you are always meeting yourself'.[122] This relates to communications theory models such as the Johari window model above, where we can see that when two people meet there are eight aspects, four in each person, interweaving. Like Jung's view, this relates to the idea of projection; it is true that if we are not especially aware we can project onto others the dynamics from our previous relationships, especially our parents. The problems of definitions of 'madness' are encapsulated here because this could also be considered 'madness'. The inability to conceive of the other as different, that is, as not possessing a valuable uniqueness through their diversity, separate from who we are, is one definition of 'madness'. If all you see is yourself in relationships then that is a significant problem and a diagnosis of narcissism could be appropriate. The rational binary mind, 'finds itself totally out of its league in dealing with things like love, death, suffering, infinity, God, sexuality, or mystery in general'.[123] By attempting to relieve the anxiety of separateness capitalist society perverts the

[116]Ibid.

[117]Ibid., p. 33.

[118]Ibid., p. 27.

[119]Epicurus, *Being Happy* (London: Penguin, 1996), p. 1.

[120]Clare, op. cit., p. 15.

[121]John Powell, *Happiness is an Inside Job* (London: Kendall, 2017).

[122]Ekchart Tolle, *Stillness Speaks. A Guide to Spiritual Enlightenment* (London: New World 2003), p. 100.

[123]Rohr, op. cit., p. 205.

meaning of equality by destroying difference.[124] As we shall see in Chap. 7, coping with separation anxiety is part of the attraction of cults where the group is supposedly united in the One.

In nineteenth century, America schizophrenia was popular as a diagnosis while in Britain manic was emphasized, but with the globalization of psychiatry diagnostic differences dissolved.[125] Despite this, a racial dimension remained when it came to diagnosis, an area examined further in Chap. 4. After the DSM began being used internationally by psychiatrists from the 1950s diagnoses multiplied in each decade, new disorders correlating with developments in the pharmaceutical industry, and these were entered into versions of this diagnostic bible as new editions emerged. An explosion in the happiness industry took off in the 1960s, along with an emphasis on new disorders. Finding yourself as a mission during the hippy generation meant a constant questioning. As well as having the benefits for treatment new diagnoses instigated forms of behaviour to conform to. This in part was to prevent the feeling of being of being separate and to alleviate anxiety. After an existential search there could be a eureka moment for the patient once the diagnosis fitted. There is an obvious danger to this. It can limit an individual's understanding of who they are. They become merely their diagnostic label to fit into and then manifest the symptoms and behaviours to equate with this, but diagnoses can also bring comfort and relief. In interviews in Chap. 5 the benefits of diagnosis are illustrated, as well as the problem with misdiagnosis.

The 1980s witnessed an increased promotion of diagnoses, including bi-polar and borderline personality disorder (BPD), sometimes mistaken for each other, and more niche ones like Capgras' syndrome. Historically and geographically specific, Capgras syndrome was overtly popular in 1990s New York.[126] Each period has had its own fashionable diagnosis, creating wealth for the pharmaceutical industry. To dismiss diagnostic frameworks entirely for understanding and treating disorders would be erroneous and part of an ignorant binary discourse, but it is important to acknowledge non-essentialist dimensions. For example, someone is not 'a schizophrenic'. They may have related symptoms bundled up under this term, but we have seen that at different times and in different locations these symptoms are framed as something else.

Developing from the hippy generation where the ills of society were seen as caused by the evils of the nuclear family, for R.D. Laing and Laingians mental illness had its roots in the sexually and economically repressive society, especially the nuclear family.[127] Laing was a psychiatrist and celebrity guru and part of the happiness industry who claimed if the 'self is not known it is safe' and this is the

---

[124]Fromm, op. cit, p. 18–19.

[125]Leader, op. cit., p. 31.

[126]This is when you believe a significant figure in your life has been replaced by an imposter, such as an alien or robot.

[127]R.D. Laing and Aaron Esterson, Sanity, Madness and the Family: Families of Schizophrenics (London: Pelican, 1970).

purpose of 'madness'.[128] It is easier to ignore the difficult things about ourselves, but this leads to a hollow and superficial existence like that of the life of the alcoholic whose focus is on one need.[129] Who really knows the self, and does the self exist? We shall come on to this in Chap. 2 in the discussion of post-identity trauma. People remain unknown to themselves in part to remain safe, whether by choice or unwittingly. The Johari Window Model makes clear all of us have parts of ourselves we are unaware of.

Laing made psychosis intelligible and viewed schizophrenia as, 'a break in the journey'.[130] Rather than interpreting 'madness' as that which is uninterpretable, this new way of thinking about 'madness' concerned recognising the unique meaning in everyone's 'madness'. This included psychosis and schizophrenia which had often been overlooked. Seeing these forms of 'madness' as a language with their uniqueness then gave a humanity to the person who was experiencing this phenomenon. We will see how film has been interpreted as 'madness', but in this context it is useful to note that with making a film, 'you are trying to learn a foreign language—it just happens to be a unique language that is only spoken by this one film'.[131]

Laing disagreed with medical sociology which argued that there was a biological analogy from the individual to the group.[132] Seeing the group as an organism, ontologically, only leads to confusion. Society was deemed insane by some Laingians, but this inaccurately continued a false binary between sane and insane.[133] A simplistic stark division between the psychiatric establishment and the anti-psychiatry movement has been contested through reference to the impact of 1960s British film and television.[134] This has included the impact of the Laing influenced BBC television play *In Two Minds* by David Mercer, broadcast on 1 March 1967 and directed by Ken Loach, about Kate Winter (Anna Cropper) receiving electroconvulsive therapy for schizophrenia. For example, leading UK mental health organisation the National Association for Mental Health were looking to the work of director Ken Loach and psychiatrist R.D. Laing as, 'models for engaging contemporary audiences as it rebranded to MIND in 1972'.[135] We can see here the power of popular culture in engaging audiences with changing perceptions of 'madness' and in driving changes in the national mental health charity.

Laing died in 1989 and a film was made about his life in 2017, *Mad to Be Normal* (Robert Mullan, 2017). The height of his fame was during the late 1960s and early 1970s. His books became best sellers, including his unique poetry collection *Knots*

[128] Ibid., p. 13.
[129] Jason Lee, ed. *Cultures of Addiction* (New York: Cambria, 2010).
[130] Laing, op. cit., p. 70.
[131] Murch, op. cit., p. 46.
[132] Ibid., p. 22.
[133] Ibid.
[134] T. Snelson, 'From *In Two Minds* to MIND: The circulation of 'anti-psychiatry' in British film and television during the long 1960s', *History of the Human Sciences*, 2021 34(5), pp. 53–81.
[135] Ibid., abstract.

(1971).[136] During the era when Laing became a celebrity guru an obsession with personal happiness arose with an industry to match. Political calls for freedom in certain groups, including those related to sex, race, and sexuality, rocketed. Laing mixed with these movements during this period of collapsing traditional boundaries where drugs were also used to facilitate an overcoming of boundaries. Not only was this about controlling treatment but controlling journeys to another non-physical world through drugs.

Coming from the medical establishment and formally an army psychiatrist, Laing was well-positioned to challenge and transgress the establishment. Edna O'Brien claimed that the James Bond star Sean Connery warned her not to take LSD after he experienced a bad trip given to him by Laing for his stress when filming *Goldfinger* (Guy Hamilton, 1964).[137] The drug was used legally and therapeutically between 1950 and 1965, then banned, with legal experiments beginning again in Switzerland in 2000. LSD became popular for individual personal inner journeys and for healing, as explored therapeutically from a contemporary perspective in *Nine Perfect Strangers* (novel Liane Moriarty, 2018, Netflix adaptation 2021). LSD reveals how the self is constructed in the brain and allows for the study of the foundations of psychology with a study in 2021 showing 80% of users reporting a lift in depression.[138] LSD enables the exploration of transrational knowledge for healing.

Prior to the industrial revolution the 'mad' were taken care of by the community and then with the rise of industrialized society an institutional approach to containing the 'mad' evolved.[139] This industrialized 'madness' situated people as units, resources, and numbers for processing, producing data as the new data-God. To place someone losing their mind and identity in an institution might give them a function and role as a patient, although it could just as easily divorce them from all that was sustaining their identity, creating further 'madness'. Thus the 'mad' industry began. The regimentation of institutions went hand in hand with, 'differentiation of different sorts of deviance'.[140] During the 1980s the UK moved towards what was termed 'care in the community' with the government closing large state-run mental hospitals. Public 'madhouses' were sold off to private property developers.

Private companies, including the well-known private equity owned Priory Group, then took over mental health treatment. The profit motive was a priority in post-Thatcher Britain. Within this ideology the market is viewed not just economically as a benign force but is positioned morally and socially as an objective higher power which it is thought, like data, has removed any debasing human influence. It is interesting to note in both contexts how the human is viewed as an evil influence, as if humans can and should remove human influence, which is preposterous. The

---

[136] It is remarkable for any book of poetry to become a best seller, so this indicates his real guru status.

[137] Edna O'Brien, *Country Girl* (London: Faber and Faber, 2012).

[138] TV show.

[139] Scull, op. cit., p. 14.

[140] Clare, op. cit., p. 17.

market then becomes God. There was now a supernatural belief in the market. This has resulted in horrendous mistakes, multiple suicides, and no follow up care. The desire for profit in the mental health industry means self-diagnosis is bowed down to, with private 'over-spill' beds funded by the taxpayer. There is no incentive to discharge people, given the profit to be made.[141] Placing people outside the walls of the public 'madhouse' may appear benign, but interviewees for Chap. 5 who worked in the 'madhouses' pre care in the community remarked on the strong sense of community felt by staff and patients. In 1977 there were 160,000 mental health beds in the NHS.[142] Ten years on 67,100 and by 2018/19 the number had dropped to 18,400.[143] An exponential growth in homelessness in the UK and America is partly explained by the closing of hospitals with then a rise in mental health problems created through people being homeless. There have been several deaths within Priory Group hospitals indicating the dangers of this profit motive approach, including that of Amy El-Keira at the group's Ticehurst House hospital in East Sussex in 2012, plus several units rated inadequate by the Care Quality Commission and closed. In 2022 there were three deaths at the Priory Hospital Cheadle Royal in the space of two months, Beth Mathews, Lauren Bridges, and Deseree Fitzpatrick. A jury concluded the hospital provided 'inadequate care' with the Priory Group apologising 'unreservedly'.[144]

'Madness' can mean the dominance of the unconscious mind but, as Surrealism found, the unconscious is not pathological—it is the 'original human quality'.[145] Grandpa Simpson in *The Simpsons Movie* (David Silverman, 2007) apparently goes 'mad' in church, but what he utters is prophecy regarding his son Homer's transgressions concerning dumping toxic waste, the film an ecological warning. Prophets historically have been accused of being 'mad', or personally thought they were, a subject addressed in Chap. 7. Jesus Christ was thought 'mad' by the religious authorities and by his own family as were his disciples when filled with the Spirit as explained in *Acts*. Muhammad needed reassurances from those around him that he was not 'mad'.[146]

Those thought 'mad' can be visionaries, artists, and prophets with these 'mad' voices functioning as a warning and a challenge by breaking through the control of everyday reality. 'Madness' can be viewed as the total inability to change which is summed up by the popular explanation that 'madness' involves repeating the same

---

[141] Anonymous, 'Woeful scarcity': NHS psychiatrist decries lack of mental health beds', *The Guardian*, 24 April 2022, 'Woeful scarcity': NHS psychiatrist decries lack of mental health beds | Mental health | The Guardian (accessed 27 April, 2022).

[142] Andrew Crowcroft, *The Psychotic. Understanding Madness* (Penguin: New York, 1977), p. 67.

[143] The Strategy Unit. Exploring Mental Health Inpatient Capacity across Sustainability and Transformation Partnerships in England, NHS Midlands and Lancashire, November 2019, p. 14.

[144] Tom Ball and Lawrence Sleater, 'Three deaths at psychiatric hospital', *The Times*, January 20, 2023, p. 5.

[145] Chris Jenks, *Transgression* (London: Routledge, 2003), p. 157.

[146] Karen Armstrong, *Islam: A Short History* (London: Phoenix, 2001).

thing expecting different results.[147] Part of the invention of 'madness' concerned the need by those in power to segregate off those threatening power and examples of this concerning gender, sexuality, class, and race are addressed in Chaps. 3 and 4. In societies that prioritize production and data over the human, the transrational reinvigorates offering breaks in an inhuman system with 'madness' part of this.

The UK wellbeing industry is worth 24 billion dollars which is roughly three times the value of the British film industry.[148] The happiness industry does not deny the importance of wealth in spiritual attainment and it is often seen as evidence of the Spirit's blessings. For one contemporary shaman who brags about his rich friends, 'Spiritual people are definitely not poor, because if you don't have anything to give, then you're not going to be very good at being spiritual'.[149] Self-styled happiness gurus attractiveness can be seen from how many of their books are in the top ten best-seller lists.[150] Popularized through television documentaries and YouTube videos and intense social media marketing, one well-known example is Tony Robbins. His philosophy teaches people to think big, to dream big, while he receives a big fee. Others such as Eckhart Tolle draw on a synthesis of Buddhism and new age style self-realization. This includes mindfulness which is a practice that has filtered into office culture indicating how mainstream it has become.

In *McMindfulness* Ronald E. Purser insightfully revealed the problem with neoliberal mindfulness which as the subtitled states is the new capitalist spirituality. Not only has stress been medicalized and pathologized but there is an ideological message that, 'if you cannot alter the circumstances causing distress, you can change your reactions to circumstances'.[151] The way Purser describes it is that this is a form of 'magical thinking'; it 'hypnotizes' people into seeing stress as their own fault, so there is no reason or need to be critical of the, 'systemic, institutional and structural causes' of stress. What this means is that stress becomes privatised in a neoliberal. The 'public sphere and body politic' is undermined.[152] Significantly, the growth of corporate mindfulness programmes began with the financial crash of 2008, with the rise of layoffs, the 'precariat', and employees being commanded to, 'do more with less'.[153] While not entirely new, the wellbeing and happiness industry flourished through the depression and stress that followed the crash with $300 billion lost to stress-related absences in the US alone.

---

[147] Often attributed to Einstein but in the following context: at quantum level the nature of reality is 'mad'; when you conduct the same experiment you never get the same result. See Chap. 5.

[148] Jennifer Colin 2019 'The $10 billion business of self-care', *Los Angeles Times*, May 10, 2019 (latimes.com) (accessed 16 October, 2023).

[149] Shaman Durek, *Spirit Hacking: Shamanic keys to reclaim your personal power, transform yourself and light up the world* (California: Hay House, 2019), p. 139.

[150] This includes books on eliminating negative thinking, mastering stress, and developing your own happiness journal.

[151] Ronald E. Purser, *McMindfulness. How Mindfulness Became the New Capitalist Spirituality* (London: Repeater, 2019), p. 38.

[152] Ibid.

[153] Purser, op. cit., p. 135.

'There is nothing either good or bad/But thinking makes it so.'[154] We might want to agree with Hamlet, but I think Shakespeare is condemning such an approach. Changing your thoughts to change your own world, as you experience it, can be helpful advice but it is problematic. Self-help guru Wayne Dyer claims we exist in a spiritual world before we are born. We choose our physical body and the parents we need for this 'trip' on earth and for him there, 'are no wrongful deaths or mistakes'.[155] Those whose loved ones have been murdered will find this problematic. In terms of sanity, philosophically, it can make sense to believe, 'what *is* could not be otherwise'.[156] But what if this were not the case? In *Sliding Doors* (Peter Howitt, 1998) Helen (Gwyneth Paltrow) is sacked from her job in London and is on two trajectories. In one, Helen arrives home early to find her partner Gerry (John Lynch) in bed with women; in another she arrives after the woman has left. For Bergson time is neither a unity nor a multiplicity, duration ineffable, and only shown indirectly through images that are not complete with science unable to measure it. This film reveals both scenarios concurrently, offering a light-hearted way of exploring this philosophical theme through a romantic comedy. For Bergson time can only be grasped through a simple intuition of the imagination, that which is part of the transrational.[157]

We know physical health can be found through exercise and diet, but personal happiness is more subjective. There is nothing essentially malign about this New Age branch of the happiness industry, unless coercive pressure is involved then certain movements can become abusive cults as discussed in Chap. 7. The trouble is with the whole of Western society geared up to commodification and with the dominance of advertising what coercive means becomes more fluid. These beliefs can lead to non-action and a total acceptance of the damaging political status quo, if all that matters is you and your perception rather than the world. To claim you can have it all, as Robbins and others do, can lead to unhappiness as it is fundamentally untrue. For example, if we consider inherited wealth not everyone is born with old money. Freud's focus on turning neurotic misery into ordinary unhappiness is more realistic but stems from a more pessimistic outlook aligned with the period in which he was born and the time he lived in, including the rise of Nazism. There is an irony when we talk of self-help when this is devotion to an ideology. The cultish behaviour that can build around these types of gurus, including figures like Robbins and Freud, is not entirely of their own making. Often people want to believe totally in these gurus, despite (or because of) gurus telling people not to so. Total belief offers a simplicity. Pushed by polished marketing, people become worked-up into a 'mad' frenzy of 'mad' belief in these new messiahs.

[154] *Hamlet* 2. ii.

[155] Wayne Dyer, *The Power of Intention* (California: Hay House, 2006), p. 121.

[156] Tolle, op. cit., p. 117.

[157] Henri Bergson, *The Creative Mind: An Introduction to Metaphysics* (London: Kensington Publishing Corps, 1998), pp. 165–168.

Elements of mainstream psychology has swallowed the ideals of the happiness industry, so it has become positively orientated. This might cause harm, a subject we shall return to in Chap. 8.[158] For example, it could lead to a stigmatization of the negative dimensions of human life which are crucial for existence and then this exacerbates mental health problems. Figures like Jacques Lacan, who built on Freud, and those before him like Lucretius, realised that the anxiety at the heart of humanity cannot be totally cured. There is a necessity to reassert the concept of negativity within psychoanalysis.[159] Negative psychoanalysis was introduced as a concept by Russell Jacoby (1972) to maintain Freudian psychoanalysis as a pillar of critical theory. But, as Duane Russell maintains, clinical and theoretical psychoanalysis is inherently negative anyway.[160]

Removing traditional gatekeepers, new media technologies have personalised the happiness industry through influencers. Popular guru figures include celebrities and influencers who sometimes have built on their pre-existing cultural capital via acting careers to promote themselves as wellbeing brands, such as Gwyneth Paltrow and Russell Brand. Consumers think they know these influencers personally and see them as their friends. This is highlighted well in Season 5 Episode 3 of *Black Mirror*, 'Rachel, Jason and Ashley Too', where Miley Cyrus plays a Britney Spears type trapped popstar Ashley O, who has her own doll that acts as a friend to her fans.

Russell Brand's informal and direct style on his YouTube channel invites the viewer in so we can be part of his experimental chatty world. In 2022 his channel was censored for allegedly spreading COVID-19 misinformation, sparking a debate over freedom of speech. Whether Brand's channel did or did not spread misinformation, on the surface it seems absurd that people take what celebrities say seriously. In Chap. 7 we shall see how the world is disenchanted so celebrity culture brings an acceptable magic and creates a fantasy so those who do not know people like Brand at all think they know him, creating a trust and bond. To trust in celebrity culture indicates society is suffering a deep sadness, with people unable to trust in close relationships. In Brand's case this trust is exacerbated by his characteristically open and blasé attitude and this apparent genuine nature means more of his endorsed products are sold. While it is easy to mock these figures and their followers, they are only passing on their apparent wisdom and making money in the process and for Brand this includes his knowledge of the 'madness' of addiction, his 2007 memoir being insightful.[161]

One problem is the branded self becomes a deified commodity which consumers become addicted to, like joining a cult. The belief is that by simply purchasing into these gurus this financial exchange deepens happiness. An initial hit and high with

[158] See James Marriott, Chap. 8.

[159] Duane Russell, Call for Papers – Negative Psychoanalysis: Nurturing Negativity, Death, and Trauma, ed. Julie Reshe & Duane Rousselle, 21 January 2022.

[160] Ibid. Negativity, death, and trauma are prevalent in the work of Julia Kristeva, Catherine Malabou, Todd McGoawn, Sabina Spielrein, Slavoj Žižek, Alenka Zupancic, and others.

[161] Russell Brand, *My Booky Wook* (London: Hodder & Stoughton, 2007).

this consumption, not unlike other addictions, may occur, then unhappiness reigns from the failure to live up to the brand. We find this conceptualized through, 'languages that are medical, therapeutic, or "spiritual"'.[162] This leads to another purchase at a higher-level, amassing wealth further into the hands of those who already have an abundance, furthering the wealth divide, creating wider social unhappiness. Happiness is dangled as just out of reach with higher levels to reach enlightenment involving the cult behaviour addressed in Chap. 7. It must remain out of reach, otherwise happiness gurus go out of business.

In these terms the happiness industry is part of the advertising industry, but there is an even darker side preying on contemporary vulnerabilities. Keith Raniere was sentenced to 120 years in prison in October 2020 for running the abusive sex cult NXIVM. On the surface this appeared to be part of the legal and lucrative wellbeing industry, but his level of control was shocking. One woman testified she was confined to a single room for two years, after she confessed finding someone other than Raniere attractive. Without the unhappiness of desire constructed by unrestrained capitalism and marketing, including excessive desires driven by gurus promoting their brands, this abusive system does not thrive. An endless cyclical process of dissatisfaction/non-satiation and unhappiness drives the un/happiness industry.

The high priests of the un/happiness industry are psychiatrists and medically trained psychologists who can prescribe 'happy' pills. While using this religious terminology may appear metaphorical, during interviews conducted for Chap. 5 it was clear that the term high priest is correct. They still possess an overarching power and are at the top of the power pyramid.[163] In *Side Effects* (Steven Soderbergh, 2013), Jude Law plays English psychiatrist Dr. Banks now based in New York making money through pushing a new drug Ablixa on his patients. His patient Emily Taylor (Rooney Mara) murders her husband Martin (Channing Tatum) while on Ablixa. The film reveals issues with the medicalization of society, how this imagined route to happiness is fallacious, and the fluid definitions of insanity that have various purposes including legal defence a subject returned to in Chap. 8.

Emily stabs Martin to death while apparently sleep walking, supposedly a side effect of Ablixa, then pleads insanity. She is found not guilty, but one condition is she must remain in a psychiatric hospital under Banks's supervision until he gets to the truth. The murder was premeditated because Emily had a pact with her lover, psychiatrist Dr. Victoria Ziebert (Catherine Zeta Jones). Dr. Banks has a partial breakdown which is an enlightening experience. As we see in Chap. 7, this form of breakthrough often occurs and can be a moment the individual learns a transrational viewpoint where they are taken outside of their own preconditioning.

[162] McKenzie Wark, *Capital is Dead: Is this Something Worse?* (London: Verso, 2019), p. 98.

[163] Visiting a mental hospital in the early 1990s, I was amused to find during one meeting with patients the psychiatrist literally sat on a high-chair raised above the group and other staff, so they could assert their authority from their God-like total view of the group.

Banks supersedes the 'mad' containment of his profit-based psychiatry, driven by the capitalist modality which had controlled his actions and made him transgress. This is morally and therefore psychologically beneficial and we see how his wellbeing is accomplished through this transrational education. Perching in his New York office in the sky, like one of his sectioned patients, Bank's was trapped. Where the incarceration is becomes part of a larger question controversially raised by Baudrillard concerning the 9/11 terrorist attacks. For Baudrillard those working in the New York offices destroyed by terrorists already had their lives curtailed due to entrapment within the system prior to the attack.[164]

American TV programmes, such as *Oprah* (1986 to 2011), popularized finding the real self for maximizing happiness, and of ridding from one's life everything that was holding you back. Happiness like 'madness' is a fluid paradigm. This stress on the real self or authentic self could lead to greater unhappiness. To highlight the complexities and absurdities of this area Richard Bentall, a highly influential figure in British psychology, argued in the well-respected *Journal of Medical Ethics* that happiness can be classified as a mental illness.[165] *Side Effects* reflects on the different approaches in American and Britain and Europe concerning the goal of treatment and psychoanalysis. Freud's goal was to turn neurotic misery into general unhappiness which was a way of managing the expectations of those in psychoanalysis. In America treatment seekers wanted an absolute cure, not just temporary relief, happiness without limits, which partially explains why the happiness industry is strongest in America. This also concerns an early American Puritan drive to literally establish heaven on earth, away from the evils of Europe and the residues of these beliefs are still strong and contribute to the messiah worship of Donald Trump.[166]

Concurrently, rather than blaming misfortune on the direct outcome of one's mistaken deeds, there is a belief in blaming an invisible presence, such as evil, which we will examine in Chap. 2. Non-medical treatment, including spirituality, competed with the pharmaceutical industry. Psychologists, psychiatrists, psychotherapists, and all manner of positive lifestyle gurus and wellbeing advisors, possessed answers to the human condition. While ancient literature showed happiness and the meaning of life to be a quest that included suffering, not an immediate fix, this was now a multibillion-dollar global industry worth over 4 trillion dollars.[167] Without sadness, often caused by over-emphasizing our want for material desires, there was no industry. You can have it all, but how much do you want it, Madchester (sic) rock group Oasis sang, self-reflexively, as a mantra in 1994. Unhappily, too much was never enough.

[164] J. Baudrillard, *The Spirit of Terrorism* (New York: Verso, 2013).

[165] Richard Bentall, 'A Proposal To Classify Happiness as a Mental Disorder', *Journal of Medical Ethics*, vol. 18, no. 2, June 1992, pp. 94–98.

[166] Jason Lee, Nazism and Neo-Nazism in Film and Media (Amsterdam: Amsterdam University Press, 2018).

[167] 2018, Global Wellness Institute (the GDP of the UK and Canada combined), FutureLearn, 27 January 2022.

1.3 Conclusions: Language and Medication

This chapter has explained how 'madness' changes over time and place, how it is not necessarily a physical or medical problem and may not even be a problem at all. We know that to a degree language constructs reality and 'madness' can be a metaphor, but it was also shown how it is not merely a metaphor. The transrational was introduced and it was explained how it has been relegated; the transrational concerns the emotional which is at the heart of psychic distress and humanity. Denying the transrational leads to mental health problems. The problem is with the reporting of emotional states which are part of the transrational. For example, it may seem a cliché that men cannot express their feelings but there is truth in this. Male suicide is the largest killer of young men in America and the UK. Being able to express emotions can help, as can an awareness of transrational knowledge as explained here which includes the emotions. Hiding emotions is still today often thought to be a good thing because expressing them is thought to be a sign of weakness.[168]

Of course, in certain circumstances being over-emotional might be a weakness and *Se7en* (David Fincher, 1995) depicts this well. Here David Mills (Brad Pitt) plays a rookie detective hunting a serial killer and Mills is over-emotional about killers. This means he fails to understand their behaviour, condemning them as psychos and positioning them beyond understanding. When Mills kills John Doe (Kevin Spacey) for cutting off the head of his wife Tracy (Gwyneth) this has an inevitability to it, because throughout the film Mills is played as over-emotional. He is manipulated by John Doe. The transrational also concerns the unconscious which is always one step award ahead of the conscious mind. We can understand the fruitful inevitability of this narrative and many others once we register that there is a popular misconception that the unconscious is an area dominated by the irrational, as if entering it too fully leads to 'madness'. We can take this in another director; following Lacan, it needs acknowledging how the unconscious has its own logic.[169] This logic is a truth that is different from ordinary thought but can be considered a form of language. Instead of existence stemming from thought in the Descartean fashion, if the Lacanian subject exists it is where it does not think; it is in the unconscious, which speaks before any subject has the illusion of thought.[170] This illustrates the authenticity of transrational knowledge and the power of these narratives.

Our autonomic nervous system is involved in facial and bodily expression, influencing our moods and mental health with any real division between the physical and mental fallacious.[171] Aspects of language, such as syntax, are 'wired into the

[168] The media vitriol Prince Harry received for daring to speak of his emotions in *Spare* (New York: Random House, 2023) epitomises this.

[169] Slavoj Žižek, *How to Read Lacan* (London: Granta Books, 2006).

[170] Seán Burke, *The Death and Return of the Author. Criticism and Subjectivity in Barthes, Foucault and Derrida* (Edinburgh: Edinburgh University Press, 2008).

[171] Richard Bentall, *Madness Explained – Psychosis and Human Nature* (London: Penguin, 2004), p. 212.

architecture of the brain', with speaking a social process with rules and conventions we learn.[172] The 'mad' do not play by the agreed common rules, R.D. Laing positing that the real problem for people with schizophrenia is that society has not learnt to interpret the language of those with schizophrenia.[173] Language then is the key defining factor; if you call a state depression I cannot disagree if for me I would personally call this anxiety.[174] This is personal, and changes over time and place, but should mental health be about self-identifying as with many other areas? There are issues with this which have been noted in private psychiatric care where the patient, the customer, is always considered right; any attempts at objective then dissipate.

Language is again key to our understanding. Placing an emphasis on the symbolic order, Lacan sees psychoanalytically driven linguistics and anthropology as the real depth science. This is a science of detailed ethnography, revealing how the structures of language are unified with and formulating social laws that regulate behaviours, all positioned in a terrain within the unconscious.[175] We can see how this functions today through contemporary mass media, such as social media, which is algorithmically established within a racially prejudiced paradigm and to generate conflict which can lead to fear, anxiety, and depression but we should be careful to not overgeneralise in a binary fashion. Social media can and does often lead to community and wellbeing but we shall come on to some of the dangers of social media in Chap. 8. In the early nineteenth century doctors labelled negative states 'melancholia', 'neurasthenia', or 'mopishness' (for the uneducated classes).[176]

As we shall see in Chaps. 3 and 4, mental health issues and their treatment are determined by media and culture in relation to gender, sexuality, race, and class. Depression was first used to describe a lowering in cardiovascular function, psychiatrists using this term as the antithesis to excitation, then the word became part of popular discourse concerning loss.[177] During the twentieth century anthropologists believed the cultural theory of emotion, that is, emotions are learned behaviours much like languages. Paul Ekman discovered the opposite; emotions—joy, distress, anger, fear, surprise, and disgust—are innate and universal.[178] There are some obvious issues with this. English has over 2000 emotion words, but some languages contain under 200; Gidjingali aborigines do not discriminate between fear and shame, with prototypical emotions that are central in Western psychopathology conceptualization absent in some cultures.[179]

[172] Ibid.

[173] Ibid.

[174] Ibid.

[175] Jacques Lacan, *Écrits – A selection*, trans. Alan Sheridan (London: Routledge, 2008), p. 80.

[176] Bentall, op. cit.

[177] Ibid., p. 214.

[178] Dylan Evans, *Emotion* (Oxford: Oxford University Press, 2001), pp. 3–5.

[179] Bentall, op. cit.

In many non-Western cultures there is no equivalent word to depression. As Bentall explains, even when there is the same word the meaning of the word might be different in different cultures. For example, in Japanese jodo means the English equivalent of emotion, plus a range of other meanings such as considerate, motivated, lucky, and calculating.[180] It also means eliminate. Just because English has more words for emotions it does not correlate that it is more efficient or accurate at describing emotional states. Psychiatrists and psychologists globally often use models for diagnosis and treatment based on English language which limits treatment where English is not the first language and in Chap. 4. it is explained how psychiatry has been part of colonialism. The words of diagnoses can in one sense create the illness, but not always. Often depression and anxiety become split because this is how the language system works but clinical studies find these symptoms correlate and merge.[181]

Post-institutionalisation of the 'mad', society became institutionalised through maximising surveillance and control. The development of 'madness' has been examined and the problems with ignoring the transrational and prioritizing the rational outlined. According to Britain's Mental Health Foundation, 50% of the population will at some point have a mental health diagnosis, the most common being depression.[182] In these attempts to be inclusive and move towards de-stigmatisation there are problems, given if everyone has a mental health problem then no one does. As explained, if the DSM is applied literally one hundred percent have a mental health problem which is absurd. Epidemiological studies show four to 12% of the UK's adult population have a formal diagnosis of personality disorder; if milder degrees of personality disorders are considered this is much higher.[183] What exactly personality disorder is varies, differing in the two main diagnostic manuals, the *International Classification of Diseases* (ICD) and the DSM. The DSM categorizes 10 personality disorders. Borderline personality disorder (BPD) alone has produced a wealth of psychiatric literature but is a problematic diagnosis. For example, Johnny Depp's legal team in his 2022 case against Amber Heard used this diagnosis to demonise her and it worked. While some clinicians and patients find BDP a useful diagnosis, two of the most respected British researchers into BPD believe it should no longer be used as it is too contentious.[184] Personality disorders are not mental illnesses. In theory, they persist throughout life and do not have an onset and time course. This could suggest treatments are in one sense useless; these

---

180 Ibid.

181 Ibid., p. 218.

182 Menta Health Foundation, 'Good Mental Health For All', https://www.mentalhealth.org.uk (accessed 27 January, 2023).

183 Linda Gask, Mark Evans and David Kessler, 'Personality Disorder', *BMJ: British Medical Journal*, Vol. 347. No. 7924, 14 September 2013 (28-32), p. 28.

184 Antony Bateman and Fonagy, 'Mentalisation-treatment training', NHS training the Anna Freud Centre, July/October, 2019.

disorders cannot be cured, just managed. If they are so much part of someone's make-up, someone's personality, curing seems disingenuous.

As explained, the medical profession as we know it today only became interested in treating the 'mad' once the financial benefits were obvious. Is it possible to move on from limited classifications, or are the powerful systems that control diagnoses and treatment too trapped in this paradigm with the income from medication too lucrative? Peter Breggin in *Toxic Psychiatry* certainly thought so.[185] With books like Elizabeth Wurtzel's cult classic *Prozac Nation* (adapted for film Erik Skjoldbjærgof, 2001), published the same year as Breggin's book, dominating public discourse on 'madness' and celebrating Prozac, Breggin's backlash against medication was necessary for balance.[186] As a psychiatrist, Breggin was correct to condemn the farfetched utopianism around New Psychiatry where drugs were supposed to heal everything. This utopianism was without the satirical irony of Aldous Huxley's soma in his dystopian novel *Brave New World* (1932). For Breggin, schizophrenia, depression and anxiety disorder have never been proven to be genetic, or even physical in origin. The drug fluoxetine (Prozac) was found to increase suicidality and not just because those on the drug were already mentally unstable.[187]

Medicalization has brought about an over-dependence on drugs on an unprecedented scale. Overtly utopian and dystopian discourse over psychiatric medication in the 1990s related to pre-millennium fears. These dreams and nightmares have consistently shaped cultures throughout history.[188] Once the medication-utopia discourse of the 1990s faded, a more nuanced approach to mental disorders and treatments developed beyond drugs. Despite some amazing success in the field of post-traumatic stress disorder with Prozac and related drugs like Zoloft, Celexa, Cymbalta, and Paxil, these did not work with extreme cases like war veterans, a subject addressed next.[189]

There are underlying intersectional reasons for the over prescription of drugs. Drugs do not get to the underlying issues. They can control symptoms providing a mechanism for further healing and treatment, but they are also a means for control. There are other dangers on top of side-effects linked to profit and those impacted most have been those on low incomes and those of colour. On both sides of the Atlantic more expensive drugs are pushed rather than the cheaper generic equivalent. The industry was out of control with the number of people under 20 receiving Medicaid-funded prescriptions for antipsychotic drugs increasing by 51% during

[185]Peter Breggin, *Toxic Psychiatry: Why Therapy, Empathy and Love Must Replace the Drugs, Electroshock, and Biochemical Theories of the "New Psychiatry"* (New York: St. Martin's, 1994).

[186]Elizabeth Wurtzel, *Prozac Nation* (New York: Riverhead, 1994).

[187]M.J. Trueth, 'Revisiting fluoxetine (Prozac) and suicidal preoccupations', *The Journal of Emergency Medicine*, September-October, 12(5), 1994, pp. 685–687.

[188]Norman Cohn, *The Pursuit of the Millenium: Revolutionary Millenarians and Mystical Anarchists of the Middle Ages* (London: Pimlico, 1993).

[189]Kolk, op. cit., p. 35.

the early and mid-2000s.[190] In 2013 Johnson & Johnson agreed to pay more than $2.2 billion in criminal and civil fines over the promotion of the antipsychotic Risperdal. Those on low incomes were four times more likely to receive antipsychotic medicines; the argument advocating their use was that they made abused and neglected children more 'tractable'.[191] Adult people of colour receive four times the recommended dose of antipsychotic medicines.[192]

Remarkably, a complex and wide-ranging review study in 2022 concluded that there is no convincing evidence of a biomedical basis to depression, and that the serotonin theory of depression is, 'not empirically substantiated'.[193] The classist, sexist, and racist medicalization of society created the culture of mental ill-health. Over-emphasizing the rational and under-emphasizing the transrational and the emotional is detrimental to wellbeing and another danger is believing the accepted myths and status of science. For example, science is commonly associated with objectivity and truth, but this is a popular misconception. As Richard Horton, editor-in-chief of the world's leading medical journal *The Lancet* put it, 'the case against science is straightforward: much of the scientific literature, perhaps half, may simply be untrue'; similarly, Dr. Marcial Angell, a physician and long-time editor-in-chief of *The New England Medical Journal*, explained that we can no longer believe much of clinical research published, or, 'rely on the judgement of trusted physicians or authoritative medical guidelines'.[194] Paper mills, where genuine research is stitched together to produce fake research, is prolific ranging from chemical engineering to artificial intelligence. Authors are expected to pay $500 to $5000, depending on the status of the journal and while work is supposed to be peer reviewed fake work is not stopped.[195]

All the major medical journals primarily publish drug treatment studies with skewered outcomes.[196] Given mental health science is dominated by the drug industry this science cannot be associated with objectivity and truth, but in popular myth science still maintains this status of truth. We have seen how one impact of the Enlightenment was to create science as an unquestionable religion, but in such a blind belief system truth does not matter. The research is designed to increase profits

---

[190] Stephen Crystal et al., 'Rapid Growth Of Antipsychotic Presecriptions For Children Who Are Publicly Insured Has Ceased But Concerns Remain', *Health Affairs*, 35, No. 6 (2016). pp. 974–982.

[191] Trueth, op. cit.

[192] David Harewood, ''I came close to death': David Harwood on racism and psychosis', *The Guardian*, 21 August, 2021 'I came close to death': David Harewood on racism and psychosis | David Harewood | The Guardian (accessed October 16, 2023).

[193] Moncrieff, J., Cooper, R.E., Stockmann, T. et al., 'The serotonin theory of depression: a systematic umbrella review of the evidence', *Molecular Psychiatry*, June, 2022, https://doi.org/10.1038/s41380-022-01661-0 (accessed 26 July, 2022).

[194] F. William Engdahl, 'Shocking Report from Medical Insiders', NEO: New Eastern Outlook, 18 June, 2016, Shocking Report from Medical Insiders | New Eastern Outlook (journal-neo.org) (accessed 4 January, 2022).

[195] Rhys Blakely, 'Journals run fake Chinese science papers', *The Times*, October 1 2022, p. 13.

[196] Kolk, op. cit., p. 38.

of the drug industry and what has resulted from this pharmacological deluge? More people than ever at risk from becoming morbidly obese, having diabetes, suffering from a multitude of mental health problems, with an exponentially higher suicide rate (this being a side-effect of some mental health medications).

All these mental health problems were despite (or even because of) self-help gurus and the happiness industry dominating the media and identity creation, instigating a further dependency on buying into their magic. A 2020 study by Radboud University found activities for transcending the self, including self-help practices like mindfulness, inflated the ego making people more judgemental.[197] During this period when the image came to dominant through a rampant media focusing on the self and the individual for happiness it created its antithesis. Idealised happiness was subsumed in the image while the self disappeared into the image until reality became the image. The media dematerialised the real leading to the impossibility of re-apprehending the world through images; the screen was screening out of any dual relation until all that remained was the screen.[198] Chapter 8 concludes on how the transrational offers hope, but next the culture and screening of 'madness' which has informed and created the reality of 'madness' is assessed.

---

[197] Rhys Blakely, 'Why the path to enlightenment is an ego trip', *The Times*, December 29 2020, p. 1.

[198] Jean Baudrillard, *The Intelligence of Evil. Or The Lucidity Pact*, trans. Chris Turner (London: Bloomsbury, 2013), p. 59.

Chapter 2
Media and Culture

2.1 Introduction: Film and Television

As with many of the British elite in the 1930s, including members of the Royal family, the BBC's first director general Lord Reith was open about his admiration for Adolf Hitler.[1] Like the Fuhrer he admired, Reith also ran a dictatorship. He believed public broadcasting was a method for resolving class conflict.[2] On top of the established pedagogic methods through education, and the monitoring of internal and external spaces, other state methods of observation and indoctrination were seen as necessary.[3] A key component of this was public broadcasting and related media. From the mid-twentieth century this became preoccupied with the shaping of 'madness' by framing normality for social control.

A shift in thinking that evil was conceived as a disease born out of post-war optimism was used to explain a movement away from framing doctors as evil.[4] Even the 1948 drama *The Snake Pit* (Anatole Litvak), which was so damning of mental asylums health professionals they wrote to the British Board of Film Censors (BBFC) attempting to get it banned, has the main doctors as compassionate.[5] The BBFC did cut the flagged scenes in response. But we will see, just as with patients, psychiatrists and psychotherapists in later films and television shows have been positioned as evil, or at least capable of transgressions giving them an affinity with their evil patients. Within the containment of the mental hospital or doctor's consultation room, so-called evil can be confessed and purged and within the frame of the camera this contains the 'madness'.

---

[1] Tom Mills, *The BBC: The Myth of a Public Service* (London: Verso, 2018), p. 210.

[2] Ibid., p. 211.

[3] Ibid.

[4] A. Karpf, *Doctoring the Media: The Reporting of Health and Mediciden* (London: Routledge, 1988).

[5] Ibid, p. 182.

J. Lee, *Culture, Madness and Wellbeing*, https://doi.org/10.1007/978-3-031-37530-9_2

An influential study in the *Journal of Forensic Sciences* published in 2014 examined fictional portrayals of mental health in popular films from 1915 and found psychopathy the most emphasised diagnosis in film. From 400 films, 126 characters were chosen based on realism and clinical accuracy by senior forensic psychiatrists and film critics and then analysed. This research discovered fictional psychopaths in films have become more realistic over time which related to the advancement of understanding of clinical psychopathy within mental health professions. While overall realistic fictional psychopaths remained in the minority, it concluded they are useful for teaching purposes in mental health training.[6] Other work in forensic psychiatry published in 2017 using survey methodology concluded that increased exposure to fictional psychopaths advanced misunderstandings, including romanticizing psychopathy, and this might have legal, practical, and ethical implications, including influencing a bias in jurors.[7]

As Malynnda Johnson and Chris Olson explained in 2021, accurate depictions of 'madness' is essential to overcoming stigma and is crucial to those living with certain conditions, and there have been improvements.[8] According to MIND's report on British television in 2018 there has been a real improvement in representation. MIND works on 70 storylines a year involving people with lived experience making sure TV stories are realistic and sensitive.[9] Depression, anxiety, and bipolar disorder are treated with understanding and sympathy, but schizophrenia and personality disorders were still stereotypically depicted as leading to violence.[10] Those with mental health problems are more likely to be victims of violence than vice versa.[11]

Just as disorders and syndromes have their nuances, what is meant by accurate is not clear-cut, plus fantastical and impressionistic versions of 'madness' can be beneficial.[12] The creation of worlds like *Joker* can reveal more to us than verisimilitude and accuracy with its transrational imaginative quality going deeper. *Joker* re-ignited debates over mental health and film and was condemned by American mental health professionals for linking mental illness to violence.[13] This attack was erroneous because the narrative unveils Joker (Joaquin Phoenix) as not mentally ill

---

[6] S. Leistedt, P. Linkowski, 'Pyschopathy and the cinema: fact or fiction?' Journal of Forensic Sciences, January 2014, 59(1), pp.167–174.

[7] M. Keesler, D. DeMatteo, 'How Media Exposure Relatest to Laypersons' Understanding of Psychopathy', *Journal of Forensic Sciences*, November 2017, 62(6), pp. 1522–1533.

[8] Malynnda Johnson and Chris Olson, eds., *Normalizing Mental Illness and Neurodiversity in Entertainment Media: Quieting Madness* (New York: Rouledge, 2021), p. 2.

[9] MIND, op. cit.

[10] Jenny Regan, 'Improving representations of mental health on TV, 19 January, 2018, Improving representations of mental health on TV | Mind, the mental health charity - help for mental health problems (accessed 26 January, 2023).

[11] Johnson and Olson, op. cit.

[12] Phil Hoad, 'Madness in the movie: in defence of going gothic', *The Guardian*, 24 January, 2020 Madness in the movie: in defence of going gothic | Film | The Guardian (accessed 26 January, 2023).

[13] Johnson and Olson, op. cit.

or 'mad'. In his own words he is sad, and he has every reason to be given the extreme abuse he suffered as a child and due to society. Joker (Joaquin Phoenix) finds he has been misdiagnosed and this partly causes his anger. His five murders are constructed as justified and nothing to do with mental illness. The three Wall Street men on the subway have been abusing a woman and then they attack Joker in such a fashion that for his own survival he has no option but to shoot them. The reading by mental health professionals who condemned the film ignores the significant political underbelly of the film, Joker a symbol of the justified rage of the underclass.

It is no surprise that Hollywood companies have dominated the market share of the global box office since World War 1, but there is a change in this trajectory. North American market share of the global box declined:

> from 52% in 2002, to 46% in 2004, and to 35% in 2008. The international or non-U.S. share of the global box office is projected to increase from 65% of the world-wide box office in 2008 to 71% in 2015 and 78% by 2030.[14]

American, British, and European films are discussed acknowledging looking forward this is problematic and sketchy, although the second part of this chapter tackles two areas of 'madness' with regards to film in depth. There are several ways to group films on 'madness', one being in the following 16 categories which often bleed into each other.[15] 1. society and 'madness'—*Now, Voyager* (Irving Rapper, 1942), *A Woman under the Influence* (John Cassavetes, 1974), *The Snake Pit* (Anatole Litvak, 1948), *One Flew over the Cuckoo's Nest* (Milos Forman, 1975), with the Netflix spinoff *Ratched* (2020); 2. possession and 'madness'—*Dr Jekyll and Mr. Hyde* (Rouben Mamoulian, 1931), *The Exorcist* (William Friedkin, 1974) with numerous sequels, prequels, and spinoffs; 3. eros and 'madness'—*Secrets of a Soul* (G. W. Pabst, 1926), *M* (Fritz Lang, 1931), *Straw Dogs* (Sam Peckinpah, 1971), *Bad Timing: A Sensual Obsession* (Nicolas Roeg, 1980); 4. murder and 'madness'—*White Heat* (Raoul Walsh, 1949), *Badlands* (Terrence Malick, 1974); 5. war and 'madness'—*Twelve O' Clock High* (Henry King, 1949), *The Deer Hunter* (Michael Cimino, 1978), *The Last of the Mohicans* (Michael Mann, 1992); 6. sanity and 'madness', as in *You Can't Take It With You* (Frank Capra, 1938) and *King of Hearts* (Philip de Broca, 1966); 7. religion and 'madness'—*The Mission* (Roland Joffe, 1986) and *Black Robe* (Bruce Beresford, 1992); 8. serial killers and 'madness'—*Natural Born Killers* (Oliver Stone, 1994), and *We Need to Talk About Kevin* (Lynne Ramsay, 2011); 9. death and 'madness' and death as sanity—*Dead Man* (Jim

---

[14] McDonnell, John J. and Silver, Jon (2009) Hollywood dominance: will it continue? In: What is film? Change and Continuity in the twenty-first Century, 6–7 November 2009, Turnbull Center, Portland, Oregon. (Unpublished), p. 9.

[15] This schemata is developed from two main texts: Michael Fleming and Roger Manvell, *Images of Madness: Portrayal of Insanity in the Feature Film* (Vancouver: Fairleigh Dickinson University Press, 1986); and C.JP. Lee, *The Metaphysics of Mass Art – Cultural Ontology* Vol. II (New York: Mellen, 1999). The limitations of a schemata are overt but this is at least functions as snapshot primarily in an American context, with American cinema arguably having the greatest global impact.

Jarmusch, 1996).[16] 10. leadership and 'madness'—*Once Upon A Time In Hollywood* (Quentin Tarantino) which explores the Charles Manson cult, plus the James Bond film series where the 'mad' villain is a leader and invariably a narcissistic psychopath; 11. Comedy and 'madness'—*As Good As It Gets* (James L. Brooks, 1998) and *Wristcutters: A Love Story* (Goran Dukić, 2016); 12. sci-fi and 'madness'—*2001* (Stanley Kubrick, 1968); 13. history and 'madness'—*Stoneyhearst Asylum* (Brad Anderson, 2014); 14. addiction and 'madness'—*Jacob's Ladder* (Adrian Lyne, 1990), *Fear and Loathing in Las Vegas* (Terry Gilliam, 1998), and *Requiem for a Dream* (Darren Aronofsky, 2000). Aronofsky has in many ways built his career tackling versions of 'madness', including *Black Swan* (2010) and the bizarre intertextual *Mother!* (2018); 15. genius and 'madness'—*Shine* (Scott Hicks, 1996) and *A Beautiful Mind* (Ron Howard, 2001); 16. similarly, neurodiversity and 'madness'—*Rain Main* (Barry Levinson, 1988), the glorious *Bad Boy Bubby* (Rolf de Heer, 1994), *Forrest Gump* (Robert Zemeckis, 1994), and *Breaking the Waves* (Lars von Trier, 1996) discussed next.

One unifying factor across these categories is the protagonist as rebel. Protagonists are invariably those that suffer the most and are therefore the deepest individuals, offering us the most transrational knowledge. We follow our central character's journey, stepping into their shoes as counsellors claim they must do with their clients and as they feel more, we too feel more. This is what I call the unified transrational journey where a character's arc, to use screenwriting terminology, is the arc of the film's narrative. The Freudian view is that the unconscious is negative, almost perverse, but for Jung this is reversed: it is the conscious mind that is perverse with the unconscious being natural. Often films reveal this Jungian transrational truth. From watching what can be described as timeless films we re-ignite an element of our self that has been repressed in the rational dominated doing world which is staggered by time. Protagonists need to be slightly 'mad' and this is what makes them appealing as they resist the status quo and have a vision of a different future. These movies reveal that the rational mind and the societies which have this rationality as their primary focus have damaging backward-looking limitations, confirming the importance of the transrational for wellbeing.

As explained in Chap. 1, following the Age of Reason philosophers such as the influential Immanuel Kant and those he influenced believed that the rational brain functioned like a scientist, claiming morality was based on objective facts. But when, 'you are confronted with an ethical dilemma, the unconscious automatically generates an emotional response'.[17] These are the moral instincts we all have, unless we have psychopathic traits which are more common than is normally accepted and are increasing, as shall be explained here and in Chap. 7. Interestingly, this contradicts an evolutionary view that humans, over time, become more empathetic. A 2010 study of 364 white-collar workers identified greater levels of psychopathy in more

[16] Ibid.

[17] Jonah Lehrer, *The Decisive Moment. How the Brain Makes Up its Mind* (Edinburgh: Canongate, 2009), p. 167.

senior levels of corporations and predicted this was increasing, which raises questions over moral accountability and has ethical implications for all organisations with globalisation spreading western oriented corporations.[18] The very traits of a psychopath, being ruthless, selfish, and taking decisions in a conscience-free fashion without any regard for anyone, have become traits regarded as commendable for leadership. Film and television characters who have these psychopathic traits are immensely popular, having become historical and fictional cultural heroes such as Hannibal the Cannibal.

With reference to film category 2., a patient quoted by a founder of psychology William James illustrates how 'madness' and possession are equated. In a letter, the patient argues that his fear of the devil equates with insanity and he is, 'defenceless against the invisible enemy who is tightening his coils around me'.[19] The issue for this patient is the invisibility of the enemy and he prefers death. A plethora of cultural texts concern the related subject of 'madness' and doubling which is close to the possession category above, a theme in this letter. Possession and 'madness' informs the uncanny, from Shirley Jackson's fiction; to Jack Finney's novel *The Body Snatchers* (1956, serialized in *Colliers Magazine*, 1954), with various versions and spins offs; to Ira Levin's novel *The Stepford Wives* (1972) and two film versions (Brian Forbes, 1975; Frank Oz, 2004); to Dennis Lehane's 2003 novel and film adaptation *Shutter Island* (Martin Scorsese, 2010), the novel and film *Echo Maker* (Richard Powers, 2006) and more, 'madness', doubling, the uncanny, and the transrational are entwined. These works can be deconstructed in terms of what they tell us about the societies within which they are set and produced where nothing is at it seems.[20] Such beliefs spawned conspiracy culture which to the outsider looks 'mad', but to the insider make perfect sense embodying T-O-T-A-L truth.

At a metaphysical and metaphorical level, mainstream film explores and can contain 'madness'. I mean this in both meanings of contain; films can offer a framework for containing and therefore curtailing 'madness'.[21] The film industry's Internet Movie Database (IMDB) in 2020 positioned 153 films as, 'the best movies about insanity' with *A Clockwork Orange* (Stanley Kubrick, 1971) coming top, Kubrick's *The Shining* (1980) second, and Kubrick's *2001: A Space Odyssey* (1968) third.[22] Originally from the Bronx in New York, Kubrick moved to Elstree, England, in 1968 shooting many sections of his films in the UK. Despite books appearing such as *Stanley Kubrick—American Filmmaker*, where his knowledge of the technical

[18] C. Boddy, R. Ladyshewsky, and P. Galvin, 'Leaders without ethics in global business: Corporate psychopaths', *Journal of Public Affairs*, Vol. 10, Issue 3, 04 June 2010, pp. 121–138.

[19] William James, *The Varieties of Religious Experience: A Study in Human Nature* (London: Penguin, 1982), p. 148.

[20] Alexander Dunst, *Madness in Cold War America* (London: Routledge, 2016).

[21] Although we shall see that there are some exceptions to this where films have 'caused madness'.

[22] Mladin Stajic, 'the best movies about INSANITY', The best movies about INSANITY - IMDb (accessed 24 January, 2023).

aspects of filmmaking is seen as preternatural, his films are extremely European and individual in their aesthetic drawing on existentialism.[23]

Films on the industry 'mad' film list frequently relate to a sci-fi genre that blends with horror, horror possessing the greatest ability to illustrate an overt reflection on anxieties than any other genre.[24] What is noteworthy is the 'technolatry' in these fictions, an area I highlight as a cause of 'madness' throughout this book; but writers such as William Gibson, while offering a credible reality, go beyond an obsession with the Apocalypse.[25] We shall return to J. G. Ballard in our conclusions to Chap. 8, and Ballard, along with other influential sci-fi authors such as William Gibson, Thomas Pynchon, Jayne Anne Phillips, and William Burroughs, utilised what Ballard called 'invisible literature' which was the 'permeating flow of scientific reports, government documents, and specialised advertising that shapes our culture below the level of recognition.'[26] Behind our everyday reality is this metanarrative that if we are not careful may predetermine reality if we allow it, so here science fiction works as offering a stark warning. In this sense, we may not believe we are physically caged like the incarcerated mental patient, but manipulation by 'invisible literature' means we are imprisoned.

Us (Jordan Peele, 2019) is a pre-eminent example of how new horror deals with PTSD, a diagnosis we address directly later in this chapter. Films in this genre often suggest child sexual abuse leads to an uncontrollable 'madness' and murderous rampage with a theological underpinning.[27] While a causal impact is sometimes provable 'madness' can be outside all cause and reason, being the unknown and unknowable. Paradoxically, this allows for new meaning, informing the essence of transrational knowledge and vice versa. Films have recurrently constructed and deconstructed the fragmented 'mad' mind, expressly cult sci-fi and supernatural thrillers, such as *The Sixth Sense* (M. Night Shyamalan, 1999), *Donnie Darko* (Richard Kelly, 2001) and *Twelve Monkeys* (Terry Gilliam, 1995) with its thought-provoking television spin-off (2015–2018). The premise of the latter is: sometimes you must just trust people, even when this is totally against your reason and even if this appears to be 'madness', confirming the necessity of 'madness' for human relationships to thrive and the importance of the transrational. These films have moved from being cult audience films to international popularity, showing transrational knowledge has transglobal relevance.

Within the illustrious history of sci-fi films on 'madness' Kubrick's work is once again pre-eminent with *2001: A Space Odyssey* (1968), inspired by Arthur

---

[23]David Micks, *Stanley Kubrick – American Filmmaker* (New Haven: Yale University Press, 2020).

[24]V. McCollum, *Post-9/11 Heartland Horror: Rural horror films in an error of urban terrorism* (London: Routledge, 2016). p. 86.

[25]Bruce Sterling, preface to William Gibson, *Burning Chrome* (London: Gollancz, 2016), pp. 3–2.

[26]Ibid, p. 4.

[27]Jason Lee, *Pervasive Perversions – Paedophilia and Child Sexual Abuse in Media/Culture* (London: Free Association Books, 2005).

C. Clarke's short story 'The Sentinel' (1951). *Solaris* (Andrei Tarkovsky, 1972), *Pi* (Darren Aronofsky, 1998), and *Moon* (Duncan Jones, 2009) are significant in the context of 'madness'. Taking a step outside what is the known can be viewed as 'madness', to go beyond, such as space travel, despite the possibility that it is only through such travel that humans will survive.

In *Moon* the uncanny double again appears and the film asks: would it drive you 'mad' to find out that a company had made multiple clones of you to maximize work potential; what if you were unclear who was the original you, with your whole history including your wife and child possibly invented? The wider questions are: are all our lives now situated in a video-streamed realm that is invented; what do we really know about who we are, memory, and how time and reality exist; could this all be constructed? There is the anxiety and 'madness' shown here from being a clone, but in an existentialist sense we are totally alone which can also cause angst and dwelling on an either/or scenario could cause 'madness'.

The sci-fi *Ex Machina* (Alex Garland, 2014) further explores this classic Frankensteinian logic of machines and monsters being more human than humans in our 'mad' pursuit of the rational and confirming wellbeing through the transrational.[28] Caleb (Dominic Gleeson), an employee of a Facebook-type company, wins a trip to meet the company owner Nathan (Oscar Isaac). Caleb initially does not realise that he is part of a Turing Test form of experiment, to determine whether an artificial intelligence is capable of being like a human being. During the process he falls in love with the robot Ava (Alicia Vikander), who then manages to break free of the compound, having a higher human emotional intelligence than her maker Nathan. The film functions as a warning against the dangers of human ambition and intelligence without humanity, and how humans can be enslaved by the myths of their own creations if they avoid transrational knowledge.

As with all these films (and 'madness' in reality) the reason why cult horror film *The Wicker Man* (Robin Hardy, 1973) is designated by IMDB as part of the 'mad' film genre is contingent on how 'madness' is perceived. The fundamentalist Protestant convictions of Sergeant Howie (Edward Woodward), investigating the disappearance of Rowan Morrison (Gerry Cowper) on a Scottish pagan island Summerisle, can appear 'madder' than the pagan practices. To the islanders Howie's blind rationally focused faith is a blinkered 'madness'. This is not simply mainland rationalism versus the transrationalism of the islanders. The scenes of Howie in the director's cut on the 'Christian' mainland reveal that his behaviour there is also thought extreme and a blinkered form of fundamentalism which like some forms of science applies a literal truth.

Lord Summerisle (Christopher Lee) and his followers have a belief that to outsiders looks 'mad', but this is based on their own convictions. Howie's Christianity might be Anglican, but his approach is Puritan in the way he condemns everything on Summerisle. Max Weber drew on the writings of seventeenth century Puritans to explain how the bourgeoisie carried out their business as calling from the God for the

[28] Jason Lee, *Sex Robots – The Future of Desire* (London: Palgrave, 2018).

elect.[29] A specific version of Christianity was spawned from our 'mad' obsession with progress which vice versa shaped capitalist society. This was not just within a metaphysical teleological framework focused on the apocalyptic end times, but within the historical and physical world.[30] A fantasy of a 'world without us' is the purest one; for Slavoj Žižek humans are so deeply implicated in the fragile equilibrium of the earth our cessation would cause 'cataclysmic imbalance'.[31] From our (re)current eco-crisis apocalyptic perspective, a theme here in Chap. 8, elements of the paganism in this film seem sane with Lord Summerisle the leader of an eco-island.

According to its director, *Midsommar* (Ari Aster, 2019) is *The Wicker Man* meets *Modern Romance* (Albert Brooks, 1981); rather than being a horror film, it is about how a break-up can feel apocalyptic.[32] The main action takes place in Sweden where a ritualistic sacrifice takes place of someone who is trying to investigate the people, but here it is not a policeman but a student anthropologist. The focus is on Danni (Florence Pugh), an American whose sister commits suicide early in the film and her relationship with her boyfriend who just does not seem that interested in her. In a telling scene in an American café, male friends of Danni's boyfriend, tellingly called Christian (Jack Reynor), think he should dump Danni because, to paraphrase the annoying Mark (Will Poulter), the sex is not great and Danni is so needy. Danni is on a popular drug for anxiety that can alter libido. These young men in her life dismiss Danni's sister's needs as mere calls for attention. The implication is Danni listens to these young men, because she has four unopened emails from her sister in her inbox who then ends up dead.

There is a ruthless capitalist acquisitiveness to these men dominated by an obstinately rational American outlook who are selfishly blind to transrational knowledge and the sacred. Their discipline is anthropology and instead of wanting to truly understand they seek to categorise and label. These young men are unable to truly speak their emotions and their lack of maturity and lack of transrational and emotional knowledge is their downfall. Given the backwardness of their approach their sacrifice for the Swedish community appears justified. In the film's promotion what is stressed is Dani's psychological trauma impacting on her relationship with Christian as the main issue, rather than his faults as a man. In one interpretation this promotes a sexist position but this positions us in a trajectory pregnant for a tantalisingly stark reversal, because it is a feminist film.

---

[29] Max Weber, *The Protestant Ethic and the Spirit of Capitalism* (USA: Start Publishing LLC, 2012).

[30] Norman Cohn, *Cosmos, Chaos, and the World to Come: The Ancient Roots of Apocalyptic Faith* (London: Yale University Press, 2001).

[31] Slavoj Žižek, *Living in the End Times* (London: Verso, 2011), p. 80. Žižek was writing pre-COVID-19, during which we even further realised due to lockdowns the benefits of human non-carbon fuelled activity.

[32] Mark Olsen, '*Midsommar* explained: The filmmakers unpack the sex, rituals and shocking ending', *Los Angeles Times*, 3 July 2019, 'Midsommar' explained: The filmmakers unpack the sex, rituals and shocking ending - Los Angeles Times (latimes.com) (accessed 20 July, 2022).

The students decide to go to their friend's Pelle (Vilhelm Blomgren) closed community in Sweden. Educated in a Western system that has deleted transrational knowledge, the Americans are unable to conceive of the sacredness of several aspects of the community. Mark urinates on the sacred tree and a sacred text goes missing. Christian who initially has no idea what his doctorate will be on and Josh (William Jackson), who is already researching this area of midsummer rituals and plans to go to Germany and England, compete on who will get the most access to the community to further their scholarship and careers. In brash American imperialistic capitalist fashion, they want to maximise their consumption of the other for their own benefit and fail to see what is happening in the community.

Their autoethnography becomes lived experience, in a performative sense, like *Antichrist* (Lars von Trier, 2009) discussed next. Christian does a mock PhD viva by having ritualistic sex with Maja (Isabelle Grill), as older women ritualistically grunt and sway approvingly. Stuck in a rationality that avoids transrational knowledge, the Americans mistakenly believe they are taking conscious decisions, acting like observers of what Mark jokingly says is Waco, as in the Branch Davidian cult in Texas. Danni is elected May Queen and, after seeing her partner Christian having sex with Maja, with Danni's blessing Christian is approvingly burnt to death in the most sacred of temples. Christian is comically stuffed inside a bearskin, the evil of the community placed upon him and banished. The film closes on Danni's approving smile, as she is finally free of her appalling boyfriend and watches his funeral pyre with the evil now banished. Danni is the embodiment of natural life, Christian literally lifeless when supposedly alive and the embodiment ritualistically of death bringing new life.

In a practical sense a certain form of 'madness' is required for making films, and for leadership as we learn in Chap. 7. This is found in *Citizen Kane* (Orson Welles, 1942) and *The Aviator* (Martin Scorsese, 2004), plus many Shakespeare plays and film adaptations such as *Richard the III* (Richard Loncraine, 1995) where megalomania is close to hubris. What is entertaining is the border between conscious and unconscious behaviour, and those who step across the line of what is established behaviour. The necessity of 'madness' is overt in *Fitzcarraldo* (Werner Herzog, 1982) where a man builds an opera house in the middle of a jungle mirroring the obsessional 'madness' of the director. Even without these extremes, filmmakers speak of the 'madness' of movie making, as if the realization of such an all-encompassing creative dream is necessarily driven by a certain 'madness' beyond their control. We shall see in Chap. 6. how this relates to wider forms of creativity.

The influential films *Taxi Driver* (Martin Scorsese, 1976) and *Apocalypse Now* (Francis Ford Coppola, 1979) have created myths feeding popular perceptions and misconceptions of 'madness'. Film can change our perceptions, and has informed the reality of 'madness', and these films are imbued with PTSD. Through the impact of *Taxi Driver*, Travis Bickle (Robert De Niro) a returned soldier has become an archetype of the alienated loner on a violent mission. He commits a massacre while rescuing a young prostitute which resonates with Lynne Ramsay's film *You Were Never Really Here* (2018) discussed here. An adaptation of the Joseph Conrad's 1899 novella *The Heart of Darkness*, in movie making mythology *Apocalypse Now* encapsulates 'madness' and transrationality. Again, the whole process of making the film was 'madness', producing one of the greatest war films of all time. Swallowing the mythologizing whole would be mistaken, as it informs the film's marketing, but it is partly accurate. As Coppola put it, 'little by little we went insane'; he personally suffered a nervous breakdown and tried to commit suicide with a priest being called, and Martin Sheen playing the protagonist Benjamin Willard had a breakdown.[33] Marlon Brando's Colonel Kurtz has perhaps not yet been surpassed in terms of the total construction of the pure sane-insane man. He tried but failed in *The Island of Dr Moreau* (John Frankenheimer, 1996) which was another 'mad' production for those involved. Unlike the stereotype of the wild uncontrolled 'mad' fool, Brando's Kurtz is a self-contained pure intelligence, a version of Nietzsche's superman beyond mere mortals.

The 'madman' as psychopath, serial killer, and spree killer, are all central to popular culture and have arguably come to dominate streaming platforms. There is an issue here, given for example with *Dahmer* Netflix was not required to consult the victims. The cousin of Dahmer victim Errol Lindsey wrote on Twitter that his relatives only found out about the series when it was released on 21 September 2022. It then became Netflix's most popular show. On the flip slide, deaf actor Rodney Burford playing Tony Hughes has been praised for his compassionate performance. In 1992 his mother Shirley Hughes won a civil court judgement allowing her to intercept $10 million of any money offered to the serial killer for movie, publication or television rights to his story.[34]

This interest is also evidenced by the popularity of films such as *Halloween* (John Carpenter, 1978) which as of 2021 had 11 sequels and the television series *Mindhunter* (2017 to 2019) based on the origin of the FBI's Behavioural Science Unit. In the original *Halloween* Michael Myers aged 23 (Michael Moran) returns to his neighbourhood for a killing spree on Halloween, after being locked up since the age of eight for killing his sister Judith (Sandy Johnson). Evil and 'madness' are once again equated with Dr. Loomis (Donald Pleasance) calling Michael literally the Devil. There is a paranormal component because Michael just will not die at the end.

A plethora of films and television series and documentaries about figures like Charles Manson and the Manson Family, including *Once Upon a Time in Hollywood* (Quentin Tarantino, 2019), where Manson is played by Damian Harriman), and *Mindhunter*, deal with this theme. Those who take the moral high ground argue such depictions glorify these figures, but often these films and televisions shows further understanding of the period they portray. Set in the late 1970s, we learn in *Mindhunter* how the FBI first came to understand the need to get inside the mind of killers with Manson (Damon Herriman again) here a pathetic chancer. In the 1967

[33]Tijana Radeska, '"The Horror": A Look Inside the Grueling Madness of Making *Apocalypse Now*', *Vintage News*, February 16, 2019.

[34]R. A. Vargas, 'Mother of Dahmer victim condemns Netflix series: 'I don't see how they can do that', *The Guardian*, 10 October 2022, Mother of Dahmer victim condemns Netflix series: 'I don't see how they can do that' | US news | The Guardian (accessed 11 October, 2022).

set American period drama *Aquarius* (2015–2016), David Duchovny plays Sam Hodiak who contends with Charles Manson (Gethin Anthony) played as a violent sex fiend.

Versions of 'madness' emerge across genres, so in this sense abnormality has been normalized. For example, the romantic comedy *As Good As It Gets* (James L. Brooks, 1998) has Jack Nicholson playing bigoted writer Melvin Udall who has obsessive compulsive disorder (OCD) which has comedic and tragic impact. While all the common clichés surrounding OCD are utilized (not stepping on lines, counting, being obsessed with hygiene, which are often actually real traits people with OCD have), the plot revolves around Udall looking after his neighbour's dog and simply learning to love with the OCD being a barrier. As we have seen, following Laing, the OCD keeps him in some sense sane and safe while being his 'madness'. When he experiences the transrational through love he is healed.

The influential cult film *Quadrophenia* (Franc Roddam, 1979) concerns 'angst-ridden' Jimmy Cooper (Phil Daniels) escaping the drudgery of his London postal job as a Mod.[35] In Chap. 5 we learn from the real experiences of interviewees how anxiety and 'madness' correlate and we saw in Chap. 1 how diagnoses overlap. Set in 1964, Jimmy returns home late after falling asleep on the tube. His father (Michael Elphick) remarks, 'it's not normal' about his scooter-boy life. Seeing his parents watching a horror film on television Jimmy's reply is a key question to us all in the context of 'madness'—'oh yea, well what's not normal then!?'

The film is based on The Who's second rock opera, the double album released in October 1973 set in London and Brighton in 1965. These themes intersect with their earlier album 'Tommy' (1969) with the film version directed by Ken Russell in 1975, and include the subjects of childhood abuse, becoming one with the group, leadership, and messiahship. The second track on the album *Quadrophenia* 'The Real Me' concerns Jimmy going back to the doctor, 'yet another shrink', trying to explain who he is. Another question raised is: is there an authentic self? This question is addressed in Chap. 8 and was touched in in Chap. 1 with reference to Schopenhauer. In the song Jimmy then goes to his mother for help, saying he is crazy. Her response is, 'I know how it feels, son, because it runs in the family'. These hereditary aspects of 'madness' move us away from 'madness' as metaphor to a biological approach which we saw in Chap. 1 many have dismissed.[36]

On the album cover Jimmy sees a psychiatrist every Monday. In trendy Laingian style, the doctor does not believe in his patient's 'madness'. This disappoints Jimmy. Being 'mad' would make him different to the rest of the Mods and offer him a sense of power. As interviewee A28 in Chap. 5 states, 'madness' is equated with evil and this can offer a sense of power and control. Instead of seeing himself as schizophrenic, Jimmy believes he is quadrophonic, which is a variation of dissociative

---

[35] IMDB *Quadrophenia* plot summary Quadrophenia (1979) - Plot - IMDb (accessed 20 October, 2023).

[36] Peter Breggin, *Toxic Psychiatry: Why Therapy, Empathy and Love Must Replace the Drugs, Electroshock, and Biochemical Theories of the "New Psychiatry"* (New York: St. Martin's, 1994).

identity disorder (DID) which includes Jimmy's four personalities, reflecting the four members of the Who.[37]

Along with *Lie To Me,* the made for television film *Sybil* was also mentioned with regards to dissociative identity disorder (DID). A prescient film tackling DID is *Split* (M. Night Shyamalan, 2017) with James McAvoy playing Kevin in treatment with a psychiatrist. Kevin has 23 different personalities dominated by one repressed personality called 'The Beast' with characteristics from the animals he looks after at a zoo. Again, 'madness' is equated with evil. Kevin kidnaps three girls, so we literally have played out the idea from Foucault that 'madness' is the manifestation of the most primitive of desires.[38] Foucault extrapolated this idea of from Freud's view on the uncanny. This involves encountering what our ancestors would have believed in literally and is now considered 'mad' and concerns the return of the repressed, encapsulated here by 'The Beast'.

The film does little for our understanding of mental health and audiences boycotted the film.[39]A spectacular display of McAvoy's acting, it is united within Shyamalan's psychological oeuvre by ending with a reference to a character from his earlier film *Unbreakable* (M. Night Shyamalan, 2000), suggesting a desire for realism is misplaced.[40] While having an entertainment value in its extremism, as with so many other films the problem is *Split* equates mental disturbances with violence. Those with mental disorders are much more likely to be on the receiving end of violence. As in *The Dead Center* (Billy Senese, 2018), these films promote the view that people with mental health problems are evil with violent acts never a choice, as if they are possessed which dismisses other factors.

As we saw with the BBC, fiction and documentary can be part of ongoing containment and control and allow for temporary 'madness', but they can also deepen our transrational knowledge. Cognitive behavioural therapy (CBT) proposes distraction as a technique, including the viewing of films and television shows.[41] The viewing experience itself can be perceived as 'mad'.[42] Film content seems possessed by the topic of 'madness', especially horror and science fiction films. Film is often a form of regression, a process of perceiving as real the represented, not the representor, film being analogous to the 'madness of dreams'.[43] While socially acceptable to a degree, cinema is a, 'loophole opening on to something slightly

---

[37]The herd behaviour that brings strength, but questions individual identity as played out in Mod culture, is the subject of Chap. 7 on cults, leaders, and groups.

[38]Michel Foucault, *Madness and Civilisation. A History of Insanity in the Age of Reason*, trans. Richard Howard (London: Tavistock/Routledge, 1989), p. 193.

[39]Johnson and Olson, op. cit., p. 5.

[40]These two films are part of what is officially known as the Eastrail 117 Trilogy that also includes *Glass* (M. Night Shyamalan, 2019).

[41]Windy Dryden and Rhena Branch, eds., *The CBT Handbook* (London: Sage, 2011).

[42]Christian Metz, *The Imaginary Signifier, Psychoanalysis and the Cinema*, trans. Celeia Britton et al. (Bloomington: Indiana University Press, 1977).

[43]Ibid., p.116.

more crazy, slightly less approved than what one does the rest of the time'.[44] The relationship between the director and editor has been called dreaming in pairs. Often it is the director who is the dreamer and the editor the listener but sometimes this is reversed and the editor, 'offers the bait to tempt the collective dream to reveal more of itself'.[45]

Film depends on the spectator's transrational ability, their willingness for 'madness' being reliant on the breadth of the imagination of the spectator. As well as being proposed as a cure for 'madness', philosophy has been known to drive people 'mad' and film has also been known to instigate 'madness' in the viewing process.[46] In *Enduring Love* (Roger Mitchell, 2004) Daniel Craig plays philosopher Joe who feels he is going 'mad'. Joe has every reason to be paranoid and to feel 'madness' is enveloping him because he does have a stalker Jed (Rhys Ifans), the film investigating post-traumatic stress disorder (PTSD) after a balloon accident that were both at. As film concerns primarily the emotions and the transrational, our enjoyment of film depends on our ability for empathy and can deepen our empathy. Ideally, film enables us to feel more, to engage with this transrational knowledge and can enable us to see the good in those we initially condemned as bad or evil. This means we then have a deeper view of the potential of the humanity, which is part of the openness of transrational knowledge previously discussed.

Philosophical questions arise concerning the moving image's ability to deal with time in the present—a subject returned to in Chap. 8—with dream, and whether this is even desirable.[47] Novelists Toni Morrison and Hilary Mantel have shown, especially in their gothic fictions that fiction provides the gaps in history. Being part of the imagination fiction is part of transrational knowledge that is necessary for a deeper knowledge. 'Madness' similarly provides the gap in prescribed meaning and established frameworks, including history. Their work, especially Morrison's *Beloved* (1987) adapted for screen (Jonathan Demme, 1998), and Mantel's *Beyond Black* (2005), which we shall return to in Chap. 6, richly explores the 'madness' of the gothic uncanny and the paranormal.[48] For now it is worth noting that like 'madness' ghosts are the 'unwelcome carriers of occluded history' and they shows us 'how we screen' and protest ourselves from the past.[49] Ghosts are 'double agents' working from the 'other side'; they, 'make us recognise another past to the one we

---

[44] Ibid., p. 66.

[45] Walter Murch, *In the Blink Of An Eye – A Perspective on Film Editing* (Los Angeles: Silman-James Press), p. 28.

[46] Michael Swallow, 'French Cinema, Audiences, and Madness', Essex Research Seminars, September 1999.

[47] Gilles Deleuze, *Cinema 2: The Time-Image*, trans. Hugh Tomlinson and Robert Galeta (London: Continuum, 2011).

[48] Toni Morrison, *Beloved* (New York: Alfred A. Knopf, 1987). Hilary Mantel, *Beyond Black* (London: Fourth Estate, 2005).

[49] Graham Huggan, 'Ghost Stories, Bone Flutes, Cannibal Countermemory', in Ken Gelder, ed., *The Horror Reader* (London: Routledge, 2000), p. 354.

might have chosen: they transform, not the past itself but our 'normal,' socialised perception of it.'[50]

Spanish director Pedro Almodóvar's oeuvre also frequently delves comically within 'madness' in an exciting gothic fashion profoundly developing the uncanny. The German for uncanny—Unheimlich—is repeatedly mistranslated as 'unhomely' (interestingly repetition is part of the uncanny, making this mistranslation uncanny), when more appropriately it means unconcealed, unhidden, or un-secret. Freud took his definition from the philosopher Friedrich Schelling: 'an experience of something which ought to have remained secret and hidden but has come to light'.[51] In Almodóvar's *The Skin I Live In* (2011), adapted from Thierry Jonquet's French crime novel *Mygale/Tarantula* (1984), the protagonist played by Antonio Banderas unethically crosses animals with humans to potentially create a cure for malaria.

He then kidnaps his daughter's rapist and gives him a sex change, creating a new version of his own murdered wife. Almodóvar's film makes this 'madness' believable with sanity and insanity merging. This then moves us beyond a binary approach within transrational knowledge. The 2018 HBO series *Sharp Objects*, starring Amy Adams as an alcoholic journalist and self-harmer who has spent time in a mental hospital, is another example where 'madness' is reality. Following Hobsbawm's historical interpretation discussed in Chap. 1, 'madness' is the new sanity, however, this 'will to transgress' which challenges all assumptions is 'impossible to ever complete'.[52]

While film and television have been dominated by 'madness' with the damaged protagonist this is an ambiguous role. The James Bond film series, especially with Daniel Craig as Bond, hinges on the idea Bond can only carry out his work because he is psychologically damaged.[53] He is an example of Joseph Campbell's wounded healer, close to the psychopathological and able to kill for our entertainment and pleasure.[54] These narratives and their characters help us to understand ourselves, often working therapeutically, addressing aspects of ourselves we may not always wish to acknowledge. This is part of the psyche known as the Jungian shadow which needs negotiating in the psyche for individuation and wellbeing and transrationality is central to this. There is a need for these partially disturbed characters like Bond who frequently function on the preconscious level. They are beyond normal reason using a different, transrational, level of intelligence which gets a higher level of results, transgressing the bureaucratic mindset.

We can also perceive this in the case of Sherlock Holmes, adapted in numerous forms with Holmes played as having something like Asperger's syndrome by Benedict Cumberbatch in the BBC version (2010–2017). This disability, or different ability, gives him special abilities which can appear super-human. Despite Homes

---

[50] Ibid.

[51] Lucy Huskinson, 'Uncanny places', *The Psychologist*, December 2021, p. 40.

[52] Chris Jenks, *Transgression* (London: Routledge, 2003), p. 101.

[53] Jason Lee, *The Psychology of Screenwriting* (London: Bloomsbury, 2014).

[54] Ibid.

here being loveably difficult for Dr. John Watson (Martin Freeman) and other neurotypical folk, this is arguably a positive celebration of difference in mainstream television. The same is true of Will Graham (Hugh Dancy), the gifted criminal profiler in the television series *Hannibal* (2013–2015), who has a deep ability to empathise with killers, including the genius abilities of his nemesis, psychiatrist, and cannibal serial killer Dr. Lecter (Mads Mikkelsen).

Understanding these characters gives us insight into 'madness' and transrationality and challenge cultures which demonize those who have different abilities, like Graham who also may have Asperger's syndrome. Before we condemn these shows as over-romanticizing those who are neurodiverse, we should consider that psychological research confirms that those with autism can integrate more information than those without.[55] Through speeded up imagery and overlaid graphics, both these shows depict this exceptional ability at synthesising information well. In this regard, these shows are then accurate and do reveal society's need for those who think and feel differently.

Surrealism is central to 'madness', imagination, and creative work, particular comedy.[56] In traditional psychoanalysis it has been linked to gratification beyond the reality principle, being part of sexuality and extending beyond the individual and securing its connection with its species.[57] Similar to what we observed with fiction and history, for playwright Tom Stoppard the imagination gets at the 'truth of a person' better than the facts.[58] The imagination is part of the transrational which brings a deeper truth. David Cronenberg's films and David Lynch's, such as *Mulholland Drive* (2001), are unique examples that explore 'madness' using surrealism.

Like 'madness', in *Mulholland Drive* the narrative is uncertain, as is the meaning. It was given the tagline by the director, 'a love story in the city of dreams' and given its surrealist qualities this could be reversed as, 'a dream story in the city of love'. A rejected television series pilot, which partly explains its broken episodic and unexplained yet symbolic sequences, it examines areas connected to 'madness' including depression and hallucinations, with its main theme being the loss of identity and doubling which are key elements of a certain 'madness' as explained with category 2. above and related films on doubling and uncanny.

When considering surrealism Terry Gilliam's films are pertinent, such as *The Fisher King* (1991). Robin Williams plays an apparently insane homeless man Parry and Jeff Bridges radio shock jock Jack Lucas. Jack's on-air comments lead to a man shooting up a restaurant, killing Parry's partner when he was known as Professor Sagan and lived the life of a professional. A variety of mental health issues are

---

[55] C. Manning, 'Researching Autism', *The Psychologist*, 17 March 2020, p. 40.

[56] Jason Lee, 'Smile, Hitler? Nazism and Comedy in Popular Culture', in Helen Davies and Sarah Illott, eds., *Comedy and the Politics of Representation – Mocking the Weak* (London: Palgrave, 2018c), pp. 223–240.

[57] Herbert Marcuse, *Eros & Civilization* (London: Abacus, 1973), p. 111.

[58] John Carey, 'Review of *Tom Stoppard* by Hermione Lee', in *The Times*, October 4, 2020, p. 27.

addressed. After the death of his partner, Sagan has a psychotic breakdown entering a catatonic state from which he comes out of with the new identity of Parry. Continually haunted by the death of his wife, his fears appear to him in psychotic hallucinations as the Red Knight. While this is a romanticisation of 'madness' of sorts, fitting the framework described by interviewee A.22 in Chap. 5, it also effectively reveals Parry's fear and psychotic terror.

Once Jack realises his comments were the catalyst for multiple murders, he becomes an alcoholic and suicidally depressive. The two main characters save each other. Williams frequently played somewhat nebbish characters who find themselves but, unlike Woody Allen who embodies nebbishness, this is not achieved through narcissism but through an emphasis on deeper transrational knowledge.[59] Gilliam was part of Monty Python's Flying Circus which incorporated surrealism and insanity, this form of comedy like 'madness' being a break in the system, highlighting the 'madness' inherent in the system.

Charlie Kaufmann's screenplay for the surreal *Eternal Sunshine of the Spotless Mind* (Michel Gondry, 2004) is an example of a comedy that plays with perceptions of 'madness' and time. He also tackles versions of surreal 'madness' in *Being John Malkovich* (Spike Jonze, 2000), *Adaptation* (Spike Jonze, 2003) and the commanding and darker *Synecdoche, New York* (Charlie Kaufman, 2009). A wider trope in these films is loss which causes 'madness' and dealing with that loss, which is part of what makes us human, just as 'madness' and the transrational make us human.

An emphasis on loss and 'madness' occurs in 'Tom & Gerri' (David Kerr, 2014), Series 1 Episode 3 of the English television series *Inside No. 9* (2014–) which often features surreal black comedy. Tom (Reece Shearsmith) is a primary school teacher and aspiring writer who loses his identity as well as losing his partner. His partner Gerri (Gemma Arterton) has died but in Tom's grief stricken 'madness' he hallucinates Gerri is alive. In his confusion about who is real Tom kills a homeless man who has been exploiting him and stealing his identity. Rather than forcing us to equate 'madness' with evil, violence, or mocking the mentally ill, this episode asks us to question our own assumptions and perceptions about what is real, the extent of our own altruism, and how we would deal with loss, all framed through a uniquely surreal horror-comic lens.

Film and television merges realism with surrealism, such as *The Lady in the Van* (Nicholas Hytner, 2015) based on the true story of Mary Shepperd (Maggie Smith) who was befriended by writer Alan Bennett (Alex Jennings) at his Camden Town home. Invited to stay on his drive in her Bedford van for three months, Mary remained for 15 years. She is shown to be full of shame and suffering from a form of religious 'madness'. Bennett is depicted as two people living in one house. One is the laid-back observer, the writerly self always at his desk about to transform his observations into dry witty prose. The other is a repressed neurotic unable to relax because a 'mad' woman is harassing him. The two play off each other well having many conversations about life and how to deal with Mary. When the repressed

---

[59] Martin Hall, ed., *The Women of Woody Allen* (Amsterdam: Amsterdam University Press, 2022).

Bennett acts out his fantasies, we later realise that his outbursts are merely in his head. The film is comical and poignant, especially when we learn Mary was an accomplished pianist who when she became a nun was banned from playing. We follow his discovery after being sectioned in a mental hospital by her brother Mary escaped. This is paralleled with Bennett's fraught relationship with his finickity mother, the exact opposite of Mary who seldom washes and defecates in plastic bags.

Being such a self-reflexive and self-deprecating writer in real life, Bennett understands what these two figures signify, Mary bullying him and controlling him. Bennett relates to Mary's brother who out of exasperation had her locked up, but he never reaches that point with her. Blurring fiction with documentary, the film finally depicts the real Alan Bennett (a third version) observing the film being made with a dedication of a blue plaque to honour The Lady in the Van at his home. And then rather than there being just three Bennetts there are as many as there are people who have engaged with this story in its variety of formats. While 'madness' is revealed to be inhibiting and disturbing, hardly Foucault's 'triumph of madness' observed in Chap. 1, the film also indicates a public acceptance of Mary and 'madness' in what is stereotypical viewed as ruthless London and despite her suffering there is a liberatory spirit to her.

Psychiatric research on the 'crazy lady' trope pushes the influence model too far with research published in 2014 on the influence of popular culture and gender roles claiming 'crazy ladies' on television influenced 'bad behaviour' in young women negatively, impacting on gender roles, quoting such areas as sexual manipulation, emotional instability, and social aggression.[60] American psychiatry still equates mental health with morality. The 'crazy lady' trope continues in a variety of forms, from the work of Alan Bennett discussed here, to the Netflix hits *Cobra Kai* (2018–) and *Squid Game* (2021). In these examples, the 'crazy lady' is not dismissed outright and condemned morally for she possesses a transgressive power which can teach others significant lessons. The same is true in the film *Donnie Darko* (Richard Kelly, 2001) with genius Roberta Sparrow (Patience Cleveland). These figures are equated with an alternative truth, with 'madness' offering a deeper transrational knowledge outside the established status quo.

In Bennett's work Mary's life is not romanticized with her history haunting her and revealed through her terrifying psychotic rantings, but the film touches on a freedom she possesses, unlike the neighbours typically obsessed with house prices. This is not black and white, so possesses a transnational deeper non-binary knowledge. Mary's ingratitude to benevolence is part of what makes her endearing, as if she will permanently stand at odds to society. Unlike Bennett's northern mother, who would be thoroughly embarrassed to have a 'mad' homeless person living on her doorstep, in the metropolitan south where difference is arguably more tolerated the community eventually accepts Mary. She is their local loveable eccentric,

[60] C. Cerny, S. Friedman, D. Smith, 'Television's "crazy lady" trop: female psychopathic traits, teaching and influence of popular cuture', *Academic Psychiatry*, April 2014, 38(2), pp. 233–241.

bringing an element of continuity and community to fragmented London, the message being even the 'mad', those who do not fit in, can here without the need for incarceration. Bennett felt he was preserving her memory by writing this memoir that goes deeper than traditional realism with the triple narration device.

Works of stricter realism, such as *Girl, Interrupted* (James Mangold, 1999) based on Susanna Kaysen's account of her 18-month stay in an American mental hospital, have also been influential. These films add to the popular understanding of what is often a taboo subject, creating impact, and instigating and furthering public discourse on 'madness' often positively changing attitudes to treatment and patients.[61] Patrick McGrath is an important fiction writer on 'madness' with a strong sense of realism born from personal experience. McGrath's *Asylum*, adapted poorly for screen (David Mackenzie, 2002), is a powerful novel. Inmate Edgar Stark (Marton Csokas) slices the heads off his victims turning them into art. The deputy superintendent's wife Stella Raphael (Natasha Richardson) falls deeply in love with Edgar who then escapes. Love is a form of 'madness' here and the question remains: is it better to risk everything for love with the 'madness' of love a higher truth. If it is this is not 'madness' at all, but the quintessence of sanity revealing these constructs are not merely a matter of behaviour and outcomes, but perceptions and goals. The higher level of realism in part stems from McGrath being raised in the grounds of British mental hospitals as the son of a senior psychiatrist. The film adaptation of his novel *Spider* (David Cronenberg, 2002), where a released mental patient (Ralph Fiennes) has an addiction to writing, benefits from being more experimental.

'Mad' sometimes correlates with eccentric, a term that has been used to describe Mike Leigh's work, Leigh being one of Britain's more influential post-war directors.[62] Many of Leigh's films, from the now classic filmed-for-television stage play black comedy *Abigail's Party* (1977), to his darker works, such as his masterpiece *Naked* (1993), explore familiar and familial insanity within the fragility of human relationships. Often the backdrop is political and social decay. Some forget that an artist is allowed to use irony, attacking Leigh for supposedly approving misogyny or classism by portraying it. If art is good, it can confuse and challenge critics and audiences alike. Assaults on Leigh's work occur for him supposedly confirming and approving the prevailing ideology, when often it is highlighting the problems within the dominant ideology. In his early period, Leigh satirized the middle classes but was then accused in his later work of mocking the working classes. This binary view is too simplistic; his body of work covers adolescent malaise, midlife crises, alcoholism, rape, depression, plus severe mental illness with an original realism.

The films are real within and to their own fictional world's reflecting on society and a highly personal take that stems from the original creative process. As with directors Robert Altman and John Cassavetes, Leigh achieves this stance by having

---

[61] Malynnda Johnson and Christopher J. Elson, ed., *Normalizing Mental Illness and Neurodiversity in Entertainment Media. Quieting Madness* (New York: Routledge, 2021).

[62] Ray Carney and Leonard Quart, *The Films of Mike Leigh – Embracing the World* (Cambridge: Cambridge University Press, 2000).

no set script, working on this in rehearsals which are longer than normal, the actors building their characters and plots personally and with more depth.[63] Stressing actor performance over narrative often goes against the grain, making Leigh's worlds unique and directly getting to the root of 'madness' as loss, be it the absence of love, trauma or, more politically, hard external conditions, such as poverty and unemployment. Apart from Ken Loach, it is difficult to find another British director in this period who has had this level of an impact. Leigh's work profoundly examines desperation within the working and underclass, which can be absent from the big and small screen in British cinema which often prefers costume dramas. By doing so, Leigh is drawing attention to parts of society the establishment wants to remain invisible.

In an American context, values have shifted. Films such as *Kids* (Larry Clarke, 1995) discussed in detail here in Chap. 3, or *Heathers* (Michael Lehmann, 1998) which comically tackles psychosis and school murders, probably would not get made today due to moral sensitivities and what some see as copy-cat killings.[64] In these circumstances the influence of media is simplistically over-emphasized as in a hypodermic syringe model of media influence, with social problems overlooked and ignored. There is an ease in blaming the media rather than government inaction. Today it is social media that plays that function in public discourse, rather than films such as 'video-nasties'. Media coverage of mass-shootings frequently mentions 'dangerous people' rather than 'dangerous weapons', creating the message mental illness is a cause of mass shootings. The powerful National Rifle Association in America which supports the Republic Party has a vested interest in promoting these fallacious myths concerning mental illness. Following cultivation media theory this then has a powerful effect on audiences through repeated exposure.[65]

More recent films, such as *Psychosis in Stockholm* (Maria Bäck, 2020), have also taken a realistic approach. Here a 14-year-old daughter (Josephine Stofkoper) is in Stockholm with her mother (Josefine Neldén). The process of the physical and metaphysical journey and the holiday are framed as partly a vacation and birthday treat for the girl, but also a time for reflection for the mother leading possibly to therapeutic healing. The mother becomes more destructive following a vivid first-hand autobiographical account of what it is like to be a child of a parent suffering from 'madness'. The daughter has the task of growing up and forming her own identity through differentiating her personality from her mother's and by being her mother's protection. The source of the story comes from the director/writer's own journey with her mother. The cinematography and framing, including how the two characters' head shots stand out, enable the spectator to feel the unconscious struggles animating the two women.[66]

---

[63] Ibid.

[64] For work on *Kids* see Jason Lee, *Film International* 2018, op. cit.

[65] Malynnda Johnson and Chris Olson, eds., *Normalizing Mental Illness and Neurodiversity in Entertainment Media: Quieting Madness* (New York: Rouledge, 2021), p. 3.

[66] Ibid.

How family dynamics shift in the context of 'madness' are enlightening, transculturally. Since the 1950s. which historically was when the period of 'madness' began as explained with reference to historian Eric Hobsbawm and the Cold War in Chap. 1, Japanese films have covered a multitude of transgressions including 'madness'. For example, *I Live in Fear* (Akira Kirusawa, 1955) stars Toshiro Mifune as businessman Nakijima fearing a nuclear attack who wants to move his family to Brazil. Given Japan's history concerning the dropping of the atomic bombs, we can see this fear might be reasonable. Once his family learns of this, they plot to have him committed to a mental asylum. His insanity increases once it is explained that, even in Brazil, he would not be immune from the fall out. There is no escape. Only 1 year earlier in reality an atomic bomb had been tested on Bikini Atoll.

The Japanese four act structure is more open to narratives that are less linear and structurally fixed offering further scope for an exploration of stories outside the cause-and-effect rational paradigm than the traditional western three act or five act structure. This is especially in the third act which can sit outside the overall structure. Looked at from a western perspective this allows for a moment of 'madness', a break and fragmentation, until we return for some form of resolution in the fourth act. This is significant in terms of transrationalism given, paradoxically, Japan stereotypically is renowned for its strict rationalism and obeying of rules; art then is the zone here for healing transrationalism. In *Shang-Chi and the Legend of the Ten Rings* (Destin Daniel Cretton, 2021), one of the largest Hollywood films ever for Asian actors, the father of the protagonist hears the voice of his dead wife. An evil that is hell-bent on destroying the universe is the cause of his 'madness'. This is not just film fantasy. We shall see in Chap. 5 Example 3 how a mental health professional equates insanity with evil. If we compare Eisenstein and Kurosawa, for example, we can see a difference between Eastern and Wester film or art. The former builds a scene, the latter removes and erases.[67] In the Western setup traditionally the master shot shows the choreography of the entire scene, but in Japanese film a small fragment can be used to suggest a whole scene.[68]

The neurotic male whose antics verge on 'madness' has been the subject of a great deal of film and television comedy in both Asia and America, such as the work of Woody Allen. Concurrently, the healer figure, normally a Freudian therapist, is satirically mocked. Often there is the clash between the public persona of the patient (such as hard gangster Tony Soprano, played by James Gandolfini), and their neurotic self which, initially at least, is only revealed to the psychotherapist (and us, the audience). Therapists have been portrayed in film since its origins, including the 1913 French film *Dr Goudron's System* (produced by the Éclair film company), where inmates kill doctors, establishing their own evil cures for illness. Shifts in gender constructions were played with macho men who traditionally needed nobody and now needed help becoming fodder for comedy at the turn of the millennium,

[67] Michael Ondaatje, *The Conversations: Walter Murch and the Art of Editing Film* (London: Bloomsbury, 2008), p. 107.
[68] Ibid.

with films such as *Analyze This* (Harold Ramis, 1999) and *Analyze That* (Harold Ramis, 2002), and television series *The Sopranos* (created and produced by David Chase, 1999 to 2007) which is frequently voted the best series of all time.

Part of Tony Soprano's character is acting out an 'addiction' to the family myth which he believes his health relies on. *The Sopranos* takes areas like addiction, suicide, and self-harm seriously and informatively, elaborating and educating on mental health issues. Rather than a celebration of family or glorification of violence, *The Sopranos* proffers a Laingian approach. The family is examined as the zone and origin of 'madness', rather than the individual. In the episode 'Walk Like a Man' (Terence Winter, 2007), Season 6 Episode 17, expectations of machoness are reversed with Tony now looked up to by his gangster buddies because he is in psychotherapy. One deep tragedy in *The Sopranos* is when Tony's son is hospitalized. Tony believes he has poisoned him by his genes, allowing the show to tackle one of the most contentious areas of psychology and psychiatry—psychobiology. The tragedy of a blind acceptance of the biological mode of human behaviour is highlighted but is here significantly subverted and framed as an excuse. The myth that science and society and culture cannot combat nature is grappled with—why attempt to change if nature dictates?

The aim of Tony's therapist is to stop him acting like an animal on instinct. The doubts raised in therapy are causing him to think before he acts.[69] Initially, he enters therapy due to panic attacks which appear to be related to PTSD. Without having met her, Dr. Melfi diagnoses Tony's mother as having a borderline personality disorder (BPD), a controversial diagnosis. In Chap. 1 it was explained that while this diagnosis is still used, significant researchers and clinicians have discredited its use.[70] Talking about what has happened to us in a psychotherapeutic setting could be of use but can be easier than entering an internal experience and might be a damaging diversion. For PTSD, brain scans reveal how, 'dread persisted and could be triggered by multiple aspects of daily experience. They had not integrated their experience into the ongoing stream of their life'.[71] According to Bessel van der Kolk, therapy for PTSD only works if people are 'biologically' in the present; only then can you revisit the trauma in the past knowing it is in the past.[72]

Having a patient discuss their inner secrets with a therapist or counsellor is an ideal narrative device for exposing the inner life of characters and driving a plot. In *Good Will Hunting* (Gus Van Sant, 1997) the client (Matt Damon as Will) learns from and teaches the counsellor (Robin Williams as Sean). This also works well in the Israeli television series *In Treatment*, adapted for an American audience and originally starring Gabriele Byrne as Paul Weston (2008 to 2001, 2021). Not only

---

[69] Jason Lee, *Cultures of Addiction* (New York: Cambria, 2010), p. 249.

[70] Antony Bateman and Fonagy, 'Mentalisation-treatment training', NHS training the Anna Freud Centre, July/October, 2019.

[71] Bessel van der Kolk, *The Body Keeps the Score: Mind, Brain and Body in the Transformation of Trauma* (London: Penguin, 2014), p. 47.

[72] Ibid., p. 70.

are the sessions with clients narrated, but those the therapist has with his supervisor so we find out the secrets behind his 'madness' which again includes the death of a loved one.

Similarly, the film *K-Pax* (Ian Softley, 2001), based on the trilogy of novels by Gene Brewer is an interesting example. Brewer has each chapter written as a psychiatrist's report on the patient. Jeff Bridges plays a psychiatrist almost obsessed with his patient Prot (Kevin Spacey), a man who believes he is an alien from planet K-Pax. Spacey's fascinating Prot character parallels Jack Nicholson's R.P. McMurphy in *One Flew Over the Cuckoo's Nest* (Milos Forman, 1976). They are saviour figures who are sacrificed for the greater good, but with Prot we are left with the belief he might be only acting catatonic and their still might be some truth in his 'mad' story.

Both these films have their hero cure fellow patients and position the insanity of the institutional machine as more insane than any human abnormality. An existential view that an individual's 'madness' is an extension of a 'mad' society is still relevant. By the early 1970s this thinking was not radical, following some of the demystification of 'madness' by R.D. Laing, Thomas Szasz and Erich Fromm, as explained in Chap. 1. Nicholson's McMurphy manipulated the system to be in a mental hospital; he is a sex offender, making his hero status even more remarkable.[73] Prot is a murderer who took on a new identity after his own family were slaughtered, loss again causing 'madness'. Following an overt Christian metaphor, their individuality is sacrificed for the greater good.

The differences between a psychologist, psychotherapist, and psychiatrist are often unknown to people outside these professions. Despite developments already mentioned in film all three can merge and are frequently seen as evil, as in *Miss Peregrine's Home for Peculiar Children* (Tim Burton, 2017).[74] Based on the Ransom Riggs novel, the film refers to Nazi's as monsters, but here there are real supernatural monsters, including the psychiatrist. Jake (Asa Butterfield) and his grandfather Abe Portman (Terence Stamp) have a peculiarity for seeing monsters called Hollows. When Jake confronts Abe about the peculiar talents of the children, he suggests the term 'special needs', only because he has heard this from adults and his classmates have mocked him for believing his grandfather's stories. This is supposed to be taboo, so the children are hidden away in a large house.

They are stuck in a loop, 3 September 1943, when a Nazi bomb was dropped on their home in Wales, reliving the same day. Jake's grandfather had to leave Poland and enter this home because 'he was special'. The Hollows look as if they have stepped out of a Francis Bacon painting.[75] Bacon was influenced by the Nazis.[76] The Bacon Nazi aesthetic comes through in the form of the monsters with Bacon's

[73]Lee 1999, op. cit., pp. 149–172.

[74]Jason Lee, *Nazism and Neo-Nazism in Film and Media* (Amsterdam: Amsterdam University Press, 2018).

[75]Ibid.

[76]Ibid.

painting expressing a form of the horrors of 'madness'. Unfortunately, critics like Macnab and Lenika Cruz writing in *The Atlantic* appeared to have only watched the film once, and then blame their lack of understanding on the plot not making sense, or the film not even having one. Cruz wants the film to continue its seriousness, with its early references to the holocaust, while at the same time saying it does not have a heart.[77]

It can be argued a film largely set in 1943 must make references to the holocaust, but what is more significant are the stories Abe tells, what is left unsaid, again suggesting gaps in history. Abe is demonised as monstrous by his own family and is thought to have dementia and be a bit 'mad', apparently making up stories to tell the young Jake. When asked follow-up questions, he does not want to talk about it and this is assumed to relate to the trauma around the Holocaust which he may have witnessed but escaped from. Jake's father is, unsurprisingly, an idiot, but his obsession with birds of prey looks back to this period in history when Nazis attacked the so-called peculiar.

The Hollywood Reporter attacks the scriptwriter Jane Goldman (co-writer of two *X-Men* and two *Kingsman*) for the third act, claiming the comic villain Barron (Samuel L. Jackson) is moving us away from the Michael Powell style romance which would create a more poignant film if sustained.[78] But this is suggesting that a film should only remain in one genre, and ignores decades of recent cinema history. Barron's funny one-liners make direct reference to Tarantino movies, and the skeleton action sequence on Blackpool pier is not the first reference in the film to Don Chaffey's 1963 *Jason and the Argonauts*. Enoch's peculiar power is to bring things back to life, the film offering a precursor to the third act when Enoch shows Jake his skills, inserting hearts in scraps of animals and dolls and getting them to fight for fun. The peculiar thing about these peculiar talents is that they appear so natural.

Myths of the evil psychiatrist have not dispersed, as exemplified again in the Netflix 2021 hit *Behind Her Eyes*, but here this myth is used to lead the audience on until they are revealed to be innocent. The psychiatrist-husband is not the totally evil man abusing his wife that we assumed, it is her friend who she was in a psychiatric hospital with. These myths serve a purpose, because even though these professionals are part of a caring profession, we should not assume they are all benign. Todd Solondz's controversial film *Happiness* (1998), which would be unlikely to be made today due to its comedy concerning paedophilia, deconstructs the myth of the psychotherapist as saint. The film also reveals mental problems can be about chosen existential angst caused by over analysing things; or, again controversially, even to gain kudos and status, as in the writer who claims she has been sexually abused because this is part of the zeitgeist to sells books and appear authentic.[79] Behind this

---

[77] Ibid.

[78] Ibid.

[79] Jason Lee, *Pervasive Perversions: Paedophile and Child Sexual Abuse in Media/Culture* (London: Free Association Books, 2005).

is the belief that the world is so banal and meaningless that the only way to make it interesting is to have an existential crisis and analyse it, fake pain being better than no pain for emotional depth, creating an entertaining personal drama.

While it is controversial, this film is still relevant today given sometimes there is a tendency for society to move in the direction of victim culture after so many years of people having to repress their pain. This then means real victims are overlooked, as all pain is then rated the same; Woody Allen's work persistently encapsulates elements of this. Rather than working in a malign fashion, these comedies express the human need for meaning in the 'madness' of the void, and for the importance of admitting you are wounded within the neuroticism whether something as terrible as child sexual has happened to you or not. As Homi Bhabha puts it, all identity is mediated; the text of ourselves is part of an intertextuality within an in inescapable law, 'a detour through the word of God, or the writ of Law, or the Name of the Father', including our confessions to an 'analyst or hairdresser'.[80]

In tune with the transrational, the black comedy starring Michael Keaton as Riggan as an actor staging a comeback on Broadway *Birdman* (Alejandro G. Iñárritu, 2014) subverts expectations concerning the rational via an imaginative leap, literally in its closing sequence. As Riggan prepares for his one man show he is mocked by a dark superhero, the uncanny return of the repressed based on an old batman-like superhero character he previously played. Is this his shadow in Jungian terms, his id, or the superego in Freudian language? We are almost certain this is his demon and his 'madness' that he is metaphorically wrestling with, and part of the actor's battle with mental health issues.

In real-life Keaton played a film version of Batman which adds to the subtext. Will Riggan be able to keep it together for his comeback performance, or will his apparent psychosis be too much? In the final sequence Riggan flies off over New York in what can be described as transrational-realism. An unexpected reversal asks us to reserve judgement, and to stop dogmatically dividing the rational from the irrational with the rational part of the transrational as explained. This is the equivalent to recognizing the 'event', as Deleuze has it by drawing on Spinoza and Nietzsche, which becomes the purpose of philosophy or, to put it another way, of the experience itself. As Deleuze and Guattari proclaim: 'Philosophy's sole aim is to become worthy of the event.'[81]

According to Guy de Maupassant all fiction is based on the reality of the author.[82] Director David O. Russell's work is significant in this context. Russell's *Silver Linings Playbook* (2012), starring Bradley Cooper as Pat Solitano who has just come out of a mental hospital after eight months, is inspired by Russell's son's bi-polar disorder. Pat was locked up after attacking his wife's lover. The film also covers mild OCD with Pat's father (Robert De Niro), plus examines how grief can be overcome, with Jennifer Lawrence's Tiffany. Russell's moving earlier film *Spanking*

[80] Homi Bhabha, *The Location of Culture* (London: Routledge, 2009), pp. 81–82.

[81] Paul Patton, *Deleuze: A Critical Reader* (London: Routledge, 1996), p. 15.

[82] Guy de Maupassant, *Pierre and Jean* (London: Penguin, 1973).

the Monkey (1994) realistically depicts a sexual relationship between a son and mother, the latter experiencing mental health issues and alcoholism.[83] Guy De Maupassant's view takes towards a postmodern understanding where fiction and reality merge and is the case in certain documentaries and TV shows. There is important non-fiction work such as the television mini-series documentary *Wild, Wild, Country* (Chapman and Maclain Way, 2018) examining the Bhagwan cult (also known as Osho) a subject discussed in Chap. 7.

Despite it being taboo, popular media culture appears dominated by 'madness' and we saw in Chap. 1 why: it delineates the boundary for what is considered normal and for social control. This dominant trajectory in the media moves from *In the Psychiatrist's Chair* on BBC Radio 4 (1982–2000), fronted by psychiatrist Anthony Clare which spawned a series of books, to global television shows like *The Oprah Winfrey Show* (1986–2011), the daytime talk show with the highest audience in history, to reality television such as *Celebrity Love Island* and its spin offs (2005–). What these various formats have in common is their confessional style, promoting a spectacle of rawness, as if hidden truths will be realised. Whether these shows were benign or malign for wellbeing is contestable, as is whether this was good television, but these formats were certainly successful and led to the belief that being open and raw was beneficial to all.

From the 1980s these shows functioned as a form of group therapy often without the strict professional boundaries of the psychotherapeutic profession, although sometimes consultants were brought in when things went wrong. There were obvious dangers. Despite attempts at after care confessional and reality television went under the regulator's spotlight. In Britain, *The Jeremy Kyle Show* (2005 to 2019) ceased production following a suicide. Two British *Love Island* contestants killed themselves, but the show continued. In July 2019 the UK's regulatory body OFCOM announced it was going to work on a series of recommendations for such shows. In February 2020 *Love Island* presenter Caroline Flack committed suicide. Was the 'madness' of being hunted by the British media just too much, after she was accused of domestic violence and was facing court case despite her partner not wanting this pursued? By 2021 *Love Island* was ITV's second most popular programme, but the regulating body Ofcom was threatening to take it off air if contestants were not looked after. Actions were taken to help contestants leaving *Love Island*, including having eight therapy sessions for exiting contestants, plus advice on handling social media.

The hit American documentary series *Couples Therapy* (2019–) features clinical psychologist and psychoanalytical psychotherapist Dr. Orna Gulranik as she treats couples. Some couples appear at first to manifest irreconcilable differences which look inevitably leading to divorce. The beauty of the show is in part due to the sensitivity of the editing and the narrative arcs revealing the problems couples face, and the problems faced by those attempting to help them. We see Dr. Gulranik with her clinical advisor explaining how hard it is to get some of her clients to face their

[83] Lee, *Pervasive Perversions*, op. cit..

reality. Once we get behind these relationship difficulties, individual personal problems caused by addiction, violence, childhood abandonment and abuse reveal how personal 'madness' inhibits adult relationship fulfilment.

The historical legacy of issues, often related to parents who were unable to parent, becomes part of the appropriate material that needs addressing now, making the psychoanalytical approach still relevant. Sometimes the expert's intervention seems tangential and random, but often it is extremely insightful and strikes home. Then the real-world narratives of the couples begin to shift, as they discover self-knowledge which will help them within their relationship. This is transpersonal knowledge because of its relationship with feelings and the unconscious and moves beyond the simplicity of a rational paradigm of 'I'm right, you're wrong'.

The therapeutic component is not merely from media that contains these processes. Cinematherapy involves group viewing practices within and outside clinical settings and work with individuals by psychologists, psychotherapists, and psychiatrists.[84] There is evidence this has helped people who are unwell, including those who are psychotic.[85] In-depth psychotherapy after viewing produces impact on those facing relationship difficulties.[86] There is filmmaking as psychotherapy, including making films with clients. Concurrently, film can both cause 'madness' and heal 'madness'. Notable films include *Juliette of the Spirits* (Federico Fellini, 1965) and *Betty Blue* (Jean-Jacques Beineix, 1986), as conduits for triggering 'madness' in the audience.[87] The making of the Portella della Ginestra sequence in the film *Salvatore Giuliano* (Francesco Rosi, 1962), using 1000 peasants to enact a massacre experienced 14 years earlier, caused a 'madness' related to PTSD through this remembering of the traumatic event for good filmic effect.[88]

2.2 Theatre and Healing

Liberation offered by what can be transgressively 'mad' art forms such as theatre matched by social control through its form of Bakhtinean release. Theatre's 'mad' zone can reinscribe the reality and sanity of everyday life once the audience leaves but could alter the audience politically and psychologically. With concerns over government use of information supplied by social media following the Cambridge Analytica scandal, the power and legitimacy of surveillance is under question more

---

[84] Also known as filmtherapy and movietherapy.

[85] J. Cohen, J. Johnson, and P. Orr, eds., *Video and Filmmaking as Psychotherapy: Research and Practice* (London: Routledge, 2015).

[86] I. Egeci and F. Gençöz, 'The use of cinematherapy in dealing with relationship problems', *The Arts in Psychotherapy*, Vol. 53, April 2017, pp. 64–71.

[87] An interviewee in Chap. 5 noted this in relationship to these 2 films causing psychotic experiences.

[88] John Dickie, *Cosa Nostra – A History of the Sicilian Mafia* (London: Hodder and Stoughton, 2007), p. 264.

than ever. Changes in technological structures impact on class structures. Chapter 1 explained that mental hospitals, like prisons, were previously zones of observation but since the reduction in the number of these hospitals surveillance now subsumes all areas of life. We are all suspects. All are observed and part of the performance.[89]

Film unites the real and the unreal and, as explained, it is a form a 'madness', plus film can be a catalyst for 'madness' and for curing 'madness', as well as deepening our understanding of the variations of 'madness' and creates 'madness'.[90] Discussing the classical period Foucault assessed their perception of 'madness' as being the inability to distinguish the truth.[91] Foucault contrasted the classical view on 'madness' with the nineteenth-century view that it is the condition where no limits are known.[92] 'Madness' is a break or an absence for Foucault.[93] Cinema is a break from everyday life. Theatre today frequently uses film as part of the performance. Technologies such as film instigate this break, making the unreal real and the past and future present, part of the necessity of 'madness', and the power of the transrational. 'Editing does for film what death does for life with both introducing the possibility of meaning. Cinema, which wants to be false, can't help being real'.[94] When we go to the cinema, we believe to be real that which is unreal, with a narrative of images and sound conjuring up life.

From 600 BC, which we saw in Chap. 1 was the same period when 'madness' was being considered by Greek doctors, Greek theatre was a mechanism for healing. Theatre is 'seductive', the 'hypnotic power of mimesis—the copying of reality'.[95] Theatre can also be a break from reality and offer a heightened reality, the two not mutually exclusive. To believe actors are real is akin to 'madness', but that is how so much of theatre works. Applause addresses, 'curious collective fantasy about the nature of exchange'; it is a reminder and disavowal of, 'the hegemony of consumerism in our capitalist culture'.[96] Shakespeare's *Hamlet*, including many film adaptations, makes use of 'madness', but in one interpretation Hamlet is suffering an existential crisis, rather than a mental disorder.[97] But the two are not distinct. Seeing a ghost might mean you are 'mad' in the sense that hallucinations are a disorder relating to psychosis, but belief in the paranormal has been ubiquitous in human history so in this sense it is normal and sane. *King Lear* has 'madness' at its heart and *Othello* reveals how to drive another person 'mad' with jealousy. Othello syndrome

[89] Helen Freshwater, *Theatre & Audience* (London: Macmillan, 2009).

[90] For Stephen Spielberg making films is his therapy, Spielberg saying this is how he avoided therapy: *Spielberg* Sky Arts 9 pm, 29 December, 2021.

[91] Foucault, op. cit.

[92] Ibid.

[93] Ibid.

[94] McKenzie Wark. *Capital Is Dead: Is This Something Worse?* (London: Verso, 2019), p. 157.

[95] L. Weaver, *Theatre and Audience* (London: Bloomsbury, 2009), p. 39.

[96] Ibid., p. 21.

[97] Robert Youngson, *The Madness of Prince Hamlet and Other Delusions* (London: Robinson Publishing, 1999).

concerns 'mad' jealousy, but his jealousy can be viewed as metaphorical 'madness'.[98] Despite his physical problem with epilepsy, Othello does not hallucinate or hear voices, symptoms which have been commonly associated with 'madness', although, as we shall see in Chap. 6 hearing voices is normal. Othello's imagination becomes possessed with false fantasies concerning his wife's betrayal until for him she is a demon (des-*demon*-a) that he must destroy for what he believes is his own sanity. If he is 'mad', or possessed with Iago's evil, then we question his culpability and guilt.

Fifteenth-century Puritan Britain was swamped in pamphlets denouncing theatre as evil. Given our post-postmodern relativism, it is easy to forget solid belief in the tangibility reality of evil during this Jacobean period was more than palpable.[99] At least Othello is acting on his feelings about evil. Despite being completely duped he is behaving authentically by seeking to destroy what he believes is evil. Anti-theatrical discourse recurs over time, in such diverse historical and geographical locations that, 'we should not look principally to social factors or economic conditions to explain it'.[100] An ontological argument can be put forward concerning the blurring of boundaries causing 'madness', hence the unconscious fear of theatre and its repression. While an ahistorical approach might not be inaccurate, we should remember theatre censorship of various kinds lasted in Britain up until 1968. Even today some topics are out of bounds for fear of not just causing offence but creating outrage akin to group 'madness'. Fear of collective 'madness', discussed in Chap. 7, can inhibit artistic exploration. This indicates the power of theatre, as is it can cause 'mad' outrage. In December 2004 British police were injured during protest over *Behzti* (*Dishonour*) written by Sikh playwright Gurpreet Bhatti, a Birmingham play that concerned sexual abuse in a religious context.[101] This reflects on the nature of group psychosis and religion as 'madness'; for Freud religion was a form of 'madness', but for Jung the reverse was true.[102]

As with cinema and literature, the power elite have seen theatre as dangerous for the masses. Even those making theatrical productions often had an overt disdain for the audience. Plato believed mimesis, 'poses a threat to sanity'.[103] This stems from an anxiety that, 'subjectivity and identity are destabilised by exposure to the unending alterity of the role-play presented in the theatre'.[104] Theatrical performance in this sense is 'madness'. Early Christian theologians, including Tertullian and St Augustine, saw popular theatre as part of a plot to ensnare souls. Before social media was continually raged over and often condemned in the popular press, cartoons and

---

[98] Ibid., pp. 120–121.

[99] Vinnie Lee-Hutala, personal communication.

[100] Weaver, op. cit., p. 40.

[101] Anonymous, BBC News Channel, 'Theatre attacks Sikh play protest', 19 December, 2004, BBC NEWS | England | West Midlands | Theatre attacks Sikh play protest (accessed January 25, 2023).

[102] Jung.

[103] Weaver, op. cit., p. 39.

[104] Ibid., p. 39.

comics were found to be an 'infection', full of 'contamination', a 'disease'.[105] What really irked social commentators was the sheer accessibility of what were known as penny dreadfuls. There was a class divide, indicating a binary approach, with the vulnerable reader conceptualized as inevitably young, working-class, and emotionally and educationally less able compared to the educated commentator, plus the young reader was believed to a blank slate in need of protection.[106] So culture was thought to spread all manner of evil, functioning as a physical malady of the mind and soul.

Stage fright has been framed in the context of mental health with the Stanislavski technique suggesting the experience is a purely modern phenomenon, 'bound up with the development of psychoanalysis and theatrical naturalism', plus the use of technology such as modern lighting and the pressures of modern urban life.[107] The industrial nature of the performance is seen as the problem. Following the industrialization of entertainment, the actor was financially dependent upon the mass audience; W.B. Yeats attacked pandering for the popular audience and the public sphere while others attempted to directly engage the audience.[108] Interestingly, we can parallel the active versus passive audience dynamic with areas of mental health therapy which have culturally specific elements. Modernists such as Gertrude Stein had a problem with the 'masses' and theatre with her work considered 'unplayable'.[109] Drama therapy is used in mental health services. There are approximately 4000 people employed in the UK's NHS as creative arts therapists out of 1.2 million.[110]

All group events have a theatricality and performative element, even within the apparently insular domestic setting of sleepy American suburbia, as highlighted by novelist A.M. Homes when she describes a party of friends which hears and sees another party in the neighbourhood. 'Through the trees they can see lights in other houses. Every lit window is like a small stage, a miniature color television where little dramas play themselves out'.[111] Theatre is normally a collaborative and collective experience, contradicting the capitalist prioritization of the individual with their focus on the 'autonomous artwork'.[112] There is the fear theatre is the place where public opinion might be formed, challenging the political order, hence its radical potential.

---

[105] Mel Gibson, 'Sick Fictions: Contamination, Disease, and Addiction in Accounts of Young People's Reading of Comics, in *Cultures of Addiction*, ed., Jason Lee (New York: Cambria), p. 123.

[106] Weaver, op. cit.

[107] Ibid., p. 43.

[108] Ibid., p. 44.

[109] Ibid.

[110] Anonymous, 'NHS Workforce Statistics', 28 October, 2018, NHS Workforce Statistics - July 2021 (Including selected provisional statistics for August 2021) - NHS Digital (accessed 26 January, 2023).

[111] A. M. Homes, *Music for Torching* (London: Granta, 1999) p. 11.

[112] Weaver, op. cit., p. 45.

Other relevant performance texts, adaptations and examples, have had significant global impact in this field, such as Peter Schaffer's *Equus* (1973) adapted for cinema by Sydney Lumet (1977). *Equus* is based on the writer's adaptation of a true story of a 17-year-old boy who blinded six horses in Suffolk. Most of the play consists of Alan Strang (Peter Firth in the film) speaking with his psychiatrist (Dr Martin Dysart played by Richard Burton). Alan develops a theology around horses, the play raising provocative questions. In becoming horse, 'the man subdues his own "instinctive" forces while the animal transmits to him its "acquired" forces'.[113] Eventually Alan's passion is shown to be a personal religion, his passion something his doctor is jealous of, showing how 'madness' and the transrational can become transgressively attractive, even to those who are supposed to be curing it.

The Blue Man Group, Punchdrunk, Living Theatre, and Blast Theory, are theatre collectives that have interestingly subverted the audience-performance paradigm to varying degrees. This could be termed the theatre of pathology where audiences are put in a position that brings on a certain level of 'madness'. Some have found this abusive, the equivalent to torture.[114] Brazilian director Augusto Boal created the term 'spect-actors', breaking the divide part of a 'rehearsal of revolution'.[115] This recalls the experiments where people faked being mental patients and were convincing mentioned in Chap. 1. The playing with boundaries is partly why the Puritans had such a problem with theatre. These groups take it a step further. As with the work of performance collective Shunt, where the audience become for example travellers on a plane crash, or part of a swingers' party (*Amato Saltone*, London Bridge Vaults, 2006), the aim is to give the pleasure of being an insider, provoking discomfort through complicity.[116]

An important play with continuing international reach which breaks down boundaries and engages with 'madness' is *Death and the Maiden*, written by Chilean Ariel Dorfman and adapted for cinema by Roman Polanski in 1994. This premiered at the Royal Court Theatre, London, on 9 July 1991 directed by Lindsay Posner, with a workshop production staged in Santiago Chile on 10 March 1991. The play concerns Paulina Salas (Sigourney Weaver in the film), a former political prisoner in an unnamed Latin American country, who has been tortured and raped by her captors led by a sadistic doctor she never sees (Ben Kingsley in the film). Years later this doctor, Roberto Miranda, apparently helps Paulina's husband Gerardo Escobar (Stuart Wilson), when his car breaks. Is this coincidence, is she psychotic, or can nothing in a country which has a repressed history be taken at face value? Paulina might be suffering from 'madness' related to post-traumatic stress disorder (PTSD). She takes the doctor captive to extract a confession. The questions remain—can you extract truth under torture, is she now indistinguishable from her torturer, or is she

[113]Deleuze and Guattari (2011), op. cit., p. 287.

[114]Weaver, op. cit.

[115]Claire Bishop, *Artificial Hells. Participatory Art and the Politics of Spectatorship* (London: Verso, 2012), p. 122.

[116]Walker, op. cit. p, 66.

insane while he is innocent? Truth and 'madness' in these circumstances are politically defined.

Death and the Maiden has been produced globally and turned into an opera by Jonas Forssell with the libretto by Ariel Dorfman premiering at the Malmö Opera on 20 September 2008. The Hindi translation opened at the India Habitat Centre New Delhi on 17 February 2002, produced by Asmita Theatre translated by Shalini Vatsa. The play returned to London and was performed at the Harold Pinter Theatre with a version staged in Nottingham in 2018. As this play shows, artistic interpretations of 'madness' as truth are translated and re-translated across time and cultures in a global context with political ramifications. The story is an example of how a person marginalized threefold (woman, torture victim, and mental health sufferer) acts to gain a voice.

In some versions of the play the ghost of the country's dictator, the gothic double, returns to the stage before the final curtain, being the return of the repressed, implying an uncanny 'madness' will forever haunt countries that refuse to face their past. Zimbabwe is one such country among many. After President Mugabe's death in 2019 people were afraid to face their history, or even properly bury their dead, the country gripped by a fearful 'madness'. As is the case historically, in several Latin American countries the official 'mad' story is so twisted, conceptions of reality are dictated to by a fictional state-authored narrative. The insanity of this reality was one reason novelists and filmmakers in the region developed magical realism.[117] This was also the case in the UK in September 2022 during the ten days of official mourning following the death of Elizabeth II when all voices of dissent against the monarchy were outlawed, one protestor arrested for holding up a blank piece of paper. With a media blackout, the country returned to a primeval mythical fairy-tale past for political purposes. Significantly, 'capital, with its conflicts, contradictions, violent history—simply with its 'history'—is ultimately just the prehistory'.[118] For Baudrillard liberation is precluded by natural predestination absolving us from original evil.[119] This is explored next by an evaluation evil in relation to the 'madness' of PTSD and depression and its significance for transrational knowledge.

---

[117] See John King, *Magical Reels. A History of Cinema in Latin America* (London: Verso, 2000).

[118] Baudrillard 2005, 41.

[119] Baudrillard 2005, 40.

2.3 Evil and Mental Health

2.3.1 PTSD

We examined how 'madness' is equated with evil and possession, and how performance has been conceived as evil. When someone is 'mad' it can appear that their behaviour is out of their own control and being driven by something other, a different performer. PTSD concerns trauma that haunts the present, so relates to evil and possession. Depression correlates with evil through the concept of loss. 'Since possession is not normative in Western cultures, it is the cultural context which determines the distinction between psychosis and the spiritual.'[120] Like unhappiness, there is a reduction of evil to misfortune and fate. This has more of an association at the lexical level in French: le mal (evil), le malheur (misfortune), and le bonheur (happiness).[121]

Evil is construed as misdeeds, accidents, and slips.[122] Therefore, given parapraxis (Freudian slips that speak the unrepressed truth), a more authentic real self can be equated with evil. 'The sovereign hypothesis, the hypothesis of evil, is that man is not good by nature'.[123] That is one biblical theological interpretation. Another is that we are good by nature and it was the temptation of evil that cast us from paradise, but without this sin there would be no human race. Adam and Eve saw each other were naked once they tasted from the forbidden tree in the Garden of Eden and were cast out, fornicated, and the rest is human history. Without the crimes of history (including original sin and evil), following Montaigne, this would destroy the fundamental conditions of life, including narrative.[124] Sin is essential for narrative and storytelling; what we are attempting is an understanding of the accidents and slips.

If original sin is the original 'madness' (to turn against God), then this spawns humanity which explains how 'madness' and humanity are endemically entwined. The hearts of people are, 'full of evil, and madness is in their hearts while they live'.[125] Alienation and alienating work are punishments for defying God in Eden, called Paradise in early translations, and it is the result of evil.[126] Life then becomes a matter of paying off the debt of original sin through good works, the Protestant work

[120] Simon Dein and Abdool Samad Illaiee, *The Psychiatrist*, Vo. 37, Issue 9, September 2013, pp. 290-293.

[121] Jean Baudrillard, *The Intelligence of Evil – Or the Lucidity Pact*, trans. Chris Turner (London: Bloomsbury, 2013), p. 107.

[122] Ibid.

[123] Ibid., p. 107.

[124] Ibid., p. 111.

[125] Ecclesiastes 9:3. *The Bible*, New Living Translation (London: Tyndale House, 2007).

[126] It is interesting to consider what depression and PTSD Adam and Evil felt cast out of Eden and being condemned, after their biting the apple and enjoying evil, but even early scholars of the Church such as Ambrose of Milan in the fourth century saw these figures as metaphors, Eve being akin to the senses.

ethic turning work into the embodiment of goodness. Arguments on original sin are akin those on genetic predispositions, such as people being born with the potential for 'madness', or the propensity for evil. Evil's demonic power is beyond human nature or actions according to *Genesis*. In *The Book of Enoch* fallen angels instigate our troubles.[127] The paradox of progress, where scientific development and growth in trade brings as many issues as improvements, is expressed by this myth of fallen angels.[128]

The aggregate of human evil is not the equivalent to the totality of evil, for evil is supernatural and of cosmic proportions. For Milton, 'madness' stems from our fall from grace, it is self-inflicted, moving us away from our real destiny.[129] Evil was so interwoven with good; 'from the rind of one apple tasted, that the knowledge of good and evil as two twins together leapt forward into the world'.[130] According to the early church fathers, God created evil and this was the only way good could arise. The Platonic origin for evil was ignorance and Jesus Christ asked God to forgive those who crucified him, killing God a heinous sin, as they did not know what they were doing, they were ignorant. In Christianity evil involves the loss of God. Depression involves loss also, so logically within this paradigm loss of God, or faith, would bring about the deepest depression. Rejecting the idea of a subject, for Baudrillard evil is automatic; 'those who practise evil certainly have no insight into it, since their act supposes the intentionality of a subject'.[131] We can see how this relates to the Christian view of evil as ignorance. Baudrillard claims we have confused the idea of evil with an objective existence of evil, and it has no more meaning than an objective existence of the Real. Building on Nietzsche's Eternal Return, in Baudrillard's paradigm evil consists in diverting things from their existence.[132] This we can parallel with a Christian view that in the grander scheme of things evil is the ultimate illusion, being convinced flesh and matter are the only reality, diverting us from the Spirit, as emphasized in Pauline theology.[133]

Evil and 'madness' can take on mystical predetermined undertones, appearing as if they cannot be prevented. This has a Calvinist ring to it and can be scripturally supported.[134] Paradoxically, this only adds to the attraction of evil and a sense of purity—evil is often thought of as false, but as we have seen evil as purity and authenticity is another interpretation. Evil can be interpreted as an accident, just like 'madness', such as a gap or slip which in Freudian terms reveals the truth. God can

[127] William Neil, One Volume Bible Commentary (London: Hodder & Stoughton, 1996), p. 29.

[128] Ibid.

[129] John Milton, *Paradise Lost* (London: Penguin, 1989), p. 269.

[130] Ibid., p. xxv.

[131] Baudrillard, op. cit., p. 123. From Chap. 1 we see how he has developed Schopenhauer.

[132] Ibid.

[133] See Galatians 5: 16–17. *The Bible*, Revised Standard Version (London: Collins, 1977), p. 977.

[134] 'For if the gospel we preach is hidden, it is hidden only from those who are being lost.' 2 Corinthians 4:3. This refers to unbelievers. The implication, at least in this translation, is this is predestined. *The Bible*, Revised Standard Version (London: Collins, 1977), p. 968.

be described as in league with the principle of evil.[135] If God created all, then God created evil and the more evil necessitates more good.[136] William Blatty, the author of the book that led to the film *The Exorcist* (William Friedkin, 1973), explained how for Jesuits evil is the crucible of goodness.[137]

There is an ongoing notion of a malign force to be dealt with, often projected onto any other or outsider. This offers a sense of power within personal and collective narratives and constructions of physical and metaphysical time, including the end of time, when all evil doers are supposed to be punished. So-called evil events have been known to cause PTSD. In 1872 Charles Darwin's *The Expression of the Emotions in Man and Animals* was published. For Darwin the purpose of emotion is to, 'initiate movement that will restore the organism to safety and equilibrium'.[138] Avoiding behaviour puts the animal at a disadvantage, stuck in survival mode where there is no room for nurturing.

For those with PTSD stress hormones do not return to an equilibrium; fight/flight/freeze continue after an event.[139] Returning to the trauma of the event, or ones like it, may bring meaning but does not bring healing. Psychiatrist Abram Kardiner's, *The Traumatic Neurosis of War* (1941) was a study of World War 1 veterans and was published because of the predicted high numbers of those with shellshock following World War 2.[140] What he called 'traumatic neurosis' we would now call PTSD with a physiological basis.[141] The problem was that psychoanalytical approaches became so dominant in America in the 1940s, that PTSD was believed to be not caused by trauma experienced in war but from early childhood. The 1946 Mental Health Act acknowledged that PTSD was a real issue, but given the dominance of psychoanalysis it had got the causes wrong.

Anna Freud's theories on the maladjusted child came dominate America during this period and this involved teaching adults to control their drives, including homosexuality. The slogans included, 'you can control the fire of your emotions, so your personality becomes more pleasant'.[142] Feeling and passions were considered the real evil, and people were taught by a deluge of social workers who entered homes, plus newly trained counsellors and psychiatrists, to conform to society and the status quo. As the argument of this book shows, with feelings part of beneficial transrational knowledge, their denial only led to a further mental health crisis and this investment in treatment was not just a waste but damaging. The other apparent solution at this period, led by Ed Bernays Freud's cousin, was to invent the consumer

---

[135] Baudrillard, op. cit., p. 122.

[136] This sounds 'mad', but it can be seen from claims of sexual abuse.

[137] William Blatty, *The Exorcist* (New York: Harper & Row, 1971), p. 318.

[138] Bessel van der Kolk, *The Body Keeps the Score: Mind, Brain and Body in the Transformation of Trauma* (London: Penguin, 2014), p. 75.

[139] Ibid., p. 30.

[140] Ibid., p. 11.

[141] Ibid.

[142] Adam Curtis, 'The Century of Self', Episode 2, 2002, BBC 2.

with Bernays also being used in the Cold War fight given his skills in public relations an propaganda. When Anna Freud's preeminent patient and case study committed suicide in Sigmund Freud's house in London the tide turned. Herbert Marcuse switched the source of evil from inward evil to the external with Martin Luther King mentioned in a speech that he was, 'proud to be maladjusted' to religious bigotry and racism.

Discussing what some considered his PTSD, Prince Harry in an interview with ITV broadcast 8 January claimed he had rather post traumatic stress injury, rather than a disorder which would suggest a lasting impact. There is also the insinuation that an injury, being more physical, is more noble that is something that is more a mental health problem. In his 2023 memoir *Spare* he claims two men who had undergone the same war exercise as him, 'had gone mad'.[143] Interestingly, Prince Harry claims he has few memories prior to his mother's death, as if he unconsciously built a wall. Our normality of personal time is the 'madness' of our reality and our memory is one way of regulating our lives, but PTSD alters this. What we think of as the same object persisting in time is several different objects, 'unchangingly locked into their own time'.[144] Except within the limit of the present, strictly speaking, time does not exist. But we must submit to it so we must be subject to 'that which does not exist'; we are bound by unreal chains of passive duration, or of organised time and in this sense time, 'which is unreal casts over all things including ourselves a veil of unreality'.[145] With trauma, such as PTSD, time operates differently, forcing us to question traditional ideas of time. Cinema can bear witness to 'external' trauma imitatively; immersed in the imaginary, it witnesses 'psychological reality'.[146] 'More problematically, it permits vicarious trauma, which can erase the different positions of the victim, eyewitness and spectator'.[147]

Media images situated in real and imagined events are used to inform ideas around mental health.[148] The image means the event and ideology constitutes an event.[149] From popular feature films, such as *The Deer Hunter* (Michael Cimino, 1979), *Born on the Fourth of July* (Oliver Stone, 1989) and *Jacob's Ladder* (Adrian Lyne, 1990), to hit television shows, like the BBC's *The Body Guard* (2018), Amazon Prime's *Homecoming* (2018–), and the BBC's *Peaky Blinders* (2013–), visual cultures have been instrumental in constructing an understanding of PTSD. Often these are traditional triumph over adversity narratives following well

---

[143] Prince Harry, *Spare* (New York: Random House, 2023), p. 231.

[144] Robert Le Poidevin, *Travels in Four Dimensions: The Enigmas of Space and Time* (Oxford: Oxford University Pres, 2003), p. 246.

[145] Simone Weil, *Gravity and Grace*, trans. Emma Crawford and Mario von der Ruhr (London: Routledge, 1992), pp. 45–46.

[146] Scott Brewster, 'Access Denied: Memory and Resistance in the Contemporary Ghost Film', in Jo Collins and John Jervis, eds., *Uncanny Modernity – Cultural Theories, Modern Anxieties* (New York: Palgrave, 2008), p. 118.

[147] Ibid.

[148] Aroyewn-Adekomaiya, op. cit.

[149] Susan Sontag, *Illness as Metaphor* (London: Penguin, 1978), p. 19.

documented screenplay formulas. In other stories there is a deliberate way characters become superhuman, as in *Fearless* (Peter Weir, 1993). In others still, what is relevant is the wider post-war political landscape. Wars have led to mental health problems for returning soldiers depicted on screen as part of a metaphoric wound for a nation.

In my discussions with British ex-army PTSD sufferers the term veteran was frowned upon; they did not want to be called veterans. The peculiarly American context needs acknowledging; 'self-perfection had long been living philosophies in the land of the free'.[150] At its heart America concerned the survival of the fittest, a Social Darwinist creed fused with manifest destiny. Any perceived weaknesses within this ideology, such as a mental problem or PTSD, contradicted the essence of a pioneering American self-reliance spirit, working as a form of anti-philosophy. PTSDs challenge the American doctrine of success. Blame was often cast on the individual for their disability and PTSD.

Notable films that have tackled PTSD reveal the weaknesses with America's ideology, both domestically and internationally and those discussed here involve the impact of PTSD on American war veterans. Etymologically war stems from 'confusion' and 'strife' which are words intimately connected to 'madness'.[151] Freud argued that war is innate to human nature with warfare being a projection of internal battles onto the external world.[152] For Trotsky war was the, 'locomotive of history'.[153] While being viewed as the heart of the human psyche and history, war has simultaneously been seen as a total lapse of reason linked to animal behaviour and anarchy, antithetical to all that is civilized. Given the latter definition it would make sense that war would lead to a form of mental disturbance as it appears to be 'madness'. Clinical work in psychology has existed since the 1980s to help in the treatment of PTSD as it is currently understood.[154] This work has been especially with war veterans, but it is via popular culture that wider knowledge of PTSD has been addressed and disseminated. As with most mental health diagnoses with PTSD there is controversy over definitions in terms of causes, diagnoses, symptoms and cures. It occurs due to, 'direct exposure to, witnessing or learning about an extremely traumatic event', and symptoms include, 'persistent re-experiencing of the traumatic event, typically through recollection, dreams and nightmares'.[155]

In the 1980s New York psychiatrists, including Chaim F. Shatan who had worked with Vietnam veterans, and Robert J. Lifton, lobbied the American Psychiatric

---

[150] Roy Porter, *A Social History of Madness – Stories of the Insane* (London: Phoenix, 1996), p. 189.

[151] Jason Lee, *The Metaphysics of Mass Art*, Vol. II (New York: Mellen, 1999), p. 95.

[152] Sigmund Freud, *New Introductory Lectures on Psychoanalysis*, trans. James Strachey (London: Penguin, 1996), p. 214.

[153] Daniel Pick, *War Machine: The Rationalisation of Slaughter in the Modern Age* (London: Yale University Press, 1993), p. 8.

[154] Michael Scott and Stephen Stradling, *Counselling for Post Traumatic Stress Disorder* (London: Sage, 1992).

[155] William Cockerham, *Medical Sociology* (London: Routledge, 2017), p. 43.

Association (APA) to create the diagnosis PTSD for inclusion in the *Diagnostic and Statistical Manual of Mental Disorders* (DSM-III).[156] Shatan had already written about what he termed Post-Vietnam Syndrome in 1973, but 'gross stress reaction' which covered areas including PTSD had been removed from the DSM. A wide number of symptoms have been bracketed within the spectrum of a PTSD diagnosis. Beyond representations of PTSD, popular culture has played a part in its scientific study. Bessel van der Kolk and colleagues conducted pain test experiments on American veterans with PTSD. Eight veterans watched clips from the violent war film *Platoon* (Oliver Stone, 1986). How long they could keep their right hands in a bucket of ice-water was measured. This was repeated with a peaceful clip from another film. Seven of the eight kept their hand in the water 30% longer during the violent film. They then worked out the amount of analgesia (inability to feel pain) produced by watching 15 min of a combat movie was the same as that produced by being injected with eight milligrams of morphine, 'about the same dose a person would receive in an emergency room for crushing chest pain'.[157] They concluded this was the result of morphine like substances being produced in the brain during the viewing of the violent film.

This experiment might mean that for those suffering from trauma re-encounters with stress offers relief from anxiety and those with existing PTSD can feel compelled to return to combat zones, or other violent situations, as observed in *The Hurt Locker* (Kathryn Bigelow, 2009). A desire to return may also be caused by medical treatment preventing those who have experienced horrendous injuries in battle realising the extent of the horror. Medication to 'wipe out short-term memory' to overcome trauma has been standard for soldiers in recent American conflicts with those injured only knowing the real details from their comrades.[158]

Using film for emotional stimuli in laboratory conditions one other study showed that the mood of fear produced by frightening films, 'has a lengthening effect on time perception'; and stimulus durations were, 'judged longer after than before viewing these emotional films'.[159] Neutral films, such as stock market and weather reports, did not impact on time perception. Interestingly, unlike fear in terms of neuroscience sadness is a poorly understood emotion.[160] Following the DSM criteria, treatment for PTSD has been focused on symptoms such as intrusive imagery, avoidance behaviour, and disordered arousal.[161] Despite success in the field of PTSD with Prozac, and drugs like Zoloft, Celexa, Cymbalta, and Paxil, in the main drugs did not work with war veterans and those at the extreme end.[162] Drugs do not get to the

[156]Ibid., p. 19.

[157]Ibid., p. 33.

[158]Jane Mulkerrins, 'The extraordinary life of Senator Tammy Duckworth', *The Times Magazine*, 17.04.21, p. 51.

[159]Sylvie Droit-Volet, Sophie L. Fayolle and Sandrine Gil, 'Emotion and time perception: effects of film-induced mood', *Frontiers in Integrative Neuroscience*, August 2011, Vol. 5, Article 33, p. 7–8.

[160]Ibid.

[161]van der Kolk, op. cit., p. 133.

underlying issues, but they can control symptoms providing a mechanism for healing. A significant body of research exists explaining how filmmaking and video-based therapy and cinematherapy helps with PTSD.[163]

The phrase 'that triggered me' has become popularised implying a mild form of PTSD correlating with common anxiety. Research on Americans has approximated between 5 and 12% experience PTSD with a clinically significant number going on to develop Acute Stress Disorder (ASD).[164] The anti-psychiatry movement have questioned the prioritising of diagnosis, medical terminology, and labels, and often with good reason. PTSD is part of our current belief system, as evidenced by the popularity of 'trigger warnings' and other factors explained here. Sexual abuse and violence, which may cause PTSD, are central to the exploitative capitalist framework underpinning Western society, underscoring much of media and culture.[165] Reflecting Sontag and Irigaray, for Žižek global capitalism, 'generates a new form of illness'.[166] Due to it being a return to life story, *You Were Never Really Here* (Lynne Ramsay, 2018) reverses Žižek's thesis of the living-dead post-traumatic subject.[167] The contemporary world both causes and is a symptom of this paradigm and in interviews for Chap. 5 PTSD was a common theme. One interviewee explained that through repeatedly working with news media content they and their colleagues suffered PTSD; news footage had a damaging long-term impact leading to a variety of mental health problems.

The film industry database IMDB gives 320 films and television shows related to PTSD, interestingly almost three times the number using the non-specific term 'madness'.[168] Here we shall address two significant and related films that are comparable yet distinct, *You Were Never Really Here* (Lynne Ramsay, 2017) and *Taxi Driver* (Martin Scorsese, 1976). Given an avoidance of events that may trigger trauma could be a behaviour associated with PTSD, both films could be criticised for accuracy. But, as we have seen, those with PTSD often desire to re-enter the trauma zone, especially a war zone literally or metaphorically, which happens in these two films and the experiment outlined above reveals this re-encounter with violence can reduce pain. The director reveals the long-term mental health impact of child abuse and war in *You Were Never Really Here* adapted from Jonathan Ames' 2016 novella. The protagonist Joe (Joaquin Phoenix) suffers PTSD both from childhood and

---

[162] van der Kolk, op. cit., p. 35.

[163] R. Tuval-Mashiach, B.W. Patton and C. Drebing, '"When you make a movie, and you see your story there, you can hold it": Qualitative exploration of collaborative filmmaking a therapeutic tool for veterans', *Frontiers in Psychology*, 9, Article 1954, 2018.

[164] E.L James, A. Lau-Zhu, I.A. Clark, R.M. Visser, M.A. Hagenaars, E.A. Holmes, 'The trauma film paradigm as an experimental psychopathology model of psychological trauma: intrusive memories and beyond', *Clinical Psychology Review*, 47, July 2016, pp. 106–142.

[165] Jason Lee, *Pervasive Perversion – Paedophilia and Child Sexual Abuse in Media/Culture* (London: Free Association Books, 2005).

[166] Slavoj Žižek, *Living in the End Times* (London: Verso, 2011), p. 295.

[167] Ibid., p. 294.

[168] Almost three times the number of those when using the non-specific term 'madness'.

adulthood experiences, confirming this point about returning to the trauma zone. PTSD here is not as simple as' Darwin's work maintains in that Joe does have close nurturing from his mother (Judith Roberts) and can nurture others. Ramsay subverts expectations, interestingly questioning the conventional mental health victim/survivor paradigm.

In its treatment, construction and impact, PTSD has altered over the period from the Vietnam War (1955-1975) which *Taxi Driver* (Martin Scorsese, 1976) reflects on, where Travis Bickle (Robert De Niro) is a total loner, to *You Were Never Really Here* four decades on. PTSD as we now know it was only starting to be fully addressed clinically in the 1980s when it entered the DSM during the immediate years following Scorsese's film. By the time of Ramsay's film in 2017 many variations of PTSD, from mild to extreme, were openly discussed and researched. PTSD was now part of the zeitgeist and it seemed if you did not have some form of it there was something wrong with you the phrase 'it triggered me' so popularized it was watering down PTSD's worth. There were also shifting cinematic styles and language over the period between the films.

In Deleuzian terms Ramsay employs the act of seeing in a visceral sense.[169] Ramsay's shots concern 'the perception of perception', looking at something through something, a theme in all her films.[170] Despite his suffering, Joe still manages to maintain relationships. Because he suffers, he can relate and have empathy with the main girl he rescues. In both films the protagonists are heroes, rescuing girls. The balletic exterior and extroverted violence of *Taxi Driver* is replaced by Ramsay with a deeper muted interior and introverted violence. Unlike Travis Bickle, who wants to get rid of all the night animals, 'whores, skunk pussies, buggers, queens, fairies, dopers, junkies', Joe is methodically doing his job as an assassin, often tenderly, even holding the hand of a dying man who may have killed his mother.

You Were Never Really Here is also the antithesis of the earlier film aesthetically and in the way night and day are juxtaposed. For Maurice Blanchot the uncanny entails the loss of the familiar leading to the intimation of death, but in *Taxi Driver* Blanchot's autre nuit (other night) is fertile via this form of cinematic dream novella, a phantasmagoria.[171] Contrapuntally, in *You Were Never Really Here* day is victorious. Far from there being an immateriality of signs, worshipping nothingness, there is a heightened signification leading to meaning. For Scorsese movies are a dream state.[172] Ramsay closes on Joe dreaming about shooting himself, then he awakes to

---

[169] Gilles Deleuze, *Cinema 2: The Time-Image*, trans. Hugh Tomlinson and Robert Galeta (London: Continuum, 1989), p. 9.

[170] R. De Luca, 'Dermatology as Screenology: The Films of Lynne Ramsay', *Film Criticism*, Vol. 43, Issue 1, March 2019.

[171] E. Bronfen, 'Night and the Uncanny', in Jo Collins and John Jervis, eds., *Uncanny Modernity – Cultural Theories, Modern Anxieties* (New York: Palgrave, 2008), p. 61. Check!

[172] I. Christie and D. Thompson, *Scorsese on Scorsese* (London: Faber & Fabert, 2003), p. 54.

the woman he has freed telling him it is a beautiful day. The nightmare was his own fantasy and ours, given the false suicidal ending is believable.

The downbeat didacticism of Scorsese's earlier film has shifted in multifarious ways. In Ramsay's *You Were Never Really Here* the psychoanalytical view on the early development of the diagnosis of PTSD in terms of the mother is disproved. Film helps us understand further elements of PTSD and this is the core paradox Ramsay concentrates on to such profound effect. Like any mental health problem PTSD has a range of severity, but what the protagonist Joe has suffered and is still suffering physically as well as emotionally manifests as PTSD. Flashbacks occur and he is on medication presumably due to his military service and his childhood trauma, although the details are not spelt out, allowing for audience interpretation and a less moralistic cinematic experience.

From *Taxi Driver* to *You Were Never Really Here*, which in aspects of its cinematography and plot has consistent parallels with the earlier film, PTSD is central to how the contemporary is experienced, perceived, and negotiated. PTSD contests the traditional American belief self-reliance. Michael High argues for the sagacity of Žižek's view that violence in American cultural texts empowers us to differentiate the antithesis of American self-reliance.[173] Travis's behaviour is not a righteous act but involves the repetition which is at the heart of PTSD. There is a transitory limited wholeness conjured up via the oft-quoted Lacanian mirror scene ("You talking to me?") and the masculinity is a 'misrecognition' which is not sustained, 'when confronting others who do not share is imaginary ideal. It is only through death that he can finalize and concretize the image of wholeness'.[174]

Paul Schrader wrote the script to 'exorcise the evil I felt within me' in under two weeks as 'self therapy'.[175] He goes on to explain he had been sleeping in his car at the time, the taxi in the film a coffin. This coffin has wider ramifications when we consider the impact of violent American imperialism which both Travis and Joe with their PTSD are victims of. While Travis's taxi functions for us as a mobile cinema, machinery in Ramsay's film functions as a backdrop offering comfort and solace. The American hammer functions as an administrator of freedom. This implement which symbolises civilization is anonymous and is an overt signifier when purchased at a hardware store by Joe with a close-up on the place of manufacturing. America is doing the damage and has the means to destroy domestically and globally. Ramsay's film offers an individually and locally specific and yet global commentary on the damage which causes PTSD. The high level of PTSD historically within American culture parallels the spreading of this disorder through American led imperialism and capitalism across the globe. The cut-throat razor that the rescued girl Nina Votto (Ekaterina Samsonov) uses to kill her abuser (Alex Manette), carried out off screen,

[173] M. High, '*Taxi Driver* and veteran trauma', in A. Baker, ed., *A Companion to Martin Scorsese* (Oxford: Wiley, 2014), p. 375.

[174] Ibid.

[175] G. Macnab, *The Making of Taxi Driver* (New York: Unanimous, 2006).

is a more individualised weapon, a form of love token despite its lethal ability, Joe previously playing with a knife at home like a child.

Joe has flashbacks to a war zone and to his childhood. Significantly, for PTSD sufferers, flashbacks can be worse than the incident of trauma, with the latter having a beginning, middle and end.[176] You cannot predict when a flashback will occur or for how long, and dissociation occurs which is the essence of trauma. Fragmentation concerns emotions, sounds, images, thoughts, and physical sensations, which then take on a 'life of their own'; fragments of memory, 'intrude into the present', and if, 'the trauma is not resolved, the stress hormones that the body secretes to protect itself keep circulating, and the defensive movements and emotional responses keep getting replayed'.[177]

When cinematography and editing plays with fragmentation and analepsis film is the ideal medium to portray and comprehend PTSD. In one flashback Joe hands an Arab boy a chocolate bar near an American compound in the Middle East. The child is then immediately shot by another boy—just for the chocolate. This parallels later action in America and is a warning. Once you help someone, you do not know the consequences. How much of a martyr will you be? The Middle East and America fuse as a unified war zone united with Joe's childhood abuse, so initially evil dominates.

An inability to rise above events like this is a symptom of PTSD, the protagonist sucked back into the traumatic moments of his life. The Middle East is no longer an anonymous region in *You Were Never Really Here*, but uncannily returns to haunt the homeland. This is more tangible than cinema's 'rhetoric of the uncanny' and the dream-like darkness of *Taxi Driver*.[178] In *Taxi Driver* we are made aware that this is not objective within the refracted gaze of the taxi driver's mobile cinema.[179] With *You Were Never Really Here*, while the gaze is still highlighted within the director's oeuvre, there is an objective documentary aesthetic, especially in the street scenes.

Phoenix playing Joe carries with him the cultural capital of similar roles, including that of PTSD sufferer navy veteran Freddie Quell who zealously joins a cult based on Scientology in *The Master* (Paul Thomas Anderson, 2012). The beliefs of Scientology can be termed 'mad' but they also claim to cure 'madness' if this is defined as a sickness of the soul. Both roles allow Phoenix to channel into the dark underbelly of American culture and feed into *Joker* (Todd Phillips, 2019), which again has flashbacks to abuse and concerns PTSD and takes full advantage of references to mental illness.

How mental illness has come to dominate popular culture is illustrated by the immense popularity of the DC comics' 'mad' character Harley Quinn (Margot Robbie), originally the Joker's psychiatrist who became his girlfriend. This is a form of revelling in 'madness', and part of her appeal is we do not know what she

---

[176] van der Kolk, op. cit., p. 66.

[177] Ibid.

[178] Bronfen, op. cit., p. 66 (accessed 16 October, 2023).

[179] Ibid.

will do next, making her exciting as well as excitable, as in the comic wedding sequence in *The Suicide Squad* (James Gunn, 2021). 'Madness' as entertainment that can be traced back to views on 'madness' as overexcitation and anarchy as propounded by the Rev. Dr. Francis Willis.[180] Willis was consulted over King George's illness in 1788, popularized in the film *The Madness of King George* (Nicholas Hytner, 1994).

As with films like *Joker*, negative critics of *Taxi Driver* claimed there was a revelling in the psychotic protagonist's 'madness', as if it was immoral to be entertained by this film, but Scorsese positions New York as the real 'madness'.[181] Contrapuntally, films of the 1980s such as *Ferris Bueller's Day Off* (John Hughes, 1986) with Cameron Frye (Alan Ruck) as the suicidal sidekick of the protagonist, position trauma as within the individual's attitude rather than the environment. This personalisation is far more conventional and less political, reducing external influence epitomising the 1980s focus on selfish non-political individualism which is film genre terms is more acceptable to mass audiences and film executive.

While PTSD in *You Were Never Really Here* is recurrently linked to wars and a brand of American imperialistic evil, what evil is (like 'madness') is questioned. *The Master*'s background is the war in Asia in the 1950s when America was asserting its role as the global police officer. American imperialistic might without boundaries made it the universal transgressor, the epitome of 'madness', as revealed in *Apocalypse Now* (Francis Ford Coppola, 1979), while simultaneously attempting to bring law and order. This is not as overt in *You Were Never Really Here*, but while America rapes the world external to itself, to gain oil for example, the film reveals domestic rape of the young, political power thriving on this inward and external exploitation. The film mirrors the evil of the Trump administration's manipulation of power at home and abroad.

Nina is the survivor of a child sex abuse brothel, The Playground, and manifests obsessive-compulsive disorder (OCD) which relates to her PTSD. We see here how diagnoses bleed into each other and what might be perceived as our insanity is often what keeps us sane, or, in Laingian terms, keep us safe. Nina counts for what appears to be distraction and this could be perceived to be mentally abnormal (OCD), but this is a way for her to maintain order while distancing herself and staying safe. Through doing so she can manage reality and fear. A focus such as this is a type of concentration, working like meditation just as a repetitive petitionary prayer (as in the Roman Catholic prayer Hail Mary, Full of Grace and so on) works, to focus the mind. This also relates to popularized techniques recommended in cognitive behavioural therapy (CBT).[182] This protects Nina from the underlying horror of

---

[180] R. Porter, *A Social History of Madness; Stories of the Insane* (London: Wiedenfeld and Nicolson, 1987), pp. 46–47).

[181] P. Kael, 'Underground Man', *The New Yorker*, 9 February, 1976, https://newyorker.com/magazine/1976/02/09/underground-man (accessed 16 October, 2023).

[182] P. Myles and R. Shafran, *The CBT Handbook: A Comprehensive Guide* (London: Constable & Robinson, 2015).

what has happened and may happen to her, functioning as a protective mental screen. Joe too has his own obsessions; both are PTSD sufferers mirroring each other and acting out.

The rescue of Nina (resurrection) and the burial of his mother merge in the funeral sequence which doubles as a baptism. Joe's love for his mother stands outside the hatred and destruction in his environment, grounding him. Like a shaman, Joe dresses his mother for the burial as if she is taking a journey to the next world and he is Charon, carrying her across the river Styx in his best suit carrying her to a lake. This is concurrently his own baptism, burial, and resurrection with strong mythical import following the wounded hero arc.[183] Humans worship the hero who has encountered death, as this brings liberation from fear with the taboo having been crossed and the hero surviving.[184]

The complexity of PTSD in terms of its impact on being is felt here. While underwater putting his mother to rest, Joe mystically encounters the lost girl, Nina. She is still alive, but this is a form of hallucination or mirroring. Nina has metaphorically been underwater, drowning in the brothel. This is a prophecy, as he shamanically exchanges one love for another, neither being primarily sexual with Joe a contemporary prophet. There are several rites of passage Joe performs on himself and others as a shaman and archetypal wounded healer. From the outside this appears to be a pathological procedure, but it is the reverse confirming the profound disposition of transrational knowledge. The poignancy of this ceremony deep in nature reminds us there is love and innocence beyond the corruption and evil of civilization. Joe has the potential to drown with his mother, entering the lake with her dead body, but at the last minute he removes the stones from his pockets. He is in all respects liminal, on the line between life and death.

As in *The Master* and *Joker*, Joaquin Phoenix plays a form of transrational shaman. Shifting from past, present, to future, his being allows for the spirits from other worlds to enter, especially when he holds the hand of the dying officer. This tenderness, in what initially was conceived as a brutal psychopath, subverts expectations. Joe rescued the girl, but it is the girl who kills her own abuser not Joe. Again, this is a major subversion of expectations. Joe's story is Homeric given when home is found, like Odysseus, he must move again, this time with Nina. Homer's *Odyssey* warriors' diaries are accounts of intense disturbances during and after battle, the being examples of ancient PTSD narratives.[185]

When in the final sequence Joe shoots himself in the head, we fully accept this as reality, more than when we realize this was his fantasy, the final subversion of expectations being a happy ending. The wounded couple are together despite or because of all the suffering and this may turn out to be a 'beautiful day' as Nina wryly notes; there is transrational hope. Joe's life as a bounty hunter, driven by an

183 Joseph Campbell, *The Hero with a Thousand Faces* (London: Fontana, 1993).

184 Ernest Becker, *The Denial of Death* (New York: Free Press, 1973), p. 12.

185 M. Scott and S. Stradling, *Counselling for Post-Traumatic Stress Disorder* (London: Sage, 1994).

unconscious need for violence due to his PTSD, is overcome. His trauma as a child and adult is vividly depicted in flashbacks, but his often-overwhelming PTSD is revealed to be not having permanent life-limiting implications.

Healthily contradicting the predetermination of puritan theologian Calvin and postmodern philosopher Baudrillard, the film reveals nothing is inevitable and offers transrational hope. This life-affirming message is not clichéd, but the antithesis to the darkness of *Taxi Driver*. Living is often harder than dying. The uncanny spell of the evil 'madness' of child sexual abuse and politics surrounding Nina and Joe is broken. The subtext is wealth and power will buy you anything and that in some positions you are above the law, but it is someone outside the law like Joe who can bring you to justice.

With its uncanny doubling, *Taxi Driver* has been interpreted as a descent into the final frontier, the night.[186] In this world the law cannot help the vulnerable and the weak with those in charge of the justice system exploiting those who need protecting. Joe as an outlaw has little to lose, but this world is not shot like the Wild West balletic violence of Sam Peckinpah, Martin Scorsese, and Quentin Tarantino. The female director captures a more sinister mood than boys' own violence through a more complex visual language, including CCTV, with the cinematographer Tom Townend often going with flow of Joaquin Phoenix's approach to scenes and his position.[187]

Ramsay's approach is normally to shoot a wide and close-up as required for editorial without much coverage, the film planned and shot mainly as a single-camera shoot with it fixed on the tripod or dolly with a brace of handheld or Steadicam shots.[188] Townend used Panavision Anamorphic lenses which 'suited the character study aspect of the narrative', giving 'extra space in frame to include the city'.[189] The camera movement was curtailed to, 'give the actors as much freedom as possible to perform without the distraction of the camera'.[190] This adds an originality to the film and power to the acting, plus it was shot 'like a documentary' without the time to storyboard and be 'over precious'.[191] Influences included 'filthy and disturbing shots of prostitutes in South East Asia' by Antoine d'Agata, 'Francis Bacon-meets-Lucian Freud style' and Townend also mentions the influences of the naturalistic-looking films of the 1970s, including the cinematogra-

---

[186]Bronfen, op. cit., p. 63.

[187]Tow Townend, 'New Shoots: Visual Storytelling Masterclass' with Tom Townend, Shooting People, 21 April 2022.

[188]Ron Prince, 'OUT OF CONTROL Tom Townend/*You Were Never Really Here*', *British Cinematographer*, 7 May 2018, *https://britishcinematographer.co.uk/tom-townend-you-were-never-really-here/* (accessed 16 October, 2023).

[189]Ibid.

[190]Ibid.

[191]Ibid.

phy of Gordon Willis ASC for *Klute* (Alan Pakula, 1971) and Michael Chapman ASC, *Taxi Driver*.

Entering a house full of drugged and abused girls, echoing the labyrinth of the uncanny, Joe methodically attacks people with the Made in America hammer. He is not sadistically reaping revenge and justice, just doing a job. Joe's victims appear all Asian, adding a racial dimension to the plot and similarly the racial politics of *Taxi Driver* are ambivalent.[192] Does *Taxi Driver* align itself with Travis's racism, or is Scorsese deconstructing the protagonist's, 'paranoid re-encoding of nocturnal New York into a violated feminine body, which must be saved from its polluting aggressors'?[193] This depends on the position of our gaze which is further complexified in *You Were Never Really Here*. The male gaze theory that the female is situated as an object is challenged through multiple viewpoints in *You Were Never Really Here*. The events Joe uncovers are being recorded and watched by cameras implying a central invisible voyeur, plus some form of exterior control complexified through the secondary layer of the gaze of the female director. The violence becomes procedural and methodical rather than irrational mapped out as embedded within a wider purpose. Sociologically, the capitalist world of exchange has led to these 'mad' events with the girls positioned within the evil milieu of The Playground being bought for sex while Joe is then paid to rescue them.

American critics thought less favourably of the film, the rawer artistic elements too much. For the *National Post* critic, the film, 'pushes the audience away at every turn'.[194] American critics appeared to want everything easy while appreciating the cinematography misunderstanding the sociological and philosophical point that often society is alienating. Neither state nor society can embody freedom and, confirming the transrational once more, following Hegel reason and rationality ultimately leading to 'unfreedom'.[195] 'If the past is just left behind and forgotten, there will be no end to destructive transgression. Somehow the progress of transgression must be arrested.'[196] The hangover from multiple wars, including those in Iraq and Afghanistan, is not something they wish to face. With a female director, the film subverts expectations with the girl ultimately saving herself and the male protagonist. The political patriarch, the essence of American capitalism, is shown to be evil itself.

Relationships between PTSD and film have been evaluated, we have seen how film is used scientifically to further the understanding of PTSD, and how aesthetically film deepens our understanding of PTSD it being the ideal medium for this. The experience of trauma is highly personal, of course. For sociologist Frank Furedi the dominance of therapeutic culture has developed a victimizing and traumatizing personhood.[197] There is some truth in this, but it is too binary to totally condemn

[192] Bronfen, op. cit., p 64.

[193] Ibid.

[194] Knight 2018.

[195] Herbert Marcuse, *Eros & Civilization* (London: Abacus, 1973), p. 91.

[196] Ibid.

the ‘snowflake generation’. Since its definition and introduction as an official diagnosis in the 1980s, when 1% of the population had PTSD, this is now as high as 12%. The framing of a diagnosis may create the disorder. More might be seeking treatment, due to greater awareness, which is positive, plus there could also be more events today traumatizing people. The constant bombardment of newsfeeds about apocalyptic scenarios can create trauma; an interviewee in Chap. 5 explains how violent images cause PTSD. This also indicates that people are not being treated successfully for PTSD, plus a broader spectrum of difficulties are bracketed as PTSD. People might self-identify with this popular disorder for many reasons, but a danger with over-emphasizing risk and trauma is that it removes ‘autonomy’, ‘choice’, and ultimately can remove ‘meaning’ and ‘humanity’.[198] Arguably the word ‘choice’ is here problematic, philosophically, historically, and psychologically; many soldiers had no choice in terms of conscription and certainly no choice over getting PTSD.

As with all mental health terminology the problem here is differentiation, definition, and purpose. Once the term triggering becomes ubiquitous and used synonymously with annoyance (the way she looked at me triggered me and so on), it loses any meaning. From its biological context in the nineteenth century, to the psychological frameworks of the DSM in the 1980s and beyond, we have chartered PTSD’s development and by 2021 the term was over-used in a variety of contexts. A review of Lily King’s novel *Writers & Lovers* claimed descriptions of working in a restaurant were so immersive, ‘I started having PTSD flashbacks to my waitressing days’.[199] This is not meant literally and is a comical aside, but does make us think what essentially is PTSD? Plus, this includes the current popularity of giving trigger warnings in the media, such as one on BBC Radio 4 on 10 January 2022 news when a warning was giving over discussing fictional deaths, including hearing a character being beaten together with a large cheese on *Midsomer Murders*.

After September 11 some mental health professionals were critical of the tendency to medicalize all responses. Labelling all stress reactions as illness and each event as triggering is unhelpful. For example, having bad dreams or being unable to sleep in such circumstances might not be signs of PTSD and could be a common reaction.[200] Simultaneously, following the non-binary transrational approach at the heart of this volume, trauma should not be underestimated. Trauma from the wars of the 1970s has not dissipated and recent wars reinterpret and reignite this often-repressed trauma, as does related phenomenon such as the American withdrawal from Afghanistan in August 2021. The relationship between *Taxi Driver* and *You Were Never Really Here* states this clearly. *Taxi Driver* (Martin Scorsese, 1976) also

[197] F. Furedi, *Therapy Culture: Cultivating vulnerability in an uncertain age* (London: Routledge, 2004), p. 129.

[198] Ibid., p. 130.

[199] L. Murphy, ‘*Writers & Lovers* by Lily King review – a novel about writing a novel’, *The Times*, May 29, 2020, p. 15.

[200] Furedi, op. cit., p. 14.

offers the screenwriter's, Paul Schrader's, 'vision of a sinful world waiting to be redeemed'.[201] Both films have wounded Christ figures as protagonists-saviours, Schrader's Calvinist education appearing influential as is Scorsese's early calling to the Catholic priesthood.

There are parallels between the clinical literature and cinema, with four major Vietnam movies: *Taxi Driver* (Martin Scorsese, 1976), *Coming Home* (Hal Ashby, 1978), *The Deer Hunter* (Michael Cimino, 1979), and *Apocalypse Now* (Francis Ford Coppola, 1978). All have emphasised: (1) the limits of stress tolerance; (2) character disorder and asocial behaviour; and (3) post-traumatic stress disorder.[202] The impact of film has been made overt in the following example. One decorated veteran was involved in drug trafficking and after showing segments of *The Deer Hunter* the defence called upon witnesses to argue the client's actions resulted from traumas of war that needed to be relived. While the defendant was found guilty, 'the relationship between screen depictions, psychiatric concepts, and the legal codes that reflect our social order was clearly evidenced'.[203]

Documentaries have vividly explored treatments that move away from a biomedical model, including the use of surfing and the environment for a deeper healing for soldiers, *Resurface* (Josh Izenberg and Wynn Padula, 2017) an exemplary example. According to seminal film theorist Christian Metz the cinematic process can be considered 'mad', a form of regression where we perceive as real the represented and not the representer (the technological media of representation), film being like the 'madness' of dreams.[204] The process of filmmaking and films have been seen as healing, but this is not binary and black and white. The process of traditional story can function not as a healing process but as maintaining the status quo which could be harmful, exacerbating the environmental factors that enable PTSD. Cinema then becomes a form of repression.

Developing Lacan, Metz promoted the idea of the need to theorise the screen-spectator relationship not just in the context of the Imaginary but also in relation to the Symbolic.[205] Metz introduced the term voyeurism where the cinematic gaze cannot return the spectator's gaze. This is part of the lack that Russian formalist Tzvetan Todorov argued all narrative was concerned with. The aim therefore is to solve the riddle, to find the answer, to fill the lack.[206] With PTSD there appears to be a return to not a more complex instant of lack and plenitude, but a moment when pain was felt. Film can function in a fashion that gives the spectator some of the

---

[201] T. Calkwell, 'Interview', in (ed.) K. Jackson, *Schrader on Schrader* (London: Faber & Faber, 2004), p. 71.

[202] Fleming and Manvel, 1985 131.

[203] Ibid.

[204] Metz 1977, 116.

[205] Ibid.

[206] B. Creed, *The Monstrous-Feminine: Film, Feminism, Psychoanalysis* (London: Routledge, 1998), p. 81.

experiences of PTSD via analepsis where the past intervenes in the present, as with Joe's experiences in *You Were Never Really Here*.

Flashbacks in real life can be more painful than the event itself.[207] There are multiple pulls on identity via elements of PTSD. Attacking the concept of lack, Steven Shaviro argued the cinematic process should concern the loss of control, fragmentation, and subversion of self-identity.[208] This is a desire for a form of 'madness' in a controlled safe environment, in the protective darkness of the cinematic dream experience as Scorsese might put it. With regards to 'madness' and PTSD within biopsychology developments there is a desire to contain the flaw in the system. What we have in *Taxi Driver* is an actor playing a man, 'ceaselessly acting himself into being by adopting various methods of selfhood drawn from the discourses of popular culture'.[209] What *Taxi Driver* documents is not only the desire of people to create authentic selves, but an impossibility of doing so, for in a postmodern paradigm all the selves that one could fashion are no more than roles that have been played before.[210] *Taxi Driver* suggests that identity is not authentic but synthetic, a customised amalgam of images from popular culture; identity must be understood more as a series of semiotic appropriations, than as a process of self-discovery.[211]

Similarly, in *You Were Never Really Here* Joe can act the assassin and the rescuer while Nina acts the assassin and rescuer. This is not controversial and is paralleled in the text, but it is controversial to argue both act as victims, or that sociologically victimhood has become a major cultural fad, despite their being some truth in this assertion.[212] When we position their victimhood, and ours, as not intrinsic to being we understand the importance of a fluidity of ontology, and the liberation this non-binary transrational approach entails. This is the politics of transrational hope explained in Chap. 8.

For Baudrillard we are unable to conceive that identity has never existed.[213] There is an over-determination of identity through a variety of presences. We have fake news and fake identities with an over-abundance of signs; it is merely a play act which we feel to the point of exhaustion.[214] His level of metaphysics removes the need for psychoanalysis and self-awareness and we can understand it as a re-balancing given the emphasis today on identity politics. We become the 'ghost of a representation of ourselves', this is an, 'obstinate determination to carry about an identity which it is impossible to exchange'; he denies objective reality claiming it is

[207] van der Kolk, op. cit.

[208] S. Shaviro, *The Cinematic Body* (Minneapolis: University of Minnesota Press, 1993), p. 89.

[209] B. Mortimer, 'Portraits of the postmodern person in *Taxi Driver*, *Raging Bull*, and *The King of Comedy*', *Journal of Film and Video*, Issue 49, Nos. 1–2, 1997, p. 29.

[210] Ibid.

[211] Ibid.

[212] Furedi, op. cit.

[213] Baudrilard, op. cit., p. 45.

[214] Ibid.

a 'parallel illusion' and an element of the, 'metaphysical cycle into which we are locked'.[215] Such a claim might make life and death easier. With such a stress on identity today this counterbalance can be seen as positive, but Baudrillard's approach itself has been considered an illusion, as it gives too much weight to signs and codes being totally powerful and existing beyond their interpretation. Work by psychologist Carl Rogers in the 1950s, who devised person-centred counselling identity dynamics along with that of Eugene Gendlin, drew on research with war veterans. This view clings to the idea of a fixed self which with respect to Schopenhauer we have seen might be illusory.

A more liquid sense of identity following Baudrillard could bring about more wellbeing and happiness. When discussing the image and fantasy, Jung accepted that the world exists outside our image of it but showed how the world is always mediated by the image so the real then was never real in the first place.[216] Despite the insightfulness of Jung's approach he is still stuck in a binary approach when he argues that men lack Eros, what he terms the relational function. He brings this down to men thinking they can replace the relational function with reason and we can see that human's do indeed prioritise reason at the detriment to the relational function which is part of the transrational. Before we accuse Jung of being sexist it should be noted that he is writing in a period and from a culture where clearly his following thoughts are correct; where men are, 'proud that they don't let themselves be controlled by affect, because this would be womanly, tantamount to weak'.[217]

The relationship between semiology and culture, how the latter defines our definitions and understandings of apparent mental irregularities, is central. PTSD is a moving phenomenon, transcending both time and place within its experience and this encapsulates unprocessed traumas. A pathological obsession with personal identity is in part to combat what I term our post-identity trauma, the wound which we all explore to a greater or lesser extent within lived postmodern narratives. This has led to the most severe ideological extremism based on personal commitment and conjecture.[218] The test of a high functioning machine was to ascertain how human it can be. Now the test for a high functioning human is how machine like it is removing the transrational. Within a myopic biopsychological approach to 'madness' there is a desire to contain the apparent 'flaw' in the system, but it is this 'flaw'—the wound—that creates the human. This apparent flaw might be the gap instigated by what some have termed evil or 'madness', but we now can acknowledge how both are necessary.

---

[215] Ibid.

[216] Michael Vannoy Adams, *The Fantasy Principle. Psychoanalysis of the Imagination* (New York: Brunner-Routledge, 2004), p. 6.

[217] C.G. Jung, *Children's Dreams: Notes from the Seminar Given in 1936-1940* (Princeton, NJ: Princeton University Press, 2008), p. 313.

[218] David Bentley Hart, *That All Shall Be Saved: Heaven, Hell, and Universal Salvation* (New Haven: Yale University Press, 2021).

2.3.2 Depression

So far it has been illustrated how diagnoses merge. Just as PTSD can be viewed as the quintessential modern illness so can depression. This is addressed in Lars von Trier's depression trilogy *Antichrist* (2009), *Melancholia* (2011), and *Nymphomania Vol. 1* and *2* (2013).[219] In *Antichrist* nature is a cause of 'madness' plus a potential healer, overcoming a dualistic rationality substantiating this books argument concerning the importance of transnationality. This was also observed as central to Ramsay's significant work. In von Trier's trilogy the female body occupies the central role, depression and despair driving women into 'madness'. Outside this trilogy other examples are illustrative.

In *The Idiots* (Lars von Trier, 1998), Karen (Bodil Jørgensen) encounters a community pretending to be mentally challenged while she has real depression. She initially hates the community then learns from living in this therapeutic community. These individuals have come together, some from broken families, creating their own new family by what they call 'spazing'—pretending to be 'spastics'. This is deliberately politically incorrect and appears to some outsiders as offensive and things are far from perfect. The large number of close-ups in *The Idiots* reveal the awkwardness of the members, deromanticizing mental illness.

Like Karen, other female characters in Lars von Trier's films, especially She (Charlotte Gainsbourg) (*Antichrist*), Justine (Kirsten Dunst) (*Melancholia*), and Jo (Charlotte Gainsbourg) (*Nymphomaniac*), possess an altruistic sufferance which has religious connotations concerning good and evil.[220] There is a transrational truth inherent in the narrative and the ultra-high-resolution digital cinematography.[221] This is far from misogyny, more a clarity of self-actualization moving beyond the need for men. This is further complicated in *Antichrist*, given the protagonist, who believers in the power of the literal equation between women and witches, is burnt like a witch. There is a relationship between PTSD and depression and depression becomes the zone that is the base point for other mental illnesses hence its primacy.[222] Prior to World War 2 depression was not of medical interest and brain activity that was damaged was known as 'neurosis' and 'psychoneurosis'.[223]

Reversing attempts by some directors to transition film away from its literary and theatrical origins, Lars von Trier constructs his films like books with chapter headings. *Breaking the Waves* (1996) is based on a picture book *Guldhjerte* (*Goldheart*), about a girl who goes into a forest and ends up giving everything away like a martyr. The film has seven chapters each accompanied by popular music,

[219] A. Muteanu, 'The aesthetics of depression in the work of Lars von Trier. Ethical considerations on "Depression Trilogy"', unpublished dissertation, University of Bergen, 2016.

[220] Ibid.

[221] Ibid., p. 52.

[222] Ibid.

[223] Ibid., p. 5.

literally seen as the devil's work in the repressed religious Scottish community in which it is mainly set. Cinema itself is also considered evil in such communities.[224]

The central character Bess (Emily Watson) is best described as pure of heart and blessed in the Christian sense. Emily Watson playing Bess was raised in a cult. Bess lives in a strict cult-like Calvinist community when she falls in love with Jan (Stellan Skarsgård) who works on an oil rig. After an accident leaves him incapacitated, she has sex with other men at his behest. Bess's relationship with God is complex and naïve, a manifestation of the *Old Testament* God of the law and judgement and the *New Testament* God of forgiveness, the dark and the light. Without a unification this gives rise to the binary conflict appearing like mental illness.

The *Old Testament* God contains traits of the Devil. The Devil along with hell is only fully emphasized in the *New Testament*. God reassures Bess constantly, but she also out-louds God's punishing and condemning words to her speaking God's voice with a denouncing tone like God's ventriloquist's dummy. For example: 'But remember to be a good girl Bess, I giveth and I taketh away'. Bess's brother has died, so God has taken him and is the part of her that knows tragedy. This is the difficult God of *Job* and *Ecclesiastes*, the existential transrational threat at the heart of us all that in its depth is often hopeless, but this hopelessness can lead in the direction of abandonment then full trust in God, not the fallen world. Whatever level of happiness can be gained on earth we understand this all can be removed, as Bess knows full well after her brother's death. Through wrestling with this fierce God, Bess is Christ-like.

Religions normalized belief in women being evil which then was part of an agreed sanity by the establishment. Lars von Trier's films, including *Nymphomania* (2013), challenge this view. Bess is a feminist, confronting the patriarchal community through a variety of methods, such as wanting to know why only men are allowed to speak. She wants to come alive and be resurrected, so her attempts to challenge the status quo are the embodiment of a real feminist Christianity which the film ends on. Bess's simplicity equates with her lack of mendacity; God is speaking through her, but despite this simplicity she is not childlike. All who know her claim she is, 'not right in the head'. She confirms *Matthew* 25:40 and *Corinthians* 12: 22-25 concerning honouring the, 'least of the brothers and sisters'.[225] Bess becomes hysterical when Jan is working on an oilrig. The nexus of the film is Bess believing she caused Jan's accident because she prayed for him to come home. Bess does have her prayers answered, but not in the way she expected because now Jan is crippled from an accident on the rig.

Would a loving God operate via a simplistic exchange system? This is more reminiscent of the God of *The Old Testament*. As Bess is raised in a fundamentalist Christian community it is easy to understand why she thinks this is God's work. For

---

[224] This film is almost 30 years old, but in some parts of Scotland these beliefs still exist.

[225] *Mathew* 25: 40 'And the King will answer them, 'Truly, I say to you, as you did it to one of the least of these my brethren, you did it to me', *The Bible*, Revised Standard Version (London: Collins, 1977), p. 810.

her and her community this not a 'mad' interpretation at all. Further Biblical hermeneutics are revelatory; in terms of the theory of atonement, where God exchanges his Son to save the world, it has been argued that this is a mistaken view based on a mistranslation.[226] Bess's view of a punishing God is not fully Biblical but fits within her community's theology and ideology. Like other Lars von Trier films, *Breaking the Waves* exposes misconceptions concerning God and prayer in the way it is viewed and used as a form of manipulation akin to magic.

'In the beginning was the Word: The Word was with God and the Word was God' (John 1:1). A profound moment happens in church when Bess asks, how can you love a word? Bess's interrogation is a feminist challenge to the fundamentalist theology of her Scottish patriarchal Christian community. Another translation is 'in the beginning was wisdom' with wisdom traditionally more associated with the matriarchy. This is beyond the rational mind, understood through a deeper transrational approach where three can also be one. Jesus is the incarnation, God's son in flesh, and as one part of the trinity Jesus is also God. He is in a transrational relationship with God and the Holy Spirit, one and the same, but different. Like us as human's we can accept our uniqueness and difference, while simultaneously through love be united with the whole. In this paradigm difference and meaning are celebrated.

Our binary system of knowledge is a recent phenomenon. According to Jacques Rancière, the word logic comes from the Greek logos which initially meant fable or fabula in Latin; this later changed to into Italian favella—speech—and in Greek a fable was called mythos, myth, from which is derived Latin mutus—mute.[227] He explains that speech was born in the mute age as mental language so therefore in Greek logos means both word and idea. However, in its development, the over emphasis on the Greek logos (the patriarchal word), that is the rational, destroys the far deeper transrational meaning.[228] This film shows how this emphasis leads to mental illness. There is only one way to silence the transrational transgressor; in Chap. 6 of *Breaking the Waves* Dr. Richardson (Adrian Rawlins) draws up papers for Bess to be detained under the Mental Health Act which Jan signs, but Bess escapes. Part of Bess's extreme behaviour can be understood by her history, including her brother's death. Once again, we find loss and grieving leading to 'madness'. There is complexity in the ending, given that her death might be interpreted as leading to Jan's resurrection—the very heart of Christian belief. But why must a woman suffer like this for a man?

In *Antichrist* death, with loss leading to 'madness' and grief, dominates again. Biblically, death was not created by God. He created human beings to be immortal,

---

[226] Gordon Campbell, 'The World's Favourite Bible – The remarkable story of the King James Version', St Mary Magdalen Church, Leicester, 25 October 2021.

[227] Jacques Rancière, *Mute Speech*, trans. James Swenson (New York: Columbia University Press.

[228] Logos: norminative masculine singular. From lego; something said; by implication, a topic, also reasoning or motive; by extention, a computation; specially the Divine Expression. From Strong's Greek in https://biblehub.com (accessed 29 March 2021).

but death came into the world through the Devil's envy.[229] In her dazzling analysis of the origins of the film, Linda Badley in *Lars von Trier Beyond Depression* explains that for this film the director turned to his most dangerous influences, including 'mad geniuses', some of whom have been mentioned here in Chap. 1. These included Strindberg, Nietzsche, and Edvard Munch, with the title to the film possibly a homage to Nietzsche's 1895 attack on Christianity.[230] The remarkable analysis by Badley shows how the film developed, story wise, from being focused on male anxiety, perhaps close to the director's experience, and then switched with Badley claiming that her students' opinions on Japanese horror films were directly used by von Trier in developing this film. Despite the Wagnerian and Nordic mythology, the film appeals to an American and global audience by drawing on cabin horror films, 'like *Evil Dead* (1981), *The Blair Witch Project*, and, more recently, *The Witch: A New-England Folktale* (2015)', and Badley notes this tradition goes back to the Salem witch hysteria, Charles Brocken Brow, Nathaniel Hawthorne, and Arthur Miller's *The Crucible* (1953).[231]

A toddler dies while his parents, He (Willem Defoe) and She (Charlotte Gainsbourg), make love. As with *Breaking the Waves*, a tragedy is confronted. The opening black and white slow-motion is accompanied by a Handel score, sex and the possible creation of life and a child falling to death an entwined aesthetic event in the Deleuzian sense. They are perfectly in the moment, transcendent beings touching the eternal now in their lovemaking. The rest of the film is regret, depression, and 'madness'. Flashbacks show the mother was aware of what occurred, but this is ambiguous and suggests false memory.

Inside the home the parents are making love, possibly planning on having another child, and apparently oblivious to the death trajectory of their first born. In this interpretation the existing child has no choice but to make an escape pushed out of the nest. There is nothing insane about this; losing oneself entirely to the sexual act is an approved insanity, and to make love without this loss of self occurring is thought to be neurotic and the cause of 'madness'. Through this approved insanity, however, further insanity beyond transgression follows. The adults can be forgiven for not considering the child will fall out. The symbolism is rampant. The child goes through the window, re-entering the womb. The boy falls to the white pure earth in the deadly silent town. The moment of post orgasm, la petite mort, the little death, brings on a real death, le grand mort. For Roland Barthes, la petite mort is the chief objective of reading literature, what he called jouissance (bliss), when we lose ourselves in the work.[232] From this large death there is no escape and only by confronting death, as meditation in Buddhism and Christianity shows, do we reach sanity.[233] When they leave the town for Eden they are then in the work of analysis in

---

[229]Wisdom, 2:24. *The New Jerusalem Bible* (London; Darton, Longman & Todd, 1990), p. 786.

[230]Linda Badley, *Lars von Trier Beyond Depression* (New York: Columbia University Press, p. 33).

[231]Ibid., p. 55.

[232]Roland Barthes, *Le Plaisir du Texte* (Éditions du Seuil: Paris, 1973).

an attempt to rationalise the transrational which will not work which underscores the central argument of this book.

As with *Breaking the Waves* voyeurism is highlighted and through the staged performance of their lovemaking the couple are stating they need no other, paradoxically recognising their son and us, the audience, by denying both. Despite the artistic cinematography this sequence is pornographic with ubiquitous pornography embedding the position of observation and surveillance as a significant aspect of the contemporary sexual act. Being superfluous, the boy has no choice but to descend to his death as his final performance. Nature draws him on to leave the Laingian cage of the family.

A washing machine where the couple make love indicates the cleansing of this act, mirroring the mechanical piston-like activity. A close-up on the penis going in-out also reveals the mechanical nature of this act which is part of Bataille's monstrously comic vision. As he explained, this follows on the one hand from plants which are animated by a vertical movement analogous to that of tides which regularly elevate water, and on the other animals which are animated by a horizontal movement analogous to that of the turning earth. The alternating movement of coitus on the surface of the earth equates with locomotive pistons. The continual movement of coitus on the earth's surface is tied to the earth's rotation as the movement of pistons to that of wheels and man appears in this system as an, 'animal exceptionally animated by the erection-movement that projects plants in a vertical direction'; this then is analogous to the male mammal, 'who raises himself on his hind legs when mounting the female, but much more categorially erect, as erect as a penis'.[234]

The film is a fairy tale with each step paralleling the other: the boy's death is the portal to entering the woods and Eden, their and our unconscious, to track down the darkest demons and evil, including the antichrist. For Franciscan Richard Rohr, evil can only be conducted by the unconscious.[235] This could erroneously assume a binary division between the conscious and unconscious, but the point is if we were fully conscious would we commit evil?[236] A move to Eden in these circumstances is more extreme than any Jungian ideal of integrating the shadow, although analytical psychology is relevant. For example, the film is similar to a dream, being 'not quite human', and just like a dream it is 'rather a breath of nature', containing, 'a spirit of the beautiful and generous as well as the cruel goddess'.[237] As with the dream we get closer to the spirit of the film through the, 'sphere of ancient mythologies, or the fables of the primeval forest' and the issue is that consciousness often forgets the,

[233] Jason Lee, *The Metaphysics of Mass Art – Cultural Ontology*, Vol. II (New York: Mellen, 1999), pp. 195–232.

[234] Bataille 2008, 75.

[235] Richard Rohr, *Immortal Diamond – the search for our true self* (London: SPCK, 2013).

[236] This of course is Jesus's comment at the point of his death, if by ignorance we mean unconscious behaviour.

[237] C. G. Jung, M.-L. von Franz, J.L. Henderson, J. Jacobi, and A. Jaffé, *Man and his Symbols* (New York: Dell, 1968), p. 36.

'deeper instinctive strata of the human psyche'.[238] This film like dream is an expression of the instinctual through compensatory symbols.

As a non-medical psychotherapist, the bereaved father is threatened by the psychiatrists who treat the grief-stricken mother and can prescribe medicine. Idealistically, ethical boundaries would not allow a contemporary patient to be in a relationship with their psychotherapist. It appears natural that a husband would treat his wife who is a young academic and nature and the natural are questioned, plus countering the popular belief we learn that what is natural is not necessarily benign. The film constantly asks what is natural anyway? Bearing in mind Milton's 'nature is the devil's church' we need to be careful of seeing this film and life in dualistic terms. Clear divisions between good and bad, such as the civilisation where the boy dies versus the uncivilised woods where the mother dies, are flawed. In a Kierkegaardian sense humans desire a world where good and evil can be clearly distinguished judging before a full understanding, but an either-or position is imperfect.

The film works against the grain which furthers its transrational significance. The town, which traditionally is the space for thought and reflection (civilisation), is the zone for pure-machine-sex. Nothing is important here other than mechanical sex. Alternatively, the woods are the space where in-depth talk and reflection occur, the therapeutic arena that blends with the unconscious. This is part of the meaning, given Christ is the Logos, the Word (although in another translation this Logos/Word means wisdom). But, as seen with Bess's criticism in *Breaking the Waves*, is this enough? In this natural zone animals talk, despite creatures traditionally denied the use of language. Biblically there is a precedent when in *Numbers* 22:28 Balaam's donkey is given the power of speech.[239] The pre-civilised becomes civilised, but the id and chaos then reigns. We are driven by these reflections back to Bess's question—the problematic worship of the Word, the purely rational which without the transrational is evil. Only the transrational can bring deeper satisfaction. Psychoanalysis prioritises speech and for the animal the mouth is the most living part.[240] Human life is that of the beast, concentrated; 'rage makes men grind their teeth, while terror and atrocious suffering turn the mouth into the organ of rending screams'.[241]

In this primal moment of horror, the mouth of the human becomes positioned in the space occupied in the constitution of animals, highlighting the mouth in animal physiology and psychology; 'the general importance of the superior or anterior extremity of the body, the orifice of profound physical impulses'.[242] When we liberate these impulses in the brain or mouth, they become violent and bestial. Overcoming the binary, the woods in *Antichrist* are an arena of the unconscious,

---

[238] Ibid.

[239] Numbers 22: 28. *The Bible*, Revised Standard Version (London: Collins, 1977), p. 117.

[240] Bataille 2008, 59.

[241] Ibid.

[242] op. cit., p. 60.

but simultaneously the sector of total speech thus rational consciousness. Any simple binary is broken down moving us deeper within the transrational. As Deleuze and Guattari note, Jung's theory of archetypes assigns to the animal an important role in dreams, myths, and human groups. 'The animal is inseparable from a series exhibiting the double aspect of progression-regression, in which each term plays the role of a possible transformer of the libido (metamorphosis)'.[243] By having animals speak and having consciousness in nature the film encapsulates equality. Deleuze and Guattari employ the term 'analogical representations', revealing how Jung brings together nature and culture within the cycle of nature-culture-nature.[244] We need to integrate archetype, part of the dream-work; in this case what can be termed the film-work. The psychoanalyst is traditionally the controller of the discourse; like a sorcerer with spells, they are the interpreter of language. Bess's point in *Breaking the Waves* that love is not a word is again significant.

In *Antichrist*, He's patient/analysand/student/wife/torturer/She is completing a doctorate and the radical reversal occurs when She declares that the women researched for her doctorate are literally witches and they should have been persecuted and burnt to death. This indicates a total belief in the occult. The psychoanalyst is aghast by this view. The film's core is his accepting She's viewpoint (by his actions at least)—unifying the male gaze with the female gaze and desire. He eventually burns his own partner, fulfilling her belief in the literary meaning of witches, and completing her desire. Behind this is a dynamic exposing victimhood and literal interpretation, the film functioning as a mediation and meditation. She acts out her thesis throughout this performance which the initial sex act and those following contribute to. By destroying the witch embodying evil (as the She, the female understands it) her thesis is completed. The whole act is performance art following on from the initial performative sex act. The discourse in the woods is her PhD viva oral examination, ending in the affirmative violence, her death being the proof of her thesis. She's sanity hangs on how good He is as a healer, but if She resists his healing, She can retain her autonomy. She calls him arrogant and there are moments when He arrogantly believes She is sane and is cured by his power. This is where the rational male technology of his psychoanalytical discourse turns, She into what He wishes She to resemble. Her insanity is her freedom from the chains of his discourse. These chains are literally positioned into his body when She captures him by placing a bolt through his leg creating her own Frankenstein's monster and sex doll that will never leave her.

The bolt is a Biblical reference to the millstone (*Matthew* 18:6 which refers to children stumbling, like their son who stumbled out the window to his death). By doing so, She enacts herself with the wound for She has been He's monster, creating the vagina by this act, uttering cries that He hopes will cure She. The boy falling from the window, the mother falling to the ground during the funeral, the objects

[243] Gilles Deleuze and Félix Guattari, *A Thousand Plateaus – Capitalism and Schizophrenia*, trans. Brian Massumi (London: Continuum, 2011), p. 260.
[244] Ibid.

falling from the sky at Eden, the man falling to the ground, mirror the Fall spiritually. This concerns consuming the low-hanging fruit from the tree of knowledge, but transrationally can be a falling upwards.[245] They also reflect on Satan's fall to earth and fallen angels which is the heart of temporal evil. Whether this is self-knowledge through knowledge of nature and death, or merely knowledge of falsity, it is knowledge that is subverting binaries and transrationally pure. The tree of knowledge of good and evil is a bifurcation, an either-or scenario, a forked tongue positioned as a choice within a false milieu of predestination. Calvin's theory of predestination found a revival in Nazism.[246] This is an ideology that Lars von Trier jokingly defended.[247] In Calvin's theology we are created unequally with those who saved and damned decided prior to birth. Nothing can stop the Fall. For something, anything, to happen in human terms and for conscious reflection on its meaning to exist, there must be the Fall. In this sense, alienation and intelligence go hand in hand. In terms of the transrational, meaning, 'is largely preconceptual and not subject to words', and 'nonrational'.[248]

There is a healing in the woods from being separated from a fixed reality where they fully self-create an alternative reality. But this is their metaphysical mistake, utilized as a warning to us all. At no point can humans get away from their human selves which are set up as a division by their very existence—desire (body) and grace (spirit). The more they run away the more they encounter difference essential for knowledge and for the human. Following Samuel Johnson, he who makes a beast of himself gets rid of the pain of being a human. In the darkness of this Eden this verdict is challenged and found to be an impossibility. Pain cannot be subverted. The beauty of the woods is nothing compared to the interior of the hut which functions as the exterior of their wounds which soon become visceral and a transrational liminality results.

The man tries to convert the woman through his language. She must bow down to his words for him to accept her, but also to be positioned within the paradigm of patriarchy despite his apparent healing nature. He caresses her with words believing, like Freud, that words are deeds. The wounds of her being must be filled and penetrated not just by his penis (the id), but via his language (ego and super ego). With the bombardment of his words, He fails to allow a gap in his reasoning for She's being. This is the gap as explained being humanity, so He further destroys She's existence. She's fixation on witchcraft and the empowerment of witchcraft threatens He's rationality. Truth is interpretation, not an eternal element to be discovered and contained and this is liberating. The battle is a battle for sanity. In this instance sanity means hope and growth, whereas insanity means depression, stalemate, and death.

---

[245] Rohr, op. cit.

[246] Erich Fromm, *The Fear of Freedom* (London: Routledge, 1989), p. 76.

[247] Badley, op. cit.

[248] Rohr, op. cit., p. 73.

Antichrist encapsulates the position of going beyond insanity sociologically, for She is positioned outside society. Society has not caused 'madness' or insanity—storytelling has. Can a story drive someone 'mad'? Of course, just as storytelling can heal 'madness'. As explained, there are instances of people going 'mad' during watching a film, such as *Betty Blue* (Jean-Jacque Beineix, 1986). Betty (Béatrice Dalle) is killed by her partner Zorg (Jean-Hughes Anglade) after she has a series of psychotic and self-harming episodes. He 'frees' her from her anguish only to have her return reincarnated in a cat, or at least she is now speaking to him via a cat. Was Zorg more alone when Betty was alive and 'mad', or did she make him at least step beyond his own horizon which enabled him to, 'question the unknown who comes', as Irigaray puts it, which can include animals and all 'strangers reaching his territory'?[249] When language gets stuck 'madness' and insanity may result. We do not create language, it exists prior to us, so in this sense 'madness', sanity, and insanity are not a choice, but part of innate structures. The skirting around language that occurs in *Antichrist* proves that language is not enough.

The speaking creatures in *Antichrist* have a seductive capacity working as an antidote. Animals here are the real self, not stuck within the interpretations of psychoanalysis, existing in and of themselves, for themselves. When we consider nature, it might be in the form of transcendent functions, 'controversion (sic) as Erich Neumann has it, or self-realization following Abraham Maslow, or individuation in Jungian terms . . . we are the instruments of Nature's quest'.[250] She says He sets himself up as Mr. Nature. 'Nature can't harm me, as it is outside. I am also within,' He says, 'I am the nature of all human beings. I am the nature that causes people to do evil things against women,' the subject of her thesis. If human nature is evil, then that also goes for the nature of the women and in these circumstances, they do not control their own bodies nature does.

Suffering in many branches of Christianity is good, but here this is connected to nature—the devil's church. Is her self-guided clitorectomy a refusal of meaning? Oedipus means swollen foot. She apparently has been putting her son's shoes on the wrong feet. She masturbates He until his penis ejaculates blood, then drills a hole in his leg so He cannot escape, feminising him. She decides her own genitals are useless, severing them with scissors making her untameable and unfixable, but in one sense free. These sequences violently challenge our preconceived conceptions of gender. Lars von Trier reportedly drove some female actors in his films 'mad', including the singer Björk, star of *Dancer in the Dark* (2000) and Nicole Kidman in the experimental *Dogville* (2003). For He/Defoe this work is sincere and personal, Lars von Trier having written it as psychotherapy when he was in a psychiatric hospital suffering from depression. While making the film von Trier was still recovering and this could be viewed as part of his recovery. While depression is not what most call 'madness' this depends on its degree and depression can lead to

---

[249] Luce Irigaray, *The Way of* Love, trans. Heidi Bostic and Stephen Pluháek (London: Continuum, 2002), p. 77.

[250] Anthony Stevens, *Private Myths: Dreams and Dreaming* (London: Penguin, 1996), p. 172.

'madness'. When She is hospitalised due to depression which is psychotic grief, we question whether this is 'madness' or sanity.

In hospital She is controlled by one man, a medical doctor, which threatens the control of another, He, her husband. He uses non-medical therapy, emphasising the word, which is a form of magical metaphysical spell meant to heal the organic and physical which is the medical. She mocks He for his know-all nature, but still follows him to their retreat, their unconscious, for treatment. Ethical boundaries in the talking cure profession are a recent phenomenon. In the realistic 1950s novels of Iris Murdoch, for example, your professional psychoanalyst was your friend and lover. The Netflix series *Gypsy* (2017), starring Naomi Watts, continues this theme and, while this show is blatantly absurd, a bisexual psychotherapist having sex with her patient also sometimes seems realistic. Here boundaries are crossed, but which partner would not endeavour to help their sick lover?

Chapter 2 of *Antichrist* is titled Pain (Chaos Reigns) with the film working as exposure therapy for the audience, given castration and genital mutilation instil fear, and we are exposed to transrationalism. 'While scopophilia is pleasurable, the object of the gaze can also be threatening, since it evokes difference, hence the issue of castration.'[251] She fears the woods so must live in them and have sex in them to feel alive to overcome her child's death, although she was planning on coming here anyway to finish her thesis, so the man is an interloper. This is also a reversal, given He and She must go to Eden to heal, to take away the knowledge of good and evil. This is carnal knowledge so this process is impossible unless castration takes place hence its implementation. For Merleau-Ponty no event in a life is externally determined.[252] Psychoanalytical discourse can easily be employed concerning this attack on genitals, but for Freud the libido is a general power not directed towards a definite end.[253] This it is what causes us to have a history. In *Antichrist* it is as if the male is almost raped. 'So the question is not so much whether human life does or does not rest on sexuality, as of knowing what is to be understood by sexuality'.[254]

Antichrist operates as psychoanalysis: of subject and object; protagonist and antagonist; and of the audience. We never truly discover what the father is thinking which is the way of psychoanalysis for the analyst must remain behind the veil, the analysand lying on the couch, not even seeing the face of their analyst. Simultaneously, the analyst through projection and transference takes on the role of everything to the analysand; nothing and everything. An enigma as a therapist, He removes himself from the equation. By doing so the client (his partner) fills the space by seeking to destroy him and is then destroyed. The secret that the film manifests is that woman can never be destroyed nor can nature. Unearthing healing

[251] Peter Brooks, 'The body in the field of vision', *Paragraph – A Journal of Modern Critical Theory*, Vol. 14 No. 1, March 1991, (46–67), p. 56.

[252] M. Merleau-Ponty, *Phenomenology of Perception*, trans. Chris Smith (London: Routledge, 2004), p. 183.

[253] Ibid.

[254] Ibid.

transrational knowledge the film asks us to question our prescribed perceptions of the natural. Is it natural that animals talk; is it natural that humans do not really talk, or at least do not disclose as in the father figure? We can answer both yes and no to these questions within non-binary transrational healing knowledge. In *Antichrist* He lectures She on what her thesis about women and witches ought to be about and He declares She is insane. For him the point about the history of witches is that they were not witches at all and not of Satan. She proposes it is more empowering for women to acknowledge their Satanic power.

'What the mind can conceive and believe it can achieve,' speaks He on the train to Eden where their cabin exists for them to play act their inner psyches. The film can be interpreted as an attack on cognitive behavioural therapy (CBT) which has become popular as a low-cost version of psychotherapeutic healing. The treatment here for deep depression leads to 'madness'. Psychotherapy may take years with traditional psychotherapy being five days a week for five years or more; CBT is just 12 to 17 sessions and tries to enable the client. The film draws from von Trier's personal experience with CBT and other treatments. 'Dreams are of no interest to modern psychology,' She states, correctly, when He says He's been having crazy dreams. In one interpretation She is emotional, the ego and id; He is the rational superego and the observer. The film struggles to overcome female sexuality that She instigates. CBT prioritises the conscious mind and is optimistic and has the core belief that direct interventions work. Regardless of their tradition, the psychotherapist and psychoanalyst have much of the power, but cognitive behavioural therapy (CBT) teaches the client to become their own therapist. We witness this in *Antichrist* so claims of misogyny in this film once again fall away. Diagnosis does not occur within this modality of therapy. CBT involves a collaborative relationship underscoring the ethical point here: what if client and therapist are known to each other?

A falsity lies in the contrast of the therapist who is the unknown quantity and the client buys time off the therapist as it is turning a human relationship into a commodity, selling time. In this film it is given freely, but we can question the freedom of these acts, emotionally, because they are embroiled in the psychodynamics of this close relationship. The experience at Eden is supposed to be therapeutic but entering Eden (the time before the Fall and evil's intrusion into and dominance of the world, along with the realisation of knowledge), healing is an impossibility hence the chaos. This is the 'mad' impossibility of achieving a pure pre-knowledge point, that is, of reversing history. There is a structure to these sessions revealing it is a problems focused technique with an emphasis on thinking patterns like CBT. This involves a movement to facing fears going from fear of death to fear of nature to fear of Satan, despite here nature and Satan being one; confronting each fear becomes a goal.

The film propounds facing such fears is dangerous with sanity gained from avoiding fears highlighting the insanity of the therapist's approach that He thinks is sane. This reflects on the Laingian notion previously discussed that we go 'mad' to keep us safe, for protection. Prolepses reveals in flashback an apparent memory when she might have stopped their child falling, but this could be a fantasy. Either way, it confirms to She women are evil. It is She that believes this, not He. If She truly believes she is evil with all women then the death of her child can easily be explained—it was her own evil fault. This offers a rational way of viewing an irrational event, enabling an understanding of the depression, devastation, and 'madness'.

The metanarrative of 'madness' and evil are an explanation for every event, allied to the words of the fox who utters 'chaos reigns'. The dualism of Zoroastrianism which had such an influence on later religions offers an explanation to the later developments within branches of monotheism concerning the good and evil bifurcation. Following a binary paradigm, heaven is the soul and earth is the body, as Jack (Matt Dillon) puts it in Lars von Trier's serial killer film, *The House That Jack Built* (2018). Christianity and Satanism offer predictions for individual and social behaviour within a wider teleological framework. With chaos and evil reigning, all is predetermined because difference and meaning are denied with no choice and free will.

We need to be sceptical about a director who constantly claims he draws on his personal depression, particularly in the period 2006 and 2007, and Linda Badley makes this point most clearly. Drawing on interviews, archival materials, and taking a transmedia approach, while interpretating Lars von Trier's work as informed by Wagner, Proust, and Marquis de Sade and Scandinavian erotic cinema and serial killer genre tropes, Badley shows how his films engage with the Anthropocene, dark ecology, and the postcinema.[255] In this chapter the two-way relationship between 'madness' and culture has been elucidated and how this relates to PTSD. The emphasis on death and loss in Lars von Trier's films illuminating 'madness' and depression has been analysed.

2.4 Conclusions: Theology

This chapter has examined film, theatre, and 'madness', including more specially conditions, such as psychosis, DID, and PTSD and depression in relation to film. We have examined how and why 'madness' and evil are equated. Following Thomas Nagel, some philosophers have viewed death as an evil because of its position as being as state that lacks existence, equating it with the unconscious. This, however, assumes that existence (nature) is benign which is undermined by the *Antichrist*. It also assumes that the unconscious is an inferior position, which is a rationalist argument that dominates post-Freudian discourse that Jung tried to subvert. Here is another reason why I maintain that the route to wellbeing is from transrational knowledge and this can come through knowledge gained from films.

Making *Antichrist* Lars von Trier knew he wanted to use the tropes of horror films but was not ultimately making a horror film.[256] Film categories such as genre were

---

[255] Badley, op. cit.

explained as not always being precise and, as with mental health diagnoses, categorisations overlap but can help people feel safe. They may offer an inaccurate and reductive rational order. Lars von Trier's work enters a depth of knowledge via transrationality. While this film may mock a form of exposure therapy what is the *Antichrist* exposing the audience to? All manner of things they/we may wish to avoid. Lars von Trier claims he wants his films to be like a stone in your shoe, not making you comfortable.[257]

The problem of false consciousness, of not understanding class consciousness, is overt, as is the fetish character of the commodity but critical theory sees through the fetish. The problem is popular works of art can make people conformist, the narrative arc being about the sole individual, rather the collective. Following Adorno, art can falsely vanquish negativity while in a utopian fashion removing class and social inequity.[258] But there is an alternative. Audiences have been so preconditioned to believe films should conform to a certain fixed narrative with a non-challenging form and standard aesthetic. Moving outside this framework is considered tasteless and deviant. Despite the success of Lars von Trier's work, for example, this can mean transrational art and knowledge ends up neglected by the wider population.

Transrational knowledge again becomes relegated confirming this volume's central argument and with this relegation the status quo exacerbated mental health problems which is a deliberate ideological process to prevent resistance. If people are unwell, they are less likely to have the strength to resist the establishment. Most texts on how to write films, for example, stick to a certain ABC format, ironing out differences.[259] Chapter 1 showed how this is also true for the happiness industry, but this is problematic given meaning only comes through difference. The American Psychology Association, the world's largest association of its type, has a stated aim to illicit what makes this profession different to those that endeavour to reach the same aim—psychological healing. Why this emphasis on difference within a well-accepted discipline? We have seen the power of the un/happiness industry and how traditional psychology is under threat from alternative healing professions working to allay psychological suffering.

For self-help gurus such as those mentioned in Chap. 1 their position is to enable people to maximise potential, hinting at a beyond, a place we can have access to if we leave our own horizons of the same behind, our own restrictive garden. Other advice is do this by accepting what you have. 'It is not in his house, including that of language, that he will find how to enter a new historical era, a new speech'.[260] As

---

[256] Badley, op. cit.

[257] Angelos Koutsourakis, 'A film should be like a stone in your shoe': a Brechtian reading of Lars von Trier', unpublished PhD, University of Sussex, 2011.

[258] Theodor Adorno, *Aesthetic Theory*, eds. Gretel Adorno and Rolf Tiedemann, trans. Robert Hullot-Kentor (Continuum: London, 2002).

[259] Jason Lee, *The Psychology of Screenwriting* (London: Bloomsbury, 2014).

[260] Luce Irigaray (2002), op. cit., p. 71.

Irigaray has it, this is a matter of discovering a, 'singularity in comparison to the animal, an aptitude—to a great extent still to be cultivated. . .human co-belonging with the other'.[261] A co-belonging such as this is the subtext to Lars von Trier's films and is overt in Lynne Ramsay's work. In Lars von Trier's so-called depression trilogy what is perceived to be insane, such as nymphomania, keeps people sane.

Have the filmmaker and the therapist done their jobs when these issues are raised in a person-centred manner? As Irigaray puts it, if the same conceals the specular or the speculative I return to myself unchanged in a closed History or world.[262] The differences analysed in films in this chapter do not close off History. In *Antichrist* there is the attempt to reconcile not just with grief and depression but evil which, as we have seen, involves loss. Most people find the traditional origin story of original sin difficult to fathom. Why did Adam and Eve listen to the serpent rather than God? One interesting explanation is the following. In Eden Adam and Eve could have debated with God and said the law to not eat any of fruit of the tree of knowledge of good and evil just does not make sense and then ask for an explanation; this would have introduced a level of dialectic. They broke God's law without understanding it. This has been paralleled with our general failure to debate with, or listen to, the God within when we take an action. Similarly, in Chap. 1 it was noted how Virginia Woolf saw the internal path as one of resistance to external pressure and patriarchy. This path might be more difficult, but it is the most fulfilling and is akin with the saying enter by the narrow gate.[263]

Evil traditionally is punished by expulsion from the garden of Eden which is highlighted in *Antichrist*. This was a place where humans were eternally at home, the opposite of the uncanny, where difference and real conscious meaning were unknown. *The Revelation to John* commences by maintaining heaven is the return to Eden. The choice then is of being at one and at home or gaining knowledge with the recognition of difference and the uncanny, recognizing the validity of haunt (ontology).[264] This is part of transrational knowledge that can lead to wellbeing. For Saint Anselm we are enslaved by sin and the devil, but within the theory of atonement Christ crucified releases us from the debt of our sin, so we then become indebted to God. The debt has been transferred, so in this sense God becomes the Devil.[265]

The transrational is central for moving us beyond this realm of debt-payment theology, and it is this deeper knowledge that is required for wellbeing. Unfortunately what we have, 'prefigured in the "linear" monotheism of Judaic, Christian and

---

[261] Ibid.

[262] Ibid.

[263] M. Scott Peck, *The Road Less Traveled: A New Psychology of Love, Traditional Values and Spiritual Growth.*

[264] The concept of hauntology is one explained by Derrida.

[265] Ryne Beddard, 'Anselm's Atonement Theory – "Unmaking" The Indebted Man', *Religious Theory*, January 3, 2017. Rethinking Anselm's Atonement Theory – "Unmaking" The Indebted Man (Ryne Beddard) – RELIGIOUS THEORY (jcrt.org) (accessed March 22, 2021).

Moslem "supernaturalism"', is then, 'violently transfigured by the "ungiving" and almost exclusively accumulative character of modern CAPITAL (sic)'.[266] 'If the implications of Anselm's theory are taken seriously, it is inescapable that God seems less and less like a loving God . . . more like a self-obsessed psychopath'.[267] There is an economic logic to the theory of atonement, but in the profounder theology of Franciscan Duns Scotus the salvation of the world is united with the creative source without a need for this blood sacrifice.[268]

In Pauline theology the Devil is the ruler of the physical world.[269] Evil and 'madness' are often framed falsely at the heart of creation theology and unfortunately this sacrificial view on atonement is popular. We have seen how God and the Devil can be one and, in this interpretation, both are the foundation and embodiment of 'madness' and here the evil debt of She and He in *Antichrist* is paid by depression and 'madness' and is easy to comprehend through this chapter's analysis. This religious logic of the individual indebtedness of evil is of no use regarding the world's structural problems, such as systematic racism addressed in Chap. 4 and our ecological crisis which we conclude on in Chap. 8.[270] The logic of demonization of marginalized groups needs renouncing by recognizing how structural evil, 'disproportionately effects certain people'; we need to see, 'suffering as a universal problem, implicated in a universal need for collective action against the principalities of darkness that threaten to consume us'.[271] Here metaphysics coalesces structurally with politics, again transcending the binary through reinscribing the transrational, leading to wellbeing.

---

[266] Stephen Pfohl, *Death at the Parasite Café. Social Science (Fictions) and the Postmodern* (Palgrave Macmillan: London, 1992), p. 129.

[267] Beddard, op. cit.

[268] Rohr (2013), op. cit.

[269] See 2 *Corinthians* 4, 'in whom the god of this world hath blinded the minds of the unbelieving'.

[270] Ibid.

[271] Ibid.

Part II
Identity and Theory

Chapter 3
Gender, Sexuality, Celebrity

3.1 Introduction: Gendered Culture

At the 2019 Academy Awards sportswear company Nike premiered an advertisement on the gender bias women face at work and in life. Tennis star Serena Williams narrated *Dream Crazier*. 'If we show emotion, we're called dramatic,' Williams claims. 'If we want to play against men, we're nuts. And if we dream of equal opportunity, delusional.' 'When we stand for something, we're unhinged,' she continues. 'When we're too good, there's something wrong with us. And if we get angry, we're hysterical, irrational or just being crazy.' 'So, if they want to call you crazy, fine,' she declares. 'Show them what crazy can do.' This illustrates the way 'madness' has been used to dismiss women, but the argument in this advert is embrace your 'madness'.

Away from the glamour of the Oscars, discussions of Charlotte Perkins Gilman's influential novella on 'madness' *The Yellow Wallpaper* (1892) expose elements of the problems of analysis. Chapter 2 examined the relationship between 'madness' and evil with the idea that women are frequently termed 'mad' and evil. The move away from the word (Logos), that in one interpretation represents the father or superego, is part of the breaking away of feminist critics including Luce Irigaray who sees all Freudian theory as suspect.[1] The difficulty is exacerbated due to the economic position of women. Comparable to *The Antichrist* discussed in Chap. 2, Charlotte Perkin Gilman's character in her story *The Yellow Wallpaper* escapes her husband's power and that of his patriarchal medicine through 'madness'.

Disappearing into hallucinations within the walls of her house is entering a nineteenth-century gothic virtual reality, but it is in part her own internal liberation. There is a sense of freedom here and paradox where:

[1] Luce Irigaray, *Je, Tu, Nous – Toward a culture of difference*, trans. Alison Martin (London: Routledge, 2007).

J. Lee, *Culture, Madness and Wellbeing*, https://doi.org/10.1007/978-3-031-37530-9_3

> the Virtual can deny its own reality only at the same time as it denies the reality of all the rest. It is caught up in a game whose rules it does not control (no one controls them!).[2]

This Virtual stems from the perpetuation of the primacy of the image as the Real, with no signifier behind it. We shall see how this relates to 'madness'. 'Madness' is shaped by fiction and the image, and this especially concerns how gender and class are shaped by 'madness', but we need to be wary of reductionism. A class analysis of culture does not mean class or some other form of social division is all we need to take into consideration; nor does it mean all forms of culture are understood in terms of social structures and conflicts.[3]

The historical demonization of the female body is well-known and the vagina has been viewed as pathological. Woman as body is a common trope with both frequently defined as evil. In *The Anti-Christ and Vagina*, we learn it is better to kill people than allow them to masturbate.[4] Castration is seen as the only hope for female patients. At least 200 million girls and women alive in 30 countries in 2021 had suffered female genital mutilation.[5] Possession has always been at the essence of ideas of womanhood, as it has with ideas of 'madness'. Women as evil witches, a subject we return to in Chap. 7, is central to these constructions and is explained by economic factors. This construction of witches is not just historical. During Donald Trump's battle for the presidency against Hilary Clinton in 2016 'burn the witch' became a popular chant. Actor and health guru Gwyneth Paltrow is satirized in the contemporary media for daring to discuss vaginal health treatments. Suggesting the vagina needs treatment in this fashion is a further demonization of the female body by this celebrity.

The popular view previously was that sexual seduction in men at an early age protected them from 'madness', but in women it insighted mental illness.[6] This view we should note has barely altered. Anything in the female sphere can become pathologized, including eating chocolate, working, and shopping.[7] How these beliefs are narrated and fictionalised are key to an understanding of both 'madness' and gender. Women at London's Colney Hatch mental hospital were sedated and put in padded cells six times more often than men.[8] The public were invited into the hospital for special events, including sports, theatre, and fetes.[9] The 'mad' in the

---

[2] Jean Baudrillard, *The Intelligence of Evil – Or the Lucidity Pact*, trans. Chris Turner (London: Bloomsbury, 2013), p. 62.

[3] Dominic Strinati, *An Introduction to Theories of Popular Culture* (London: Routledge, 1995), p. 175.

[4] Elaine Showalter, *The Female Malady: Women, Madness and English Culture, 1830–1980* (London: Virago, 1985, p. 117.

[5] UNICEF data.

[6] T. Szasz, 1988, 111.

[7] N. Prowse, 2018, 3.

[8] Showalter, op. cit., p. 81.

[9] My maternal great-grandparents both worked at this hospital, taking my mother to see the patients' shows. Most people in the area worked there, or at Standard Telephones, indicating how important the local mental institution was for the local economy.

flesh became part of entertainment. Divisions between worlds were not clear cut. Chapter 1 explained how public mental institutions can offer a higher level of community than that outside their walls and protection unavailable in the outside world. As recently as the 1990s UK hospitals contained women incarcerated for having children outside of wedlock.[10] On top of this came what was termed the moral management of appearances in the female sphere. This can involve plastic surgery creating the ideal superwoman with no fissures. The construction of mental health is tied to this construction of what it means to be the perfect woman, the perfect image controlled by the media and being culturally defined.

The image was used therapeutically with the staging of 'madness' central to the constructions of 'mad' women and gender with photography a therapeutic tool. Female patients posed while incarcerated in mental hospitals. Women were considered sad rather than 'mad', but these terms merged.[11] Fiction and the image shaped reality. Art and literature framed the reality of insanity so powerfully that in Victorian Britain the style of insanity for women came from portraits and interpretations of Shakespeare's Ophelia in *Hamlet*.[12] John Everett Millais's 1851 to 1852 painting *Ophelia* is the best known. The model is 19-year-old Elizabeth Siddall. In the play Ophelia is driven 'mad' when her father Polonius is murdered by her lover Hamlet. The scene depicted in the painting is not seen on stage but is discussed by Queen Gertrude and Ophelia's brother Laertes.

Ophelia fell into the river while picking flowers and drowns slowly while singing. The model Elizabeth Siddall became ill posing for Millais in a bath of freezing water. Stories about her nearly dying in the process added to its romantic myth. This image of a romantically doomed woman combined with legends of yearning, nature, and mortality, had an enormous influence on the nineteenth-century's conception of female 'madness' and beyond. It became an inspiration for artists' models in the twentieth and twenty first century.[13] As with today's culture, image was reality. Psychiatrist Hugh Welch Diamond's photographs of female mental patients in the 1850s were used in films such as *The French Lieutenant's Woman* (Karel Reisz, 1981) because they were viewed as authentic.[14] Diamond's work was used to record mental disorders, but he also claimed they worked in the actual treatment of patients. The science of observation and the technology of reduplication of the image merged with healing, mental health, and wellbeing.

In an earlier age 'madness' was considered satanic, insanity equated with insecurity.[15] Women who did not conform were simply equated with evil and 'madness'. What was happening outside the asylum challenges some well-established myths.

---

[10] This comes from my personal experience of working with hospitals in Merseyside.

[11] Showalter, op. cit., p. 8.

[12] Ibid., p. 92.

[13] Kelley Swain, *The Naked Muse* (Valley Press: Scarborough, 2016), pp. 14–17.

[14] Showalter, op. cit., p. 97.

[15] Masters 1977, 31.

'The success of moral management for women may have had less to do with the humanity of the asylum than with the dreariness of life beyond the walls'.[16] Women continue to be diagnosed with some form of classified mental disorder in greater numbers than men. 20% of women and 14% of men in England have some form of mental illness, panic disorder being the only category where there is an equality between the sexes in terms of number of diagnoses.[17] The myth that women are hysterical, difficult, fickle, and contradictory (the patronising cliché—it's a women's prerogative to change her mind) has not dissipated. In 2022 8.3 million people were on anti-depressants in England with 5.5 million of these women.[18] In the 5 to 16-year-old age group boys have a higher rate of mental illness than girls with the exception of 'emotional disorders' such as anxiety or depression; among 5- to 10-year-olds 10% of boys and 5% of girls had a mental disorder. Men are almost four times likely to commit suicide than woman and it remains the biggest killer for young men in the UK. There is not only a need for better mental health care, but a reformulation of how we analyse what mental health is.[19] Given the differences between neurosis and psychosis, the statistics are inaccurate and the dangers of the deification of data has already been explained.

For Marxist sociologists power is constructed as the result of the class structure of societies linked to the modes of production rather than the will of individuals.[20] The idea of the sick role is a highly contested one, not merely because it can deny cultural differences, sexism, racism, or social inequalities. This has contentiously been framed as a role that some groups use to cope with social failure.[21] There is also an argument that the insane are outside the sick role further positioning the 'mad' as lack and absence being defined as deviant. Those in authority are frequently white middle class men and those in the sick role are often women. What is required is a breaking of 'automatisms', to borrow from Hélèn Cixous, so surpassing the dominating discourse of philosophical-theoretical-phallocentrism. Narrative is central to wellbeing.[22] Fiction has been used prolifically in this context and can theoretically be considered a subversive activity bringing about the possibility of change. A focus on 'madness', gender, and class, in the work of Daphne du Maurier and other writers as explained here is enlightening in terms of this subversive disruption. In 2018 *Rebecca* was voted the UK's favourite book of the last 225 years.[23] The work has had many spinoffs and influences, including literary sequels Susan Hill's *Mrs. de Winter* (1993) and Sally Beauman's *Rebecca's Tale* (2001), plus Taylor Swift

[16]Showalter, op. cit., p. 98.

[17]Barks, op. cit.

[18]Kat Lay, 'Antidepressant use rises by a fifth', *The Times*, 8 July 2022, p. 20.

[19]Ibid.

[20]Patrick Athony Leiba, 'Caretakers and the Rights of the Insane: An Historical Sociology', Unpublished PhD thesis 1997, University of London, p. 30.

[21]Ibid., p. 30.

[22]Psychology of Wellbeing Routledge.

[23](REF The Conversation).

claimed her song 'Tolerate It' on her 2020 album *Evermore* was inspired by the novel. In Daphne du Maurier's 1938 novel *Rebecca*, adapted for screen (Alfred Hitchcock, 1940; Ben Wheatley, 2020), Mr. de Winter narrowly avoided a breakdown. Paradoxically, 'madness' can also come from being too focused as an avoidance and, ontologically, doing battles with being or having as Eric Fromm has explained.[24] Derrida's concepts of hauntology and the revenant are also relevant here, given all is haunted in *Rebecca* with hauntedness part of 'madness' with there being a latent and blatant insanity in these texts.[25]

According to Maxim de Winter's sister Beatrice, he is prone to fits of temper which are 'mad' rages akin to possession, but the rest of the time he keeps these repressed. Monsters lurk within. This character embodies the dark repressed side of British upper-class masculinity moving in and out of a fury bordering on psychosis. At the heart of this upper-class patriarchal power is this threatening moneyed menace. Violent abuse is legitimized and promoted via a hunting culture. These fits have been witnessed by his sister his entire entitled life. They are unrelated to specific traumatic events, such as the death of his first wife or any known early abuse. His petulant personality originates in his biology and class.

This is mirrored in the description of the wildlife and flowers that surround Manderley operating as intrinsic omens, part of the 'madness' of fate and a timelessness that cannot be resisted. Fate is also embedded within the utopian cult in du Maurier's 'Monte Verité', part of her story collection *Don't Look Now* (1971) the paranormal titular story adapted for cinema by Nicolas Roeg in 1973. In *Don't Look Now* a blind woman knows a couple's dead illustrating the uncanny and the paranormal intrinsic to 'madness' and the transrational. The paranormality that dominates narratives of 'madness' involves the inability to cope with otherness, difference, and loss. Rather than an acceptance of the transrational which would be healthy there is rejection leading to horror and insanity. We understand from this that wellbeing comes through an engagement with the transrational.

Time is presented as a non-linear phenomenon which is part of a transrational reality; past, present, and future coalesce, as with dreams in deep time. This is central to our understanding of new forms of transrational knowledge. The uncanny concerns repetition as we saw with PTSD in Chap. 2 with ghosts transcending linear chronology while simultaneously haunting the present from the past. The quintessential film director of 'madness' Stanley Kubrick utilises this non-teleological approach to 'madness'. Transrationally, the upper-class father in *Don't Look Now* witnesses his wife and the uncanny twins returning to the city as he is leaving. He is unaware this is a moment after his own death. This permits us to question our own narrative constructions within this text and our own text—our life. A deep uncanny shifting of time such as this may be more real than linear processes with the blind female twin in touch with this foresight. In this narrative industrialised time, as is commonly known and understand, is inverted.

---

[24] E. Fromm, *To Have or To Be?* (London: Routledge, 1976).

[25] J. Derrida, *Specters of Marx* (London: Routledge, 2009).

As we know from Bergson and research on PTSD examined in Chap. 2, often the past can seem more present than the present.[26] This involves being haunted and Roland Barthes's five codes relating to the paranormal enigma enable us to understand this further. The hermeneutic code concerns the part of the story that is not fully explained. The proairectic code involves the action and guessing what happens next. The semantic code includes connotation which relates to additional meaning over the denotative meaning the literal. The fourth is the symbolic code where new meaning is created out of opposing ideas. The cultural code is that which cannot be challenged, such as science, religion, and magic; this is also part of the gnomic code, including sayings, proverbs, and clichés. Narrative can systematize chaotic and random events to offer a sane order and as with psychotherapy this gives life purpose and meaning. Some of these codes go unchallenged making them unbreakable. But Daphne du Maurier uses her narrative to break apart rational processes, offering deeper insight into the transrational truth of 'madness'—the break in the system.

The hero's journey involves an encounter with 'madness' and the transrational and this is in the form of externalized demons representing inner fears, including a journey, initiation, and return which is the path to wellbeing.[27] Without encountering this movement the inner and outer danger is permanent and 'madness' may result and the fragmentation can be so splintering there is no individuation. Daphne du Maurier elucidates in *Rebecca* how avoidance and repression create 'madness' with fear dominating. Driving with Mr. de Winter in Italy the narrator of *Rebecca* wants to cling on to the singular moment forever, timelessly avoiding death by creating eternity from memory. She employs an elaborate technique attempting this again when they walk to the bay near his house. In both events it is impossible to stay hold of a benign moment and this pattern, swinging from one mode of being to another, is akin to bi-polar disorder, or more precisely borderline personality disorder (BPD) where people feel they only exist via the other. To only be able to exist if one is validated by another puts one in the control of another, but could be a common female experience at this time, or at least was the part of social pressure for females who were continually being forced to find a man to marry.[28] This deep psychological understanding is explicated in this text 50 years prior to BPD becoming popularized.

The famous opening line reveals this is the invisible narrator's retrospective narrative and her position as an outsider enables a more objective narration with alienation class-based and bound. She has been rescued in Europe by Mr. de Winter from being a travelling companion. British class prevails over the crass American wealth. *Rebecca* focuses on the problems of being poor and female, the narrator stating she may have to return home to a boarding house. Julia Kristeva's 'deject' has been used to frame this alienating place, the position many women were in during

---

[26] Bessel van der Kolk, *The Body Keeps the Score: Mind, Brain and Body in the Transformation of Trauma* (London: Penguin, 2014).

[27] These terms have been popularised by Carl Jung, Joseph Campbell, and James Joyce.

[28] This was true in 1920s England. See Ursula Bloom, *Rosemary for Frinton* (London: Robert Hale, 1970).

the 1930s which is a zone occupying an in-between space.[29] The battle with Manderley is the battle with patriarchy, 'a domestic setting that necessarily disrupts the narrator's concept of gender and femininity rather than accommodating it'.[30] In this upper-class world you are defined by the sports you do, including hunting and shooting. The new Mrs. de Winter does none of these, so in this world she equals nothing; she is a non-person, far more invisible than the ever-present ghost of Rebecca. Silence is key to her experience, along with the unspeakable secret, there being multiple phantoms. The novel was written in the late 1930s when Freudian ideas were taking hold in America. Borderline personality disorder (BPD) has been explained in previous chapters and here the narrator's neuroticism might be termed Freudian, verging on mental illness in its level of anxiety which relates to BPD. She must tread carefully, to not set off 'madness' in others and this is central to her mental instability.

Other than her brief backstory given through the time with her American companion, it is unclear who the narrator who becomes the new Mrs. de Winter is. Nameless, she has gone from being one paid companion to another and is invisible—a modern-day slave. This is where gender and class are paramount in terms of control and 'madness'; like being in the 'madhouse', the narrator is trapped within the place that is supposed to bring her security, haunted by the dead woman who had autonomy. The fact she cannot write well in terms of the conventions of Manderley is symbolic. As with many women, education was unavailable in this inter-war period during economic crisis.[31] A rebel, the autonomous Rebecca challenged patriarchy resulting in the ultimate punishment—death.

One odd argument is the female independence of works such as *Jane Eyre* and the ambition and potential independence of the previous two centuries are negated in *Rebecca*.[32] This ignores the obvious historical context. Following the World War 1, certain freedoms were rolled back with an uncertainty concerning women's roles which is perfectly conveyed in *Rebecca*. As with *Jamaica Inn*, which again has an unnamed narrator, these works 'mirror the situation' of some women in the post-war England.[33] There is suffrage for women in the inter-war period, but this is a transitional moment of shifting identity and this transitory position is underscored in du Maurier's work, offering a haven from 'uncertainty overwhelming the inter-war period'.[34] Rather than negating female independence, *Rebecca* viscerally illustrates how mental problems are caused by not seizing independence and by the denial of the transrational.

[29] N. Laouar, "Ghosts Within Us": A Study of Women of Gothic Modernism, Unpublished PhD thesis, Canterbury Christ Church University, 2019, p. 166.

[30] Ibid., p. 167.

[31] Ibid., p. 174.

[32] Ibid., p. 182.

[33] Ibid., p. 183.

[34] Ibid., p. 184.

Rebecca's mass readership was further popularized by Hitchcock's adaptation. There was a turn to consumption studies in cultural studies and by feminist theorists and for Jackie Stacey in her work on cinema and female spectatorship of this period, 'the meaning of femininity within cultural production . . . is not synonymous with the uses and meanings of commodities to consumers'; women are subjects as well as objects of cultural exchanges in ways not entirely reducible to subjection.[35] There is a role for negotiated meanings, resistance, and 'appropriation' as well as 'subjection' and 'exploitation'.[36] Despite this, the call for a celebration to mark the new bride is the celebration of an object in *Rebecca*, the narrator. Mr. de Winter has chosen his new bride because she is more easily manipulated than Rebecca and her sense of inferiority comes from her belief in her being useless which his exacerbated by other class-based issues. Just as the second Mrs. de Winter is haunted by the ghost of the first, as the narrator she is a form of ghost, remaining uncannily invisible despite her narrative presence. Along with many other du Maurier stories, *Rebecca* is a commentary on how women are foolishly yoked to men which creates a living death, and this foolishness is a form of 'madness'. The best break free into sanity, as in the short stories 'Monte Verité' and 'Don't Look Now'. The self-willed woman is always more insightful than the man she is initially tied to. In the latter story it is his belief in the 'foolish woman' archetype that keeps the male protagonist from recognizing the truth of the transrational twins and his wife's reality. He cannot go beyond his own rational belief system, the masculine tied to a blinkered cause-effect rationality, whereas the transrational has a deeper healing knowledge.

The true uncanny 'madness' that du Maurier reveals is the 'madness' of patriarchy, stuck within a myopic framework of class and blind rationality. This 'madness' is the 'madness' of priapic civilization also revealed so expertly by her contemporary D.H. Lawrence.[37] 'Monte Verité' concludes with the so-called civilised world at war and the remote country within which it is finally set only now able to do battle with a once peaceful utopia led by women possibly destroyed by men. But, radically for the period, the author argues against the inevitability of patriarchal class driven war. Even at the start of 'Monte Verité' the female protagonist goes against feminine stereotypes; unconcerned with clothes and normal domestic life she has a higher aim. Writing 30 years before R.D. Laing, du Maurier contends worshipping the rational leads to insanity and the end of life, confirming transrational knowledge. The uncanny and the irrational will break through if denied, but the transrational is more than this. This approach is subtler and less binary, more transrational and mythological, and allows for nature and the human to flourish. In 'Monte Verité' the importance of environmentalism linked to the female is stressed before environmentalism became a global concern.

In *The Birds*, a novella adapted for screen by Alfred Hitchcock in 1963 and like *Rebecca* deeply focused on class, the servant class survives the longest, as it is most

[35] Stacey in Strinati, op. cit., p. 218.

[36] Ibid., p. 218.

[37] Lee 1999a.

respectful of nature and most aware of survival. There is a strong moral and practical lesson in this. The wealthy farmer who the protagonist works for is over-confident and does not believe nature can be a threat. The privileged farmer believes he is in control, a classic human mistake when it comes to nature. Alfred Hitchcock, arguably Britain's most internationally successful and psychological filmmaker, considered du Maurier to be his favourite writer. In *The Birds* he unfortunately shifts this class focus which is one reason why the film fails artistically. Constructions of gender and women as the object are at the heart of this mistake. The director's ideas of the perfect human form, especially concerning the feminine, also means the film fails artistically. The original screenwriter argued that the problem with the story was that nothing in it was real. 'In real life, birds don't attack people and girls don't buy lovebirds to shlepp 60 miles upstate for a practical joke'.[38]

Class was a significant issue with Hitchcock hiring a realistic novelist from New York to change the working-class people in the novel into his perception of beautiful, sleek, sophisticated characters. Hitchcock eventually worked on the script with V.S. Pritchett, changing the ending and the reaction of critics and audiences at the time is entertaining. 'A stunned silence greeted the final complicated mosaic of what appeared to be 3,407 pieces of bird film,' the audience reacting with a form of 'is that it?'.[39] The original screenwriter left the cinema before anyone recognised them as the culprit. In the novella *The Birds* the landowner does not believe anything strange is afoot which is his downfall. We can compare this with the way the upper-classes believe they are superior to everything, including nature, and nothing can touch them, such as those within the British government led by Boris Johnson who ignored the original threat of COVID-19 in 2020.

In *Rebecca* nature is the threat and civilizing activities involve taming nature, for example, cutting flowers to be arranged in a certain manner in the main house. Civilization does what it can to tame nature, but it never manages to do so entirely. As we saw in the previous chapter, this is a theme examined by Lars von Trier following Milton's notion of nature being the devil's church. The concept of evil is tied together with this problematic relationship with nature which has profounder resonances when we consider the evils of human-made climate change and global warming.

The chaos of the sea has frequently been associated with 'madness' and on the trip to the bay, where the first Mrs. de Winter drowned, her successor the narrator once more meets Ben which initially does not seem as sinister as it had done previously. Ben, however, is shaking with fear and begs her not to take him to the mental asylum, the theme of insanity now overt. Repeating what happened between him and Rebecca, he explains that Rebecca told him to deny he had seen her and if she caught him again looking at her, "'I'll have you put in the asylum," she said. "You wouldn't like that would you? They're cruel to people in the asylum," she

[38] E. Hunter, 'Evan Hunter (Ed McBain) remembers with with Hitchcock on *The Birds* and *Marnie* – the complete journal', *Sight and Sound.*, Vol. 7 Issue 6, June 1997, p. 26.

[39] Ibid., p. 34.

said'.[40] Ben is known as a harmless simple fisherman with learning difficulties, but any sniff of impropriety such as him stealing a fishing line from the cottage makes him believe they will lock him up forever in the 'mad' house. Here class, disability, and transgression, are directly connected to 'madness'. While the dead Mrs. de Winter uncannily haunts Manderley, the real 'madness' is a deeper repression which is the part of the English upper-class character, servants of this class mimicking their behaviour. When this breaks through into expressed rage the danger is so blatant it is overwhelming and psychopathic.

A psychopath is far more dangerous than any other person.[41] One reason for this is they often manage to function in society exceedingly well. This is explained in Chap. 7 when we examine 'madness' and leaders. Following Derrida's work on hauntology, the spectre is part of the trauma that uncannily haunts culture and which plays with 'madness'. In *Rebecca* we get a taste of Mrs. Danvers' psychopathic traits in Chaps. 14 and 15 when she shows how much she is trying to keep the dead Rebecca alive. Even after Rebecca's death, Mrs. Danvers can, 'catch the sound of her dress sweeping the stairs', and she thinks she is watching over them.[42] Rebecca's presence is ubiquitous, making the new Mrs. de Winter sick with an anxiety verging on 'madness'. Mr. de Winter's 'madness' is marked with rage expressed by his whole face metamorphosing.[43] The 'madness' here is so innate it is part of the indivisible class divide.

The second Mrs. de Winter is constantly being told she is inferior, not just to Rebecca, but to all around her. She does not hunt, ride, or sail, meaning she does not have the physical skills and breeding of the upper-class. Not only is she thought of as inferior due to wealth, education, behaviour, and social upbringing, but due to her physical lack. She is perceived to be an inferior species, the true other. To borrow Julia Kristeva's terminology, this is part of the abject and it is this that makes her monstrous to the group.[44] However, her invisibility makes her the perfect narrator, free from the trap of the upper class who still exist in a fallen state. Because of her outsider status she sees through the charade of Manderley with its theatre of domestic bliss, all functioning as actors in a charade. The ghost as metaphor adds to the disjointedness of history, ontology, and ideology. The novel is re-entering this psychotic nightmare. Whenever anything is going well disaster and 'madness' strikes. A parallel with a certain 'madness' is clear; in 'madness' metaphoric demons are not dealt with and confronted or absorbed and in Jungian language the shadow is divorced rather than integrated. Facing the demons, as the protagonist puts it, is the only way to peace. This novel is a process of catharsis, of dealing with demons, re-entering the nightmare for the purpose of transrational knowledge and wellbeing.

---

[40] Daphne du Maurier, *Rebecca* (London: Pan, 1981), p. 163.

[41] Anthony Storr, *Human Aggression* (London: Penguin, 1970), p. 137.

[42] du Maurier, op. cit., p. 181.

[43] Ibid., p. 198.

[44] Barbara Creed, 'Kristeva, Femininity, Abjection', in Ken Gelder, ed. *The Horror Reader* (London: Routledge, 2000), 64–70, p. 65.

Having money is normally associated with freedom, but what is remarkable here is how the wealthy are revealed to be dictated to and trapped, their class and status creating a zombified culture. They must carry out tasks for the delights of others, such as the ball, despite not caring for it in the slightest. An underlying all consuming 'mad' rage possesses them with 'madness'. With the ghosts and history so heavily on the backs of the upper-class this is weighing them down so much that they cannot self-actualise in a Jungian sense. In fact, they are totally unconscious in their actions, with following Rohr implies their deeds are evil as they exist without recognizing they have choices.

We see also find this is the case in Daphne du Maurier's 1957 novel *The Scapegoat*, adapted for cinema (Robert Hamer, 1959), which again concerns the hypocrisy of the upper class, this time in France. The uncanny cage of the past, along with the chains of in-bred toxic family and associates, and the necessary rituals involved, are highlighted by the protagonist-narrator who is an outsider, originally from a servant class. The novel offers the narrator's moments of unease which functions as a feminist warning regarding 'madness', men dominating her existence fed by the overpowering ghost of Rebecca who is everyman's fantasy accentuating how life is a mask for the upper classes. As explained, *Rebecca* is the most popular novel in Britain and given Britain is still so divided along class lines this class factor in part explains its contemporary popularity.

3.2 Historical Nexus

A further germane component of this work and its adaptations is its engagement with the visual which has philosophical import concerning transrationality and transgressive culture. Significantly, the wealthy grandmother in *Rebecca* is as blind as the visionary in the short story 'Don't Look Now', and her mistaken belief that Rebecca is alive has some veracity. Although dead physically, metaphysically as well as metaphorically Rebecca is profoundly alive offering resistance highlighting how ghosts can uncannily influence the living more fully than those physically incarnated. Lacan's revision of Freud has been influential from political theorists like Louis Althusser to film critics such as Christian Metz. Even those opposed to the gendered aspects of his work like Irigaray have not furthered his critique of the visual constitution of subjectivity.[45] In the novel *Rebecca* the protagonist is always secretly watching and observing, just as she too is being watched and observed and Freud's work on Charcot's observational skills is significant here. Freud believed the desire to know (in Austrian Wisstrieb) was not innocent but stemmed from the infantile desire to see which has sexual origins. Infantile scopophilia (Schaulust) could result

[45] M. Jay, *Downcast Eyes: The Denigration of Vision in Twentieth-Century French Thought* (University of California Press: Berkeley, 1994), p. 331.

in adult voyeurism or other perverse disorders, including exhibitionism and scopophobia (the fear of being seen).[46]

In *Rebecca* the mimicking that Lacan used from the animal world to develop the mirror stage is extended by the protagonist. Mimicry causes a loss of psychic energy known as 'psychasthenia'.[47] 'Here visual experience meant a crisis of the boundaried well-informed self, which invites comparison with Bataille's idea of *informe'* (formlessness).[48] In one you developed by Lacan the difference between animal and human infants could be demonstrated via their behaviour in front of the mirror; animals fail to recognize themselves. This process instigated the visually constituted idea of self with children identifying with the pain of others, crying when another child felt pain. Known as transitivism, psychologists Charlotte Bühler and Elsa Köhler developed the belief that it was healthy to confuse self-image with the image of the other.[49] This is important with regards to Mrs. Danvers and the narrator of *Rebecca*. Human consciousness emerges over time in response to a primordial desire to overcome a lack, 'a felt sense of incompleteness on the part of the biological proto-subject'.[50]

The key nexus here is when Beatrice asks the new Mrs. de Winter to re-join the party, after her mistake of dressing up in the same outfit the dead Mrs. de Winter wore, historically resurrecting the already ever-present past. 'She had not understood. She belonged to another breed of men and women, another race than I'.[51] Class is not just a social boundary here, it is racial. 'I had not the price, I had not the guts. I was badly bred'.[52] She keeps seeing Maxim's blazing eyes and the others, 'standing like dummies, staring at me'.[53] When she does finally join the group, Maxim is automatic, a hyper-mechanical machine. The order of events is even more predetermined than a play, and here her husband turns into an automaton which is directly described by Freud in his work on the uncanny. What lies behind this need to carry out this theatre is not spelt out, but it obviously concerns control and power to assert their ruling class. The intrinsic horror lies in the fact that the upper-class is not actually in control of their actions hence their need to control others and, like animals, they cannot see themselves in the mirror.

This moment of transgression is nothing of the sort, however, more it is a moment where power in and of itself rules most thoroughly, even the band playing endlessly like clockwork, again like robots with the evil of civilisation overt and obscene. Flippantly, the new Mrs. de Winter claims this, 'situation was mad, unreal', when she finally approaches Mrs. Danvers, believing she has set up everything in her

[46]Ibid.

[47]Ibid., p. 332.

[48]Ibid., p. 343.

[49]Ibid.

[50]Ibid., p. 345.

[51]du Maurier, op. cit., p. 228.

[52]Ibid.

[53]Ibid.

hatred for her. But there is no getting through to Mrs. Danvers, who goes on, 'raving like a mad-woman, a fanatic'.[54] There is an underlying specific pathology. In a popular context it is an example of how 'madness' is central to behaviour and an element of a central emotion that motivates. Rebecca's life and death has led to various forms of 'madness', Mrs. Danvers's typology being just one.

Maxim de Winter confesses that Rebecca's behaviour drove him so 'mad' he often wanted to kill. His murderous hatred is pathologically obsessive. Mrs. Danvers' blind love of Rebecca is also pathologic with a form of 'mad' possession here by the dead. Chapter 2 explained how theatre can be used to examine and cure 'madness'. The trouble that du Maurier is exposing is the 'madness' from living a double life, pursuing acts for the semblance of normality stemming from prioritising class and 'breeding' as the Gran puts it.[55] This causes the repressed tension resulting in 'madness'. And it is not just the dead Rebecca who is the focus of this 'madness', but the whole attention and audience around her—the performance and the spectacle, the observing and the observed.

The questioning Maxim receives by the coroner almost drives him 'mad' as he puts.[56] An underlying theme is that you cannot escape facing your situation or your actions. While du Maurier is popular for her uncanny fictions that touch on the paranormal, as in 'Don't Look Now', a core element to her stories is their humanising and moralising impact. This is essential for our mental health, recognising that what others think is not central to our existence. Shrugging off hypocrisy for reality is also critical, part of the path of wellbeing which has political implications for gender and society. This is also revealed in Daphne du Maurier's work such as 'Monte Verité'. The hyper-rationality and repression of the patriarchal upper classes, a driving mechanised behaviour, is exposed as a 'madness' that needs overcoming. Not being able to cover up the past, it reaps vengeance and dominates everyone's psychic lives.

In Freudian terms neurotics are unable to deal with sexual repression which is necessary for civilization. Rebecca de Winter was far from sexually repressed, nor is her cousin and lover Jack, being the antithesis to the orderly Maxim de Winter. Simultaneously, the dead Rebecca is still the most revered in their society. Is this then contradictory to Freud's theories, with du Maurier writing at a time when these theories took hold? In one interpretation this confirms Freud given the attempt to destroy Rebecca, a form of repression, does not finally work. Maxim de Winter sinks her boat, as if you can sink and repress the id like this into the unconscious, the sea. The physical and the metaphysical combine here, as does the psyche. The community and coroner function as the super ego, critically questioning Maxim. The whole externalizing of inner psychic mechanisms is overt. When Rebecca's cousin arrives after the inquest and confesses his affair with Rebecca, presenting a note that might prove she has not committed suicide, he declares that all husbands with lovely wives

[54] Ibid., p. 254.
[55] Ibid., p. 284.
[56] Ibid., p. 332.

are jealous, and cannot help 'playing Othello'.[57] This reference to a play about 'mad' jealousy is perfectly apt. Maxim even has his own version of Othello's fits. While not epilepsy like 'the Moor', they are moments of pure rage making his actions irrational, what some might term insane, as when he calls Colonel Julyan to the house.

A possible witness to Rebecca's murder is deemed to be of 'crazed brain'.[58] 'Madness' has paradoxically often been considered a zone of truth beyond the conforming repressed rationality that skewers reality.[59] In du Maurier's short story 'A Border-Line Case', which suggests a mental patient on the edge, political and class-based issues are interpreted again that relate to the novel *Rebecca*. We have the 'madness' of play acting, but in *Rebecca* the penultimate victory with Dr. Baker is not long-lasting. Maxim de Winter has bribed Dr. Baker to say that Rebecca's appointment with him in Barnet the day before she died concerned cancer not pregnancy. When the significantly nameless narrator and her husband return to Manderley it is on fire, as if the dawn is early. The truth will always be denied, the ultimate repression but, no matter how hard the ruling classes try, there can always be revolution—this is epitomised in this instance as the narrator who has her voice. What is so captivating about the novel *Rebecca* is that the ego of the narrator is obtuse while her antagonist Mrs. Danvers lives her life only through the deceased Rebecca, the living dead.

For Lacan ego psychology was the problem not the cure and from the clinical point of view the ego, 'represents the center of all the resistances to the treatment of the symptoms'.[60] The trouble for the protagonist is her weak ego that only comes fully alive once she is informed that Mr. de Winter hated his first wife. She lives under a cloud of 'mad' depression and deception, falsely believing Maxim is thoroughly in love with his dead wife. Her precursor Rebecca was promiscuous and incestuous. The difference with *Othello* is that Desdemona is innocent. There is no justification for Othello's jealousy and 'madness', his paranoia played with by Iago. Given Rebecca's behaviour there is reason for Maxim's 'madness'. Unlike Othello, who also kills his wife, when Maxim kills his wife, it is not represented as irrational or 'mad'. In *Rebecca* Daphne du Maurier reveals the corruption of an innocent women through her association with a man, exposing patriarchy and class as the central paradigms that dehumanize us all.

In *Jamaica Inn* (novel 1936, film directed by Hitchcock, 1939) du Maurier begins by addressing one of society's centrals myths, that women without men go 'mad', and then deconstructs and challenges this. To be individuated involves our species. For example, we could not achieve it, 'were it not for language, which belongs to me only because it belongs to the species first'.[61] In both these texts a woman tries to fit

---

[57] Ibid., p. 341.

[58] Ibid., p. 348.

[59] Lee (1999b), op. cit.

[60] du Maurier, op. cit., p. 348.

[61] Terry Eagleton, *Trouble with Strangers: A Study of Ethics* (Wiley-Blackwell: Oxford, 2009), p. 96.

in to find a new happiness and then must learn the new language to do so. In *Rebecca* she is extremely false to herself. To always perceive the other as a threat creates anxiety, but the prevailing ideology of Western capitalism insists on this 'madness'. This is fed by an overt belief in a rationalism that avoids deeper transrational knowledge and healing for wellbeing. There is a political choice here: encountering the real via transrationalism or denying it furthering 'madness'.

Due to patriarchal class oppression women are thrown into the position of having to conform to others and confirm others which can remove a sense of being leading to 'madness' akin to diagnoses such as borderline personality disorder (BPD). Daphne du Maurier's writings interrogate and contest this patriarchal approach, plus there is a healing process proffered via her fictions that furthers wellbeing. The protagonist Mary Yelder in the novel *Jamaica Inn* (film adaptation directed by Alfred Hitchcock, 1939) is acting on instructions from her mother. She wants to remain on her family's farm after her parents' death, but her mother's guidance is that this is no place for a young woman on her own. This of course would not be said had she been a man and she is wrenched from the bosom of home into the hell of Jamaica Inn. Following Foucault, we have seen how 'madness', 'even if it is provoked or sustained by what is most artificial in society, appears, in its violent forms, as the savage expression of the most primitive human desires'.[62] This is part of its transgressive attraction; human free-will is substituted for animalistic instincts working on an unconscious level which, as explained, is always one step ahead of the conscious mind. This also explains why the 'mad' can have gifts of foresight as they function more within the unconscious where past, present, and future and less demarcated. One problem with 'madness' is when only one position is maintained with the answer to this problem the non-binary approach where we become free from the entanglement and tension of opposites without agitation.[63]

3.3 Narration, Politics, Sanity

Transrationality subverts normalized perceptions of time that which philosopher Simone Weil has shown are unreal.[64] Both *Jamaica Inn* and *Rebecca* tackle 'madness' by displacing time to an eternal point within their transrational knowledge. This playing with time is freeing and horrifying, both being horror stories along with 'Don't Look Now'. By suggesting that narrative frameworks always offer sanity there is a danger given each era invents, 'new masks, new screens, displays, or

[62] Michel Foucault, *Madness and Civilization. A History of Insanity in the Age of Reason*, trans. Richard Howard (London: Routledge/Tavistock, 1989), p. 193.

[63] C.G. Jung, *The Psychology of Kundalini Yoga: Notes of the Seminar Given in 1932 by C.G. Jung* (Princeton, NJ: Princeton University Press, 1932), pp. 82–83.

[64] Simone Weil, *Gravity and Grace*, trans. Emma Crawford and Mario von der Ruhr (London: Routledge, 1992), p. 45.

artifices in order to not advance in this new speech, universal in its diversity'.[65] Is it impossible to approach the other without being already restricted in a zone that reduces differences to the same offering a tautological exchange for which there is an, 'already programmed scenography, a monologue in two voices?'.[66] This hellish scenario propagated in both versions of *Jamaica Inn* involves purpose and meaning, but should not lead to despair given there is an excessive optimism behind this voice. Irigaray has an ambitious set of demands for language that goes way beyond how we use it to satisfy our needs and approach the other. This is not situated in an anthropological or sociological methodology but is partly drawn from a higher-level metaphysical aspiration.[67] This is where the relevance of the transrational for wellbeing is once more reinscribed.

How then does it constitute and unveil the human? It would be obvious to purport that 'madness' is this second guessing concerning an unveiling, ripping, or ploughing through the postures of meaning which correlates non-transrational knowledge to a metaphoric stamp collecting (fact collecting). Knowledge should be far more than collecting parallels of meaning, but often with a rational discourse it ends up being no more than this. We can understand why Irigaray is disappointed by the lack of forgetting of 'man' and the lack of questioning of what 'man' is.[68] There is no agreed definition of what the human is, but frequently we act as if there is. Behind this is also an attack on male-led science which wants to know what is external for the purpose of dominating and not caring about the internal. This confirms the argument maintained here concerning the importance of transrational knowledge which has often been ignored.

Self-knowledge and self-will have not been greatly advanced despite the venturing across the planet.[69] The fault then is the turn outward, to rationally control external environments, rather than inward, where emotionally transrational knowledge is found. We have seen how Carl Jung, Virginia Woolf, and Richard Rohr all confirm this. Conversely, against their wellbeing, Daphne du Maurier's characters are compelled to externally act out their own anxieties. The scientific method accentuates distance and offers a split with nature.[70] The key criticism by Irigaray is the pursuit of universals, moving us away from specifics, namely that which is most near to us, ourselves. We are chained to a priori constructions and pre-programmed artifices.[71]

There is a possibility, however, of some form of gap. 'In the dimension of ourselves where Being still quivers, identity is never definitely constituted, nor

[65] Luc Irigaray, *Key Writings* (London and New York: Continuum, 2004), p. 46.

[66] Ibid., p. 47.

[67] Ibid.

[68] Ibid.

[69] Richard Rohr, *The Universal Christ* (London: SPCK, 2019), p. 47.

[70] Luce Irigaray, *Je, Tu, Nous – Toward a Culture of Difference*, trans. Alison Martin (London: Routledge, 2007), p. 38.

[71] Ibid., p. 92.

defined beforehand'.[72] Irigaray claims illness is caused by civilization destroying our immune system.[73] What exactly is a healthy living body, and does technology obfuscate our understanding of the body and mind?[74] With the reification of data, of storing and processing information concerning our behaviour and desires, monitoring's role supersedes function. Collation and assessment of data deletes origin as does the virtual. Irigaray positions a series of illnesses together, from cancer to AIDS, suggesting even sterility is caused by the, 'constant stress caused by noise'.[75] Conversely, curing, she argues can remove people of their voice situating them in a particular diagnosis.[76]

This is specifically accurate in the context of gender and Irigaray is correct when she situates the cause of malfunction on the over-valorisation of perceived masculine attributes.[77] While the second Mrs. de Winter prays Maxim loves her, she can only fully accept he does upon learning that he killed his first wife. It is only in his later neediness, suspected of Rebecca's murder, that he turns to our narrator. As soon as 'madness' is understood it might be thought to be contained; Maxim's odd behaviour, which he admits verges on 'madness', is self-explanatory once full knowledge of his murderous actions are revealed. The work of artists and writers like Edvard Munch, August Strindberg, and Franz Kafka, for example, suggest fear in the male of 'feminine inconsistency'.[78] This dread is of feminine hysteria, which traumatized these men with the multiple masks of the feminine, is still based on masks.

Birth anxiety causes a trauma which echoes Derrida's hauntology, yet this anxiety is essential for ego formation, giving individuals an opportunity for independence. Wisdom is often paralleled with sanity, but the antithesis is also correct. In Belgian television series *The Forest* (Julius Berg, 2017) a 6-year-old girl is found on a doctor's doorstep. He then raises her, and she spends 2 years in a mental hospital overcoming what happened to her. Nobody, including herself, has knowledge of what has occurred. This lack of knowledge helps keeps her sane. As she grows up, she is promiscuous and does not want attachments, but conducts religious ceremonies with her adopted Jewish father and is a successful French teacher. Her experience means she is more sensitive to the needs of the adolescents she teaches than some of the 'normal' local people.

The stereotype view is that people condemned as 'damaged goods' through having been abused in childhood have less empathy, but in reality the reverse is true. Those who suffer childhood trauma, known to create poor mental health, have

[72] Ibid., p. 93.
[73] Ibid., p. 56.
[74] Ibid.
[75] Ibid., p. 57.
[76] Ibid.
[77] Ibid.
[78] Slavoj Žižek, *Living in the End Times* (London: Verso, 2011), p. 150.

greater empathy as an adult.[79] In this instance, instead of a television show conforming to stereotypes and myths, a more accurate portrayal is given. Concurrently, a traditional story of an outsider with a secret wound entering a traditional village bringing an almost supernatural healing is played out in a contemporary context, paying close attention to the clandestine and womanhood. For Munch there is hysterical theatre concerning the concept that behind the mask there is nothing, no 'ultimate Secret'.[80] The 'ultimate Secret' here is part of the pursuit and what occurs is the explication of the relevance of existentialism.

'Madness' develops through the absenteeism of engaging in the 'mad' principles of society.[81] In working out the true purpose of psychoanalysis Habermas claims the 'I' of the patient recognizes itself in its other represented by its illness, that is, its own alienated self it identifies with.[82] Illness can equate with and create the self, or it can be an over identification with civilization, as we saw with Irigaray. If we are certain that all forms of difference are part of our illness, then to cure the self is to cure the other. For Badiou, 'the only ethics is of processes of truth, of the labour that brings *some* truths into the world'; he follows Lacan's ethics of psychoanalysis, so ethics is not pre-existing, but there is an 'ethic-of' (of politics, of love, of science, of art).[83] This leads to a deeper consideration of the ethical.

Behind the truth of 'madness' is the truth of avoidance and repression which is the essence of desire and, in this sense, Freud is correct. The dishonesty of humanism which then developed into Rogerian person-centred psychotherapy is that it too simplistically states the self-actualizing tendency is undeniably at the core of being. Once we consider the nature of the human to be both destructive and constructive to suggest otherwise is fallacious, but this dialectic does not need to be binary. The importance of love, which is often actually a battle for supremacy and ownership as we see in 7.2.1, perfectly sums up this conclusion, and *Rebecca* illustrates this well. The unknown protagonist grows up the moment she hears about hate, in that she then knows that any love her husband has for her is not limited by a previous wife, so ownership of love is central. Idealistically, love is about enabling the freedom of another. But this ignores other forms of love, including possessive love and jealous love.

The Lord your God is a jealous God states *The Old Testament*.[84] This is part of the framework of many relationships, including culturally, such as in *Othello*. In this play on race, gender, and class the protagonist is always about to make love with his new bride, considered by those who truly know her to be a virgin. The paradox is this

---

[79] Greenberg DM, Baron-Cohen S, Rosenberg N, Fonagy P, Rentfrow PJ (2018) Elevated empathy in adults following childhood trauma. PLoS ONE 13(10): e0203886. 8.

[80] Žižek, op. cit.

[81] Ibid., p. 22.

[82] Ibid.

[83] Alain Badiou, *An Essay on the Understanding of Evil*, trans. Peter Hallward (London: Verso 2012), p. 28.

[84] Deuteronomy 4:24. *The Bible*, Revised Standard Version (London: Collins, 1977), p. 133.

can never happen, as it is the eternal and infernal fantasy of her, be it virgin or whore, that must prevail. For Othello, he may mouth-off about his victories in battle, his words considered magical spells, euphemisms for his sexual prowess, but he never actually gets to prove his virility or strength in battle during the play, in or out of bed. This is part of his racialized 'madness', the fantasy of him having sex with a white woman part of the 'madness' of others which it can be argued is at the core of the play.

Following Lacan's gloss on Freud, 'in the field of the dream, you are at home'.[85] The central Western idea of science as a disinterested pursuit of knowledge is, 'a sublimated version of other desires which have been repressed in Western culture'.[86] This sublimation is a form of 'madness' in its denial, or a way of combating 'madness'. 'It is in our relations with other people that we gain a sense of ourselves; it's that, pretty much, that makes relations with other people unbearable'.[87] 'Madness' is the torn position of lived rupture. Once the space between us is thoroughly deleted then there is no room for our existence. Within 'madness' there is no space for anything other as it is fully other.

Psychopathy can be considered 'madness' and is very attractive to audiences of theatre, fiction films, television series, and documentaries. Is this a form of 'madness', or a means to sanity? For example, a psychopath traditionally has little to no empathy therefore the psychopath has no real feelings of jealousy which taken to extremes, as in *Othello*, can lead to a form of 'madness'. One form of 'madness', including psychopathy, can enable high-functioning people such as CEOs to succeed, preventing another form of 'madness'.[88] We speak of a craze, a fad, which is group 'madness'. In these circumstances capitalism's key players, including advertisers, attempt to create a craze, a crazy 'madness' of purchasing.

'Madness' then is at the heart of capitalism, and our constructions of gender and class. This is unsurprising given, as we have seen, 'madness' is close to savagery.[89] Capitalism and the savagery of the market highlights this where the market exists as an apparently eternal uncanny, an entity deified as the god without limits that is always right. Simultaneously, the ideology of the boundless market is the essence of transgression.[90] Sanity concerns boundaries and limits. Whatever feeds the market is part of the ritual of transgressive worship and this blind ritual is 'madness'; the market is everything, 'madness' is everything. Behind this is the myth that everything is as it should be which paradoxically makes any action that challenges this view a version of 'madness'.

---

[85] Žižek, Slavoj, *How to Read Lacan* (London: Granta Books, 2006), p. 144.

[86] Ibid., p. 145.

[87] See Michel Houellebecq in Julian Barnes, *The Sense of an Ending* (London: Vintage, 2012), p. 89.

[88] See Chap. 7. for a more detailed analysis of this subject.

[89] This point was made in Chap. 1. with reference to several historians of 'madness'.

[90] Stephen Pfohl, *Death at the Parasite Café. Social Science (Fictions) and the Postmodern* (London: Palgrave Macmillan, 1992).

As we saw with du Maurier, what role and identity a woman should play is central to her 'madness'. Analysis that employs semiology or explicates ideology from a Marxist or feminist perspective needs to acknowledge its own limitations.[91] Gender and class constructions have been found to be factors when it comes to what is 'madness'. In one interview discussed in Chap. 5 with someone who had worked in the British health system for 30 years, it was found far more women than men would be brought for electroconvulsive therapy (ECT), a subject Plath utilizes in her fiction. Through an exegesis of Plath's ironic semi-autobiographical *The Bell Jar* (1963, originally published under the pseudonym Victoria Lucas) and other texts the verdict is overt: treatment for 'madness' is a punishment for women who did not fit in, for women being who they are, for women not being men. Overall, a diagnosis of 'madness' is a method to curtail difference.

The silencing of female voices is a popular trope, but the complex dialectic of the demotion and promotion of the female voice, philosophically and culturally, is not new. Historically it has often been tied to prophecy in England.[92] In the seventeenth century the way to be listened to was to frame utterances as prophecy.[93] The church, state, and university, denied women a voice. During the English Civil War (1642–1651) when there was less censorship there was a change. Lady Eleanor Douglas, for example, published thirty-seven known tracts between 1641 and her death 11 years later.[94] Regardless of gender, speaking out against the church or state was criminalized, so this was often framed as direct prophecy to legitimize it. This meant for such a religious people it had to be listened to, whether these were the rantings of the 'mad' or otherwise.

The politicizing of 'madness' should not be overlooked in any century with 1950s and 1960s America like the Russia and China of today with psychiatric treatment enacted for political purposes.[95] The various houses of the mental hospital in Plath's 1950s-set fiction function like a boarding school having crossovers with the early treatment of the mentally afflicted discussed in Chap. 1. Socialization and surveillance were and still are key to not only these environments, but also to society outside the asylum walls so once again divisions are blurred. Paradoxically, in *The Bell Jar* it is the normality of the other women that Esther finds so abnormal and this is the key nexus of the narrative we must consider. Surely, if this is truly a mental asylum the women within it would be 'mad'? Not necessarily, indeed, not at all. 'Madness' is the gap that makes society function with the insanity of normality being obfuscated by the asylum like Disneyland existing to make the rest of America look normal.[96]

[91] Dominic Strinati, *An Introduction to Theories of Popular Culture* (London: Routledge, 1995), p. 210.

[92] Which many would consider 'madness'.

[93] Keith Thomas, *Religion and the Decline of Magic* (London: Penguin, 1978), p.163.

[94] Ibid.

[95] See Chap. 8.

[96] This is a line followed by postmodernist such as Baudrillard, amongst others.

Irvin Levine's 1972 novel *The Stepford Wives* reveals a small-town world of wealthy men who cannot handle difference who turn their wives into conforming robots and the accusations of 'madness' abound. As with Margaret Atwood's 1985 novel *The Handmaid's Tale* (with its film and television sequels and imitations, plus its second volume, *The Testaments*, 2019), *The Bell Jar* is a similar seminal text. Plath's work involves the slavery of women, both inside and outside the asylum. Like the institutions in the nineteenth century discussed in Chap. 1, the twentieth-century mental hospital magnified and paradoxically dignified the dynamics already existing, being both a macro and micro political lens. Tellingly, in *The Bell Jar* men are physically unwell rather than mentally sick. Interestingly, the current suicide rate for men is three times higher than that for women in the UK and even higher in America.[97]

As with *The Stepford Wives*, Plath reveals what is going on behind apparently perfect lives. Esther is not an especially appealing character, far from it, but that is the point and like the narrator of *Rebecca* she just wants to fit in. Her problem is she cares too much about people liking her, but unlike the narrator of *Rebecca* she is no prude or wilting violet. The desperate need to belong is part of this modern slavery to the external. If you cannot fit into the machinery of work, marriage and motherhood, there is the other machine—the insane asylum. Fitting in means you do not challenge the machine. Anyone outside the system is a problem, a difference that must be eliminated. To go insane is to not communicate within the system where language compliance is everything. The writer's creation of the manuscript itself is a voice of defiance. Language is a tool for freedom, but it is also a trap. Losing the ability to communicate sanely means forfeiting the right to live in normal society and gain the rights that entails given you are a threat.

Women, who had only gained the vote under three decades earlier, had taken male jobs during World War 2. When the men returned this threat was dealt with by the asylum. The end point includes being in a padded cell, where no one can hear you scream; ECT treatment, which can discombobulate you and stop you screaming; and then lobotomy, as in the film *One Flew Over the Cuckoo Next* (Milos Forman, 1976). Many other cases can be given; in 1961 America's future president John F. Kennedy would learn of his sister Rosemary's disastrous lobotomy two decades earlier that left her severely disabled.

Whether on a real or metaphoric level, outside the asylum, excessive consumption of alcohol, drugs, false religion, and popular entertainment lobotomise the citizen making them more fully integrated within the system and more easily manipulated. Self-medicating via the drugs and alcohol of personal choice became a catchphrase in the early 1980s, but Plath's novel plays with this. At least it was felt to take control away from the doctor and psychiatrist giving it back to the patient to a degree. The relationship between mental health and alcohol consumption is

[97] Samaritans, 'Latest Suicide Data', 2021, Latest suicide data | Suicide facts and figures | Samaritans (accessed 30 January, 2023).

well-known.[98] In *The Bell Jar* there are moments when Esther's entirely loses consciousness after drinking and this appears to bring on her mental illness. Betrayal at the deepest level is at the heart of the story. Esther is looking for a benign mother and thinks she has found one in the doctor who tells her she will be warned before she has any ECT. The moment she is aware she will be receiving ECT and the doctor has not yet warned her is a moment of clarity. From then on, she cannot trust anyone. Her anger is set aside for zombie-like compliance which is a real moment of defeat. If no one can be trusted then why go through with this, why go through with living?

At first *The Bell Jar* initially seems an obvious text, but there are gaps in the text, moments when reasoning shifts beyond language, offering deeper transrational knowledge. 'Madness' can be defined as a place outside language that challenges the rationality of language or 'delanguization'.[99] This novel is important not only because of its content, but due to what it has come to represent—a holy text for young women, as the pilgrimages to Plath's grave still testify. It encapsulates the fear and dread and terror of young women across generations. In Esther's first session the therapist mentions all the pretty girls he once knew at her college. This is an indicative sign as to how the overall system is set up within a patriarchal framework, despite the other doctor who leads her to ECT being a woman. It does not matter what sex you are; if you are complicit with the system, you are one with the system. The ongoing Plath industry continues to deconstruct her father.[100] Esther's father is absent, and the boys and men in her life are virtually absent.

Doctors see her as a sex object. As we saw with 'madness' and Virginia Woolf, could suicide then be the only option by removing herself as a subject from their objectification? There are parallels here with Chap. 2 and *Antichrist*; killing the body to protect the mind and soul in this instance is a form of resistance. Esther has been objectified by the system and turned into a piece of meat. ECT's origin stems from the slaughterhouse. The method is Frankensteinian, as if zapping someone who has lost the will to live will bring them back to life, electricity offering the victim a way forward. Esther is destined for great things and ends up in a lunatic asylum with people she already knows as if this is another university campus. Another woman who was dating one of Esther's boyfriends is with her in the asylum and is now a lesbian. The asylum mirrors the outside world in its organization and offers a rite of passage, including ECT which is almost Egyptian in its mythological depth with the ritual of ECT crossing the Styx and back. Paradoxically, that which we may wish to extirpate and annul, our anxieties, our depressions, our worries, and fears, are intrinsic to what makes us original and unique—they make us human. In a Kierkegaardian sense, existential worries are the core of our being. So, the temptation here

[98] See Jason Lee, ed., *Cultures of Addiction* (New York: Cambria, 2010).

[99] Wouter Kusters, *A Philosophy of Madness – The Experience of Psychotic Thinking*, trans. Nancy Forest-Flier (Massachusetts: MIT, 2020), p. 213.

[100] Jason Lee, 'The Zoo Keeper's Strife: Will Self's Psychiatric Fictions', *Philosophy and Literature*, 36(1) (2012): 196–208.

is to destroy the self to enable a semblance of life. Is a semblance of life better than a living hell, or are the two identical?

As in Chap. 1, we see how the happiness industry is the unhappiness industry. In all major faiths the hero becomes disillusioned by events of the everyday world and sees through the veil of appearances. Joseph Campbell called this the hero's journey, where death is transfigured, and this is identified in many myths through various cultures.[101] The problem for Esther Greenwood and those like her is that instead of going through the pain, confronting the monsters in both the internal and the external world, there is a fixation. The journey is the process of actualization via integrating transrational knowledge. And it can be more than this, part of the suffering unconscious reaching out to communion with, 'infinite life in the countless forms of existence'.[102]

Characters like Esther get transfixed on death seeing it as annihilating all. This is where she is mistaken and many have followed the suicide cult of Plath. The secret for followers of Campbell is that death is not a finality. Insanity can be described as an unwillingness to allow this journey, pre-empting it, or bringing it on too soon by suicide. Maeve O'Brien turns traditional analysis on its head concerning women finding their voice, maintaining that women writers have a proximity to silence throughout history. Plath made conscious decisions concerning her isolation to enable her writing. Silence in her writing is used poetically to problematize horror. Her radical departure into silence was to break free from the restrictions of Standard English to restore an autonomy.[103]

The Bell Jar subverts traditional narratives, as does another book involving female suicide, Richard Yates' novel *Revolutionary Road* adapted for cinema by Sam Mendes in 2008. In these types of fictions there is often the 'mad' prophet figure, like Mose Harper (Hank Worden) in *The Searchers* (John Ford, 1956).[104] In *Revolutionary Road* it is John Givings, Jr. (Michael Shannon), son of estate agent Helen Givings (Kathy Bates) who finds the perfect couple (April and Frank Wheeler played by Kate Winslet and Leonardo Di Caprio in the film) a house. John is a genius mathematician who has had a breakdown. Once he has left an insane asylum, he confronts this apparently perfect couple seeing through their lies. Like a soothsayer in a Greek tragedy, his role is to warn us of the horror about to unfold.

All April wants is to live in Paris which Frank agrees with initially, but when he receives a promotion Franks sees France as a pipedream. Like Plath in real life, April sticks her head in their oven gassing herself. Both Plath and Yates are writing from the position of white privilege that goes wrong embedding their narratives with

---

[101] Joseph Campbell, *The Hero's Journey* (London: HarperCollins, 1990).

[102] C.G. Jung, *Psychological Reflections. An Anthology of the Writings of C.G. Jung*, ed. Jolande Jacobi (London: Routledge & Kegan Paul, 1986), p. 270.

[103] Maeve O'Brien, 'The courage of shutting-up: decisions of silence in the work of Sylvia Plath', unpublished PhD, University of Ulster, 2017.

[104] Jason Lee (CJP Lee), *The Metaphysics of Mass Art, Vol. II* (New York: Mellen, 1999b), p. 25–35.

autobiographical elements, exposing the American dream as an American nightmare; the false happiness and obsession for perfection a drive to avoid the void. There is tangible despair following a period of war with the growth of existentialism. Many died for what they thought was the sake of their country, but then started to question their allegiances. The children are now carrying the aftermath of post-traumatic stress disorder.

There is another way to examine the criticism of Plath's work and women positioned within this genre, those 'crazed' authors who are known to have mental illnesses such as schizophrenia, bipolar disorder, and depression. A non-psychoanalytical view argues that such a reading is positioned by patriarchal norms.[105] Areas of mental illness are then linked to disabilities studies. A patriarchal approach means disabled women are undermined. 'Madwoman theory' prioritizes a disablist view arguing that any diagnostic terminology is wrong including that which is used to examine fictitious characters and authors.[106] This approach promotes a future that enables the voices of disabled women taking a priority over the reductive diagnostic patriarchal paradigm.

Evidence from group therapy treatment centres for sex offenders shows that repressed hostility towards the mother is one of the most common unconscious motivations for violent rape.[107] Writing originally in 1973, in her 1986 collection of essays and journalism *The Madwoman's Underclothes* Greer is over optimistic given little progress has been made since. There is for Greer a need for authenticity in sexual relationships, but she in part blames the media and what she calls 'the permissive society'.[108] She claims masturbation and fantasy have got in the way of reality.[109] Greer's central fictional example comes from *The Bell Jar* originally published in 1963, explaining how the protagonist Esther Greenwood has an encounter with a man called Marco who has brought her, 'to the beginning of the end'.[110] Marco sees all women as sluts who are uniform, merely identical playing cards in a pack. Greer and Plath do not blame him for this—this is the way of the world; men are not to blame in general according to Greer. Esther absorbs this psychopathology of oppression, unfortunately, and this is the deeper danger many women can fall into that Greer rejects.

Conceptions of transgression and the uncanny have been applied to Plath's work with Jacqueline Rose's *The Haunting of Sylvia Plath* instrumental in increasing attention to the way in which Plath transgressed boundaries in her writing.[111] This is

---

[105] Maria Rovito, 'Toward a New Madwoman Theory – Reckoning the Pathologization of Sylvia Plath', *Journal of Literary & Cultural Disabilities Studies*, 2020, 14(3), pp. 317–332.

[106] Ibid.

[107] Germaine Greer, *The Madwoman's Underclothes: Selected Journalism 1963–1985* (New York: Atlantic Grove, 1986), p. 163.

[108] Ibid., p. 164.

[109] Ibid.

[110] Sylvia Plath, *The Bell Jar* (London: Faber & Faber, 2010), p. 165.

[111] Jacqueline Rose, *The Haunting of Sylvia Plath* (London: Virago, 2013).

in the modernist and populist approaches and also the boundaries between those fields of work marked as 'masculine' and those viewed as 'feminine'.[112] Feminist writers like Plath highlighted the divisions between writing and typewriting.[113] Literary skills then established strategic affinities with women in the expanding pink-collar proletariat.[114] The sexual division of textual labour is expurgated by such endeavours, and we also find mental health at the heart of the work of one of the most influential feminists since the 1960s, Germaine Greer. Her main issue is with women who have internalized their own pathology making themselves a victim which correlates in part with a Jungian view and that of sociologist Frank Furedi previously discussion. Contradicting the stereotype of a feminist Greer, especially in *The Female Eunuch*, does not primarily blame men for gender inequality.[115]

Due to Greer speaking out on issues since 2017 she was no-platformed at UK universities which could be framed as part of group psychosis discussed in Chap. 7, a form of 'madness' driven by the fear of a different opinion. We have seen 'madness' is the impossibility of dealing with difference, internally and/or externally, and part of this difference is the acceptance of the transrational. Greer is against victimization and victimhood and is optimistic when it comes to feminism and the rights of women. Part of the arguments against Greer in the public domain stemmed from a complex historical context regarding developments of feminism, and her attempts to continue to distinguish between sex and gender. It is obvious why feminists wanted to escape perceived biological determinism and the historical myth that women were destined for home life rather than the professional or intellectual life.[116] What was less obvious was how this was in part resolved.

The work of French feminist theorist Monique Wittig and American philosopher Judith Butler in the 1980s could lead to the observation that it is the division between men and women that naturalizes a social phenomenon of oppression so there is a clear solution; go beyond biological determinism by overcoming biological necessity and within this logic gender and sex are one.[117] But there is also a more ambitious approach that Butler recognises on a revolutionary front which can get overlooked when identity politics usurps intersectional class struggle. Calls for a feminist strike in Central and Latin America and globally by Verónica Gago unifies the praxis of international revolution through attacking patriarchal finance under

[112] A. Jernigan, 'Paraliterary Labors in Sylvia Plath's *The Bell Jar*', *Modern Fiction Studies*, Vol. 60, No. 1, Spring 2014, pp. 1–27.

[113] Ibid.

[114] Ibid.

[115] Germaine Greer, *The Female Eunuch* (London: MacGibbon & Kee, 1970).

[116] Kathleen Stock, *Material Girls – Why Reality Matters for Feminism* (London: Fleet, 2021), p. 15.

[117] Ibid.

neoliberalism.[118] The latter within this framework is positioned as a form of state terrorism directed against women and indigenous cultures.[119]

3.4 Sexuality and Adolescence

Controversies regarding childhood and sex are arguably as volatile as wars between transgender activists and critical feminists. Controversy has followed screenwriter and director Harmony Korine since he wrote the film *Kids* (Larry Clark, 1995) which focuses on New York teenagers having sex. The film encapsulates moments of sexually transgressive transitions from childhood to adulthood, the 'madness' of youth, and poignant transrational knowledge. In what ways can we understand enjoyment and pleasure in relation to *Kids*? This returns us to Chap. 1 and the happiness industry, film in one sense being part of this industry. How does this film function in terms of morality, an area that we have seen throughout is closely allied to framing 'madness'? What are the ethical implications concerning youth culture in relation to Korine's work? Immoral behaviour often involves duplicity which relates to evil discussed in Chap. 2, and this film reveals endemic duplicity. How does this relate to cultural studies, film theory, aesthetics, and further approaches to gender studies and sexuality? This approach reveals nihilism in American culture can be considered optimistically with regards to difference, presence, and becoming, as conceived by Luce Irigaray through an awareness of transrational knowledge.

Since the release of *Kids* there has been an ongoing obsession with children and sex and as James Kincaid has shown this is nothing new and is the foundation of recent popular culture. The excessive, simultaneous, media worship and scorn, in the mid-1990s, of Harmony Korine, the 21-year-old screenwriter of *Kids* (Larry Clark, 1995) indicated Korine was powerfully unearthing divisive issues of the period concerning youth culture and boundaries. Interviewed by *The Guardian* in June 2015 in preparation for the twentieth anniversary screening Korine claimed there was no way the film could be made now. People would see the film as far too dangerous, so it just would never get off the ground. Since the 1990s and an American teen obsession with sex and weed as revealed in *Kids* the data indicates this obsession was depleting over time. For example, teen birth rates hit a record low in 2017, *Time* reporting in 2018 a drop in American students claiming they have ever had sexual intercourse from 47% in 2005 to 41% in 2015.[120] This film is therefore significant in our wider context due to it tackling youth, sexuality and 'madness' and

---

[118] Judith Butler's introduction to Verónica Gago in *Feminist International – How to change everything*, trans. Liz Mason-Deese (London: Verso, 2020).

[119] Ibid.

[120] Alexandra Sifferlin, 'Fewer High School Students Are Having Sex', *Time*, January 4, 2018, https://yahoo.com/news/fewer-high-school-students-having-180241040.html (accessed 26 January, 2023).

transrational knowledge, but for Korine the film depicted normality. Overall, this was far less contrived than ordinary filmmaking with Clark not having directed before and the actors not having acted.

Given the depiction of sex and drugs it received an NC-17 rating. Miramax paid $3.5 million to distribute the film worldwide, but because they were owned by Disney they could not release it. Miramax started a new company to release the now unrated film. The film created moral panic, with Rita Kempley writing in her 25 August 1995 review for *The Washington Post* that *Kids* is, 'virtually child pornography disguised as a cautionary documentary'.[121] While being condemned with Clark as the devil incarnate, Korine was simultaneously feted as the new messiah figure of film. Following his directorial debut *Gummo* (1997), Bernardo Bertolucci claimed Korine could create a revolution in the language of cinema.[122] Cary Woods of Independent Pictures compared Korine to Sam Shepherd and figures such as Oliver Stone and Martin Scorsese proclaimed they wanted to work with him.[123]

Kids' apparently shocking nature has been emphasized by many critics, but other elements, such as its deeply moral stance have been overlooked, due to a typical binary discourse that dominates the media. As part of the audience, we can hopefully dialectically enjoy and even learn from the so-called immoral and the moral elements and this is the essence of the analysis here. *Kids* was inspired by real events in New York City when primarily due to AIDS condoms were being handed out to adolescents who wore them around their necks. Some chose to not use them and just have sex with virgins instead.[124] For Korine the activities in this film are normal, but writing for *The Washington Post* Kempley claimed people would not recognise their own kids here, and that the central problem of the film was the lack of characterisation and communication, Clark being compared to the character Jennie (Chloe Sevigny).[125] In this context the director cannot win; because he does not preach he is attacked for seemingly not having an opinion. The film might be viewed as a purely masculine trajectory in terms of the protagonists' development, but the nihilism of the sex is non-gendered.

At Steven's party, Tally (Leo Fitzpatrick), aged approximately 16, has sex with the virgin Darcy (Yakira Pequero) aged 14. Given the age of consent varies globally this might not be considered controversial, but this is constructed as abusive and not morally correct, so the film is condemning this action. The film takes place within 24 h, opening on Tally having sex with another virgin who may be just 13. Jennie,

---

[121] Kempley, Rita. "Review of *Kids*." *The Washington Post*, 25 August 1995, available online, http://www.washingtonpost.com/wpsrv/style/longterm/movies/videos/kidsnrkempley_c029f5.htm (accessed 23 March 2018)

[122] Elayne Taylor. "Script Comments." *Creative Screenwriting*, Vol. 7 No. 1., January/February (2000): 14–15.

[123] Ibid.

[124] Jason Lee, 'Are You Kidding? Reassessing morality, sexuality and desire in *Kids*', *Film International*, Volume 16, Issue 3, September 2018, pp. 16–26.

[125] Kempley, op. cit.

Tally's previous conquest, tests positive for HIV. She tries to confront Tally, takes a pill in a nightclub, and by the time she arrives at Steven's party she is nearly unconscious. Discovering her former sexual partner and virus spreader having sex with a minor, she says nothing. Falling into a comatose-sleep Jennie is raped by Tally's best-buddy Casper (Justin Pierce). This blatantly controversial content, along with the documentary style combined with elements of expressionistic and naturalistic cinematography, produces a powerful and disturbing film.

There are mesmerising moments when time appears to standstill, functioning as a backdrop to the frenetic lives of the 'lost kids' and *Kids* raises important ethical questions. What is permissible, how can we tackle such material, and is there a boundary? Director Larry Clark was accused at the time of its first release of being a voyeuristic, like a 'dirty old man', along with the film's audience. Simultaneously, in an age that claims to have seen everything, the artist needs to delve further into darker areas and, as Jean Luc-Nancy explained, the reality of our time, the actuality and necessity of our present, is to present the limit as such.[126] There is no proven reason, as Mulvey assumes, that we project our repressed desires onto these performers.[127] Psychoanalytical approaches such as this myopically ignore the moral content and the transrational dimensions that shall be explained here. An adaptation of a Freudian view is at fault because it demonises the unconscious as a repository of repressed material banished there due to it being unacceptable.[128] In this volume we have seen how the transrational and the unconscious are not merely a trash can and incorporate far more than repressed material that is deemed unacceptable and to some evil.

Arguably, there is no subject more heated than child sexual abuse and it is behind innumerable narratives of 'madness' and often given as the cause of 'madness', but *Kids* operates in the nebulous world of adolescent children having sex with adolescent children. These might be kids, but they are also adolescents, many having gone through puberty, often making deliberate choices enjoying consensual sexual relationships. Since the early 1980s many American and European films have dealt with the subject of child sexual abuse. The story of abuse is ideal because it offers numerous scenarios for triumph over tragedy, for secrets to be exposed and for the truth to be made manifest. Plus, it allows for the nuances of doubt, given truth and memory can never be fully equated, which reflects on the whole nature of storytelling and narrative.

As with stories of 'madness' child sexual abuse discourse often involves 'mad' monsters who are defined and delineated then supposedly ejected. But, as with all discourse on evil, to split the abuser off, to place him or her elsewhere as a foreigner is to place them nowhere offering the other a dangerous omniscient power. Are we right to even think about this film in the context of child sexual abuse? According to

---

[126] Jean-Luc Nancy. *The Gravity of Thought*, trans. François Raffoul and Gregory Rocco. New York: Humanity Books, 1999.

[127] Laura Mulvey, 'Visual Pleasure and Narrative Cinema', *Screen*, `6:3, Autumn 1975, pp. 6–18.

[128] Anthony Storr, *The Dynamics of Creation* (London: Penguin, 1993), p. 263.

David Finkelhor, the most cited expert in the field during the 1980s and early 1990s when this film was made, sexual victimization of children takes place when there is a sexual encounter between children under the age of 13 with a person at least 5 years their senior, and encounters of children 13 to 16 with persons at least 10 years older.[129] Within this definition Korine's screenplay is not about abuse, but it clearly is not all about consensual intimacy based on equality. The film moves beyond the binary didacticism many critics called for entering an arena of transrational ambiguity where art operates at its highest making it highly appropriate for our analysis.

The film is concerned with homosocial bonding Casper having sex with Jennie the closest he will get to sex with Tally.[130] Neither of the boys allow their sexual partners enjoyment, eliminating equality, but also situating sex as death. The final shot of the film is Casper waking up at daybreak and there is a point of view shot, but the exact horror of what Casper views is not presented so this ambiguity accentuates the film's power. His exclamation, 'Jesus Christ, what happened!' may lead to the conclusion that, like Jennie, he was unconscious when he raped her. Whether this is child sexual abuse or adult rape is debatable given both participants are of the same age, unaware of their actions due to intoxication. The UK was the only country to censor the film with forty seconds being cut due to a law that states it is illegal to have a child in the same room as simulated sex. During the scene when Casper rapes Jennie a boy wakes up just as Jennie observed Tally 'take advantage' of Darcy and did nothing. Jennie does stir here, as Casper pushes her legs up, and may be taking comfort in sex after the nightmare of discovering she is HIV positive. Within this trajectory, despite her failed attempt to warn other girls, at least Jennie is aware she has HIV. For Tally and the rest of the boys this realization would be impossible. They are too young, or just too lucky, to have HIV. For Irigaray **the spread of all illness has an economic motivation, and she questions why during our period diseases of the immune system proliferate blaming the 'madness' of everyday life.**[131]

Philosophically, *Kids* is an existential work, and its 'mad' nihilism is tinged with a romantic poignancy, functioning as a moral warning. Despite Jenny being unconscious there is a question over revenge; through have sex with Casper she may possibly give him HIV subversively attacking Tally. Another more plausible scenario is that Casper upon awaking sees the results of his abuse of Jennie, her possible suicide, hence his extreme reaction. On a deeper level the statement may also be a question, as in 'Jesus Christ, what happened?' This is the final interrogation of and for the film's audience. The audience is placed in Jennie's position during the final shot—unconsciously molested—when Casper almost addresses the camera. Will we, like Jennie, be raped if we do not stop rape in general the larger questions being are we unconsciously undergoing rape, has society already been destroyed by such

[129] David Glasser and S. Frosh. *Child Sexual Abuse*. London: Macmillan, 1988, p. 5.

[130] Jesse Engdahl and Jim Hosney. "Review of *Kids*." *Film Quarterly*, Vol. 49 No. 2, Winter (1995/6): 39–42.

[131] Irigaray, Luce, *Je, Tu, Nous*, trans. Alison Martin. London: Routledge, 2007, p. 56.

behaviour? These questions are embedded in ambiguity in the film functioning at a deep metaphoric and moral level as a warning. Whether Casper was fully conscious or not, Jennie is over the age of consent. Tally is illegally committing child sexual abuse, in terms of the most current legal frameworks, with his apparent addiction to virgins, although again this is debatable within Finkelhor's definition above. According to Irigaray doctor-patient relationships may have a power element akin to sexual relationships.[132] Like some energy charged doctor, Tally sees the 'pleasure' he is giving as the 'cure'. With regards to civilization, the arrogant war-like bragging conquest nature of sex clearly situated as an invasion within the element of harm is condemned by Irigaray.[133] In her 'I Won't Get AIDS' work, a response to the claim that AIDS would instigate a more responsible and sophisticated form of desire, improving love-making, she claims it is irresponsible to assert illness will resolve problems; sexual repression, denial and nullification, is not the answer, but respect is.[134]

Despite the uproar, paradoxically is *Kids* too moralistic? The trajectory of the two central main protagonists dominates but while pushing homosocial bonding this queer reading leaves out the position of the young women who are articulate and show their clear need not just for relationships, but sex. Young women here are less nihilistic while simultaneously in need of male affirmation. It is fallacious to claim sexual behaviour equals identity but *Kids* takes this premise to an extreme, acting moralistically as a stark warning. Casper, as a young man, is constructed as the most violent, and the most addicted to drugs; but Tally's addiction to sex is shown as far more vindictive, and he leads the way. Importantly, *Kids* closes with Casper, but the central character is Tally whose voice-over narrates the two most important scenes in the film, the opening and the penultimate. Here he repeats himself: 'when you're young nothing matters, all you dream about is pussy'. Korine moralistically reveals the obsessive and damaging nature of adolescent lust which is equated with uncontrolled capitalist greed and domination without boundaries and limits. Despite being made in 1995 this is fundamentally relevant for our times. The paradox is that sexual freedom here functions as a trap to everyone involved, but everyone is already trapped, a theme Charles Bukowski makes abundantly clear in *Tales of Ordinary Madness*.[135]

Narratives are concerned with curiosity directed at the concealed and the hidden body, 'with the concomitant suggestion that the source and meaning of the story is somehow hidden on or within that body'.[136] Jennie's body after being raped by Casper is concealed from view with the source and meaning of this story found mirrored in Casper's face. As Toril Moi observes, 'Freudian theory posits the drive

[132]Ibid., p. 57.

[133]Ibid., p. 58.

[134]Ibid., p. 59.

[135]Bukowski, Charles. *Tales of Ordinary Madness*. London: Virgin, 2009, p. 11.

[136]Peter Brooks, 'The Body in the Field of Vision', *Paragraph*, Vol. 14, No. 1, March (1991), p. 60.

for knowledge (epistemophilia) as crucially bound to the body and sexuality'.[137] But this drive is always inherently frustrated and, 'in the dynamic of narrative, we are always approaching that body, moving toward it, circling it without grasping it'.[138] Is Jennie dead for, at one extreme, the body must be killed before it can be truly represented?

> The body held in the field of vision is par excellence the object of both knowing and desire, knowing as desire, desire as knowing. But since the epistemopholic project is always inherently frustrated, the body is never wholly graspable as an understandable, representable object.[139]

Along with specifying the developments from realism into its modernist phase where, 'the frustrations of knowing produce a questioning of the very epistemophilic project', Peter Brooks correctly claims the, 'observer/knower is put into question, the very principle of knowing—as of possessing—another body comes to appear hopeless'.[140] With regards to relationships between psychology, gender studies, and queer theory this is a revelatory point for even the 'observer/knower' is put into question so the performative construction of identity, ontologically, is just as nebulous. We recognised this previously in Chap. 2 through an analysis of PTSD and identity and this ambiguity concerning identity is an overt aspect of adolescence. This is conspicuously the case with Joey, the son of Walter Berglund one of the three main characters in *Freedom* by Jonathan Franzen.

> The angry words he'd spoken to his father felt pre-formed, as if there were an aggrieved second self inside him 24/7, ordinarily invisible but clearly fully sentient and ready to vent itself, at a moment's notice, in the form of sentences independent of his volition. It made him wonder who his real self was; and this was very disturbing.[141]

Aspects of the cinematography, the long fight sequence, along with the inter-cutting sequences between girls discussing boys and vice versa, plus the coarse dialogue, all add to the film's brutal veracity. This juxtaposition into gender groupings can be seen as a weakness; where, for example are the homosexuals, transsexuals, post-sexual beings? But this is not merely fictional realism. Here the film is a drama that appears as a documentary, particularly in the following sequence which could be used as a sex information broadcast to inform both adults and teenagers about sexual behaviour and beliefs. Both girls and boys brag about their sexual experiences, one girl proclaiming she first had sex with an 18-year-old when 14, but she does not remember his name. This 'bragging' stereotypically accepted as a male behaviour is subverted here by the girl because the fact she does not remember his name is liberating. One traditional reading is that it is a conservative condemnation of the

---

[137] Toril Moi, 'Patriarchal Thought and the Drive for Knowledge', in Teresa Brennan, ed., *New Directions in Psychoanalysis and Feminism* (London: Routledge, 1989), p. 203.

[138] Brooks, op. cit., p. 60.

[139] Ibid, p. 55.

[140] Ibid.

[141] Jonathan Franzen, *Freedom* (London: Fourth Estate, 2011), p. 299.

girl—you were not even aware of who you had sex with! Another interpretation is more liberal—all men are the same, sex is just sex, it is about the sex and personal pleasure, not the relationship.

Gender construction is exemplified in the level of discourse within the groups. The girls' conversation is more mature than the boys, Jennie stating that the beauty of sex is foreplay, another theorizing on the differences between making love, having sex, and fucking. The boys do not believe AIDS exists, as they think they know nobody with AIDS, while the girls realize it does, but one girl admits to having had sex eight to nine times, four of which unprotected. Through revealing the immaturity of the boys, Korine manages to underscore how powerless the girls must really be. The fact that young girls feel compelled to do acts they often find repellent, as they admit just for some semblance of love, is typical yet still shocking. In the language of the film, some girls just suck cocks because they are expected to, but others enjoy it. Lesbianism is noticeable by its absence. This tentative acceptance and expression of pleasure, despite the heteronormativity in terms of sexual acts, might be the most radical element of the film. In some instances, girls are taking control of their sexual pleasure but, like the boys, it is their same-sex non-sexual bonding that is paramount and empowering.

Korine's screenplay emphasizes more differences in opinion in the group of girls than the boys who must outwardly at least agree to set beliefs and behaviours but essentially the girls desire to be desired rather than desire the other. Korine reveals the stereotypical gendered power relationships that are already formed at this significant age; the gullibility of the girls matches the manipulative authority of the boys. The power of the film comes from the deep tragedy of Tally's lovers who are so desperately in need of feeling cared for. Korine's script emphasizes this with Tally's two sex scenes possessing identical dialogue. 'I think if we'd fuck, you'd love it,' is the film's opening line. With this line Tally is trying to convince a girl who only went through puberty a year ago, her love-object teddy bears voyeurs along with us. This is an uncomfortable position to be in, and leads us to question who is 'perverse' here, those watching in the darkened cinema? At least that viewer is situated within a public environment where autonomy is limited; is watching at home even more perverse? Clearly, the real pleasure of the other is not on the protagonist's agenda. It is conquest. Tally repeats this phrase later to Darcy at Steven's party, and once again it works. While the behaviour is chosen and deliberate and carried out with overt will, in a non-binary fashion it also appears 'mad' and uncontrollable.

Despite the various legal definitions Korine makes it clear that Tally is sexually abusing children to assert a masculine identity. His mission to have sex with virgins is so over his personal identity, including his gendered identity and identification, is ambiguous. After Casper smells a 13-year-old on his hand for the second time Tally declares he wants to 'fuck little babies', meaning Darcy. The girls only want to be cared for, as they put it, but Tally gets what he wants by muttering: 'I love you so much; I think you are beautiful, I think if we fucked you would not believe it, you would love it'. The response is: 'I am scared, and I do not want it to hurt'. The answer to this is: 'I just want to make you happy'. This form of child sexual abuse is positioned as masculine exploitation with the opening and closing of the film repeating the same deceptive behaviour.

Whether all the virgins Tally has had sex with are now HIV positive is another question. He is seemingly unaware that he is a carrier of the virus but he does not care. In scene 13 at Paul's flat Tally attacks the use of condoms and others declare that the AIDS scare is an invention made up by adults, and if they had AIDS and were dying, they would go out and fuck. They claim to not be concerned by death, potentially spreading death in the process. For Foucault, who has been accused of child sexual abuse himself and was an age of consent abolitionist, we demand of sex that it tells us our truth, so in these terms these kids are acting out their truth.[142] The sexual instinct is that which is supposed to be natural, and we often assume natural is good, so Korine plays with the fundamentals of our belief system.

There are several pleasures in *Kids*, including its subversive fictional-documentary format and the variety of genres it ties into. This is a western vampire story, Tally and Casper suck the blood of the young, Tally already being the 'infected' Count Dracula scouring the neighbourhood for his prey and counting his conquests. This is also a mythic buddy movie where the intense love and destructive relationships between Tally and Casper is overt. At Steven's part, Casper sings the theme tune to the cartoon *Casper the Friendly Ghost* reflecting that he may be in many ways already be dead and, in his annihilation, he is destroying everyone and everything else in his path. Tally's diction and pronunciation almost contain a speech impediment with his phraseology akin to a hero in a Western calling his sidekick 'kid' furthering the frontier by his sexual conquests. Casper (the ghost) epitomises the insane 'mad' figure of the West, a living dead phantom, always desiring more experience, more dangers, whatever it takes.[143] The sexual conquest here, by literally raping virgins, functions as a metaphor for the conquest necessary for capitalism's excess growth and unnecessary waste, these two young men literally trying to go beyond all frontiers. Again, paradoxically they question their masculine positions by asserting them.

The sex scenes are less explicit than the violence; for example, in the first scene breasts are shown, but genitals appear nowhere in the film. In American culture observation of sex is a spectator sport. This film is not sexually graphic while managing to capture the blundering and awkward aspects of youth where bodies that are not fully grown are engaging in adult activities. The boys think they are being adults through having sex, asserting themselves aggressively in general, but paradoxically their behaviour is shown to be stunting their development. This is highly moralistic, in a film that has been condemned for being immoral. The opening long kissing scene emphasises the passion of adolescence, while the sex scenes show immaturity and unimaginative sexual behaviour. Again, within a queer reading this can be construed as revealing the limited nature of heterosexuality.

[142] Foucault, Michel. *The History of Sexuality*, trans. Robert Hurley. Paris: Gallimard, 1978, p. 69.

[143] See Jason Lee, *The Metaphysics of Mass Art – Madness and the Savage*, where this figure is explained in some detail, especially in relation to films such as *The Searchers* (John Ford, 1956).

There was a furore upon the release of *Kids*. Among other publications, *LA Weekly* panned the film. *LA Weekly* condemned the film, along with the films of Todd Solondz, for supposedly being part of a new nihilism portraying senseless brutal stories.[144] This is a superficial stance on this film and this style of storytelling. It reveals a resurfacing of moral panic in America concerning sex, after a decade of relative calm and scepticism concerning child sexual abuse claims from 1985.[145] Rather than a form of promotion of nihilism, *Kids* is a condemnation of such senselessness, raising complex questions concerning the construction of gender and sexuality, identity and society. By its denial of queerness, it makes such a reading overt. Tally and Casper are revealed to be ruining lives with Tally betting Casper he can have sex with two virgins in one day, the first girl apparently taking only 15 min to agree.

Importantly, just prior to the bet, a significant subplot momentarily becomes the dominant narrative. The lost life around them causes abusive behaviour—society itself is beyond repair, uncared for, just as these children have nobody that cares. A competition takes place between the boys, but this is not merely nihilism for, as W. Trotter put it, there is, 'reason to believe that the sex impulse becomes secondarily associated with another instinctive feeling of great strength, namely, altruism'.[146] This is where Korine's screenplay becomes deeply profound. As with all good screenplays scenes mirror each other. Just prior to the bet made on a subway car a legless man on a skateboard begs and Casper gives him change. After Casper rapes Jennie a blackout is followed by what at first seems an incongruous sequence shot from a bus, presenting images around New York, mainly homeless stray people. The implication is that this decline into destitution, alcoholism and insanity is a matter of course for Casper, who has sniffed glue since ninth grade, and continues to do so, taking everything possible, urinating in the street, raping girls, and savagely attacking people, but still giving to the poor and being aesthetically sensitive and offering us pleasure.

The paradoxical nature of Jasper's characterisation reveals the complexity of all humanity. The film was based on real experiences. The destructiveness was not contained by the film; Justin Pierce who played Casper and was twenty when the film was made died 5 years later of suicide. This beautiful reflective sequence emphasises the comforting surroundings the kids find themselves in. Despite Tally stealing from his mother, and Casper thieving from a shop, they are middle-class children, whose parents and fathers are noticeably absent. The only adult in the film of any significance is Tally's mother, who smokes while she breastfeeds, lies to her son, and is depressed. The absence of non-kids is profound; adults do not exist, other than mentally ill tramps who are behaving as children. The gendered adolescent groupings therefore construct the gendered behaviour, rather than the construction

---

[144] Taylor, op. cit., p. 14.

[145] Jason Lee, *Pervasive Perversions – Paedophile and Child Sexual Abuse in Media/Culture* (London: Free Association Books, 2005).

[146] W. Trotter, W. *Instincts of the Herd at Peace and War*. London: T. Fisher Unwin, 1917. 51.

through traditional family dynamics. American culture is that of perpetual mindless adolescence. The unfashionable writer and poet Robert Bly elaborates on this insightfully in a comprehensive and lucid fashion.[147] Such behaviour can only limit development, and lead to collective psychosis, 'madness', disease, and premature death.

For African American critic bell hooks the film allies itself with phallocentrism and patriarchy being deeply racist and sexist, but she does add, 'if there is any crime *Kids* exposes it is that this is the culture that white supremacist capitalist patriarchy produces'.[148] The film reveals a collective mentality that appears robotic within a culture of isolation suggesting that there might be a choice, but this choice leads even further into isolation. The sequence where Casper and the gang attack a young man for accidentally barging into Casper reveals the power of group pressure in youth culture, the gang already having verbally abused a mixed-raced homosexual couple walking in the park. Again, this can be seen as repression and denial. Importantly, it is not any explicit homosexual sexual act that causes anger. This brief public display of tender innocent homosexuality (holding hands) is the trigger. There is a self-conscious recognition by Casper that tenderness and love are the other and this must be destroyed. Despite being a film of the 1990s, the film still asks us to question what is acceptable and should be accepted in society today.

If Tally et al. had not had sex at Steven's party Casper would not have been compelled, mechanically and unconsciously, to rape Jennie. Likewise, without the bet and the admiration of Casper, it is certain Tally would not be so rampant his rap-style bragging about sex typically giving him more pleasure than the event itself. The group is observed with the cross between documentary, realist, and expressionist styles, widening the film's perspective. As W. Trotter put it, 'the only medium in which man's mind can function satisfactorily is the herd', which is not only, 'the source of his opinions, his credulities, his disbeliefs, and his weaknesses, but of his altruism, his charity, his enthusiasms, and his power'.[149] The mass of stoned sleeping bodies on Steven's floor is a frequent image towards the film's dénouement. This herd emphasizes their physicality as a congealed mass, the bodies functioning in supposedly adult ways with their minds and emotions stunted and is a subject we examine further in Chap. 7 when we tackle group psychosis.

Over twice the age of Korine and significantly older than his cast, born in 1943 the director Larry Clark was condemned for being a perverted voyeur, but he claimed he was non-judgemental. Despite this criticism, *Kids* is a condemnation of this damaging behaviour. Whether this is a wakeup call to adults is another question. In hooks' opinion when the camera returns to Tally and Darcy and, in soft lighting, focuses on their naked sleeping bodies, this suggests bliss and positions them like innocent children, undermining the violence of their encounter, just as Casper's voice distracts from the violence of rape.[150] A close study of this mass of sleeping

---

[147] Bly, Robert. *The Sibling Society*. London: Penguin, 1997.

[148] bell hooks, *Reel to Real. Race, Sex and Class at the Movies* (London: Routledge, 1996), p. 65.

[149] Trotter, op. cit., p. 42.

bodies suggests that in this form gender differentiation is difficult to ascertain. This is flesh without the other. The boys feel forced to act, but this does not overcome their alienation. And hooks would be correct if the film closed on a romantic framing of Tally and Darcy but, significantly, it ends on Casper's possible awareness of his heinous deed. Does Casper have a final revelation of what he has done and, if he does, is this too late for Jennie anyway? Whatever we personally conclude within this apparent nihilism there is a high sense of morality. There is an acknowledgement of the horror of rape.

Korine's follow up film, now as director as well as writer, *Gummo* (1997), explicitly tackles constructions of gender and includes themes of child sexual abuse. Again, the complete absence of adults, other than as shopkeepers, is palpable. One of the boy's mothers does steal a scene, dancing in the dead boy's father's tap shoes in front of a mirror, her buffoonery suggesting she has failed to enter adulthood. The point is with a 'mad' mother like this the son has no chance. These two films depict 'madness' and sexually active minors within a framework of violence and despair, the absence of adults leading to a borderless zone. Children act uncontrollably on nihilistic desire, trapped in destructive behaviour, and the films function as moral warnings. An interpretation that utilises approaches from gender studies and queer theory is beneficial, revealing such behaviours are not inevitable but socially constructed, with a more flexible gendering less dangerous and draconian.

The work of Allen Ginsberg, central to the gay liberation movement and the sexual revolution, is relevant here. Ginsberg explained that gay politics had not dealt with disillusionment with the body and that the gay liberation movement would have to come to terms with the limitations of sex. He criticized the movement for its emphasis on overt 'gayness' which he believed took away the beauty of the lightness of love. He explained that Hindus, Buddhists, Hare Krishna's, and even Christian fundamentalists, all offered a warning about the body, a warning about attachment itself. His homosexual friend William Burroughs had written about sex being another form of junk, 'a commodity, consumption encouraged by the state to keep people enslaved to their bodies . . . filled with fear and shock and pain and threat, so they can be kept in place'.[151] These are counter-intuitive radical observations connected to the sexual revolution and 1960s counter culture, already highlighted in Chap. 1 as part of a movement to non-binary transrational knowledge. *Kids* unveils this to be the case with the male protagonists captive in a competitive destructive battle that however transgressive it may appear at first mirrors the state embodying state control.

In *Kids* the consequence of this behaviour is extreme. The young and supposedly healthy become diseased, growing old dying before their time. Child sexual abuse is equated with familial and social dysfunction, annihilation, and death. For hooks,

[150] hooks [sic], op. cit., p. 63.

[151] Allen Ginsberg, *Spontaneous Mind. Selected Interviews 1958–1996*, ed. David Carter. New York: Perennial, 2001, p. 309.

Kids is reactionary acting, 'complicity with those cultural forces that view the dilemmas in teenage life as solely a function of the absence of coercive control and authority'.[152] According to Judith Butler there is no gender identity behind the expression of identity.[153] The lack of adult men, the main conductors of abuse, leads to children carrying out abuse, mimicking the father figure even in his absence. When Tally finally completes his mission and has sex with Darcy her pain is depicted. This is not love or enjoyable sex, but torture. Casper observes this and is spurred on to rape Jennie by voyeuristically partaking in Tally's actions with Darcy. Given her sex-death wish, Jennie could be considered a form of 'willing victim' as Lydia Lunch put it, one that prefers pain to nothingness.[154] And it is useful to consider this style of victimhood in general, as the girls in *Kids* do little to avoid exploitation with pain being better than the void.

Shots of people in parks and on the street, some exercising or ranting insanely, reveal the external world that Tally and Casper must face up to. Tally does question Casper's brain-damaging behaviour and Casper may finally question his own behaviour and therefore Tally's. The central characters name Tally refers to the phrase tallying up, as in counting his conquests with the activity of sex portrayed as the gathering of units in a capitalist fashion. In this sense these conquests equate with Irigaray's position that people are looking for 'an identity-space' which tallies with accumulation, such as the number of 'matches played', or 'miles covered', in a masculine sense, other than a human one.[155] *Kids* is one of many popular narratives concerned with traces of abuse that reveal the horrific outcome of apparent child sexual abuse with death and destruction and 'madness' depicted and child sexual abuse becomes symbolic of the wounded nature of humanity; it is the, 'cry of our own collective pain at the loss of our own social identity'.[156]

While Korine focuses on the life of these kids the whole outside 'mad' world is reflected upon and clearly examined; capitalist ideology situates people as units, objects for possession, consumption, and exploitation. Capitalism and sexual transgression become natural partners and there is nothing shocking or unusual about this. In cultures where sex is situated as aggressive self-fulfilment within competitive capitalism the sexual abuse of children, and the resulting 'madness', should not be surprising. In *Kids* external social fragmentation is proffered as the reason why children sexually abuse other children. Nihilism has been central to this analysis, but this concerns a feasible future incorporating the transrational, a subject we shall conclude with in Chap. 8. The paradoxes extrapolated through this analysis of *Kids* can be further explained via Luce Irigaray's work on love; nihilism is useful here

[152]hooks, op. cit, p. 167.

[153]Judith Butler, *Gender Trouble: Feminism and the Subversion of Identity* (London: Routledge, 1992).

[154]Lydia Lunch in Jason Sergeant, *Deathtripping. An Illustrated History of the Cinema of Transgression* (London: Creation Books, 1999), p. 180.

[155]Luce Irigaray, *Je, Tu, Nous*, trans. Alison Martin (London: Routledge, 2007).

[156]Chris Jenks, *Childhood.* London: Routledge, 1996, p. 109.

because in order, 'to meet with the other, I must first let be, even restore, the nothing that separates us'.[157]

From this perspective *Kids* can be seen as an attack on Western culture which positions all as the same within the world, not allowing for, 'the strangeness of the other, the recognition of a nothing in common calling into question the proper of each one'.[158] The characters in *Kids* are all striving for some form of pleasure, but the challenge is fundamentally to the audience and there is a basic understanding of this in the voice-over. Being so far away from death chronologically, but embodying death in behaviours, these kids can take risks and position themselves on the limit feeling more alive. They act out violence against difference, such as the brutal attack on the homosexuals, but this is constructed as an attack on the Real, implying a queer position on *Kids* is valid. Deeper than a manifestation of frustration and repression it leads us to question why such violence has taken hold at such a young age, given there is still beauty and charity in these characters, especially Casper.[159] The binary opposition is not just of the gendered worlds, but the physical worlds. The adolescents have their parties, clubs, and mainly interior worlds of bedrooms; the street people possess their alcohol and 'madness', functioning as a barrier and zone that is a transit to the exterior adult world. Both worlds contain strong romantic elements where freedom and liberty are physically and metaphysically embodied, aesthetically represented as beauty itself. The non-binary approach is in the cinematography, combining fictional and non-fictional footage. These worlds clash and merge raising deeper questions about the future providing transrational knowledge, making us consider our position as an audience and our responsibility. The nihilism is a challenge to our traditional binary thinking. The undertaking of the creation, 'will no longer result from the homologation in the same but from a relation to which difference remains the condition of presence and the source of becoming'.[160]

3.5 Conclusions: Feminism and Celebrity

The use of the term objectification became a type of Esperanto in feminist media studies but is highly problematic and under problematized.[161] The term implies a natural authenticity exists framed within white middle class discourse and that further issues over race and class are inferior, but intersectional discourse has

---

[157] Luce Irigaray, *The Way of Love*, trans. Heidi Bostic and Stephen Pluháek (London: Continuum, 2002), p. 168.

[158] Ibid.

[159] Justin Charles Pierce, the London born actor playing Caspar, died by hanging July 10, 2000, in Las Vegas aged 25. Termed suicide, this can be a sexual act; the binary of fiction and fact was once more transcended.

[160] Irigaray, op. cit., p. 171.

[161] Feona Attwood, 'Sex on Stage: Rethinking the Sexual Vocabularies of Objectification', Research Seminar, University of Northumbria, 5 May, 2021.

attempted to address this. Similarly, the success of the #MeToo movement has been situated in a 'me, not you' zone which involves policing the borders rather than equality.[162] Looked at historically, little has changed. In the 1990s we were informed we had the self-objectification by women that resulted in women having a negative self-image which in turn was supposed to be dictating men's behaviour. None of this particularly complexified any male and female experiences and was explicitly and unfortunately binary. From 2000 we then supposedly had the pornification of society.[163] This was not merely through sex, or even addiction to pornography, but through addiction to every form of behaviour imaginable from video games to best-seller lists to the extremes of commodification. Media consumption now became overtly pathologized and gendered. For example, in 2007 the American Psychological Association issued a damning report on sexualization and how girls see themselves in narrow terms as objects and the theory of objectification was used in a blanket manner overlooking nuances. Sex and related areas that did not fit within regulated norms and standards were seen as exploitative and damaging to men and women which filtered into all areas including fashion.[164] This brokered the defining paradigms of permitted external and internal spaces for so-called respectable femininity.

Simultaneously, from Britney Spears to Miley Cyrus alternative spaces of discourse were played out in media culture. Contemporary public images of female transgression are even more problematical, the theme of addiction blurring the boundaries between normal and pathological, self and other, life and death, and male and female, in the cultural imagination of second-order modernity.[165] There is an attraction, an addiction of sorts, to images of female celebrity as 'damaged goods', especially the transgressive image which functions by drawing the reader and viewer into the intimate and tragic regions of celebrity as click-bait. On a deeper symbolic level the theme, 'pronounces and reflects certain aspects of gendered identity roles'.[166]'The female body, transgression, and addiction operate in the narrative landscape in which the fascination for repulsiveness works in a way similar to Julia Kristeva's idea of abjection'.[167] Culture is then divorced from the threatening world of animalism and from 'primitive instincts'.[168] This transgression is an exception to the male ideal so the pathologically addicted female body 'doubles' the transgression, 'embodying not only the female body and the cultural norms

[162] Ibid.

[163] Ibid.

[164] Ibid.

[165] M. Hellman and V. Rantala, 'Codependence, Madness, and Glamour,' in J. Lee, *Cultures of Addiction* (New York: Cambria, 2012), p. 177.

[166] Ibid.

[167] Ibid.

[168] Ibid.

associated with it but also the primeval processes of addiction'.[169] This is also at the core of a certain constructions of 'madness', simultaneously repulsive and attractive.

With Britney Spears we have a breach from earlier gendered roles by an acting out of an asexual 'madness'.[170] This includes tom-boyish head shaving as a form of resistance, and the acting out against prescribed stereotypes of the apparently sane caring mother, all within a co-dependent performative media landscape. There is the breaking down here of heteronormativity and an attempt to move beyond being a commodity for all to touch. As we saw in Chap. 2 since its origins the BBC has been self-proclaimed arbiter of health and normalising arm of the government regimenting acceptable class-driven behaviours. In this instance the BBC judges that the, 'once virginal pop star has crossed the line of what will be tolerated'.[171] Rejecting the ideals of female beauty not only equates with 'madness', but a dismantling of the sacred myths of her celebrity concerning purity and youth, acceptance, and what the public should tolerate. This is according to BBC parameters which is the embodiment of the hetero-gender-normative establishment. Here we have the media as judge, jury, and executioner. There is resistance in this removing of the symbol of her prescribed femininity which none of the mainstream media seemed to understand.

The media judges Spears as woman, mother, child, and pop star 'mad' freak and along with other women like Amy Winehouse, in terms of the performance of their roles, condemns them. Their failure in the media's eyes is a failure to conform. Spears was a child star, her manufactured image playing into a Lolita myth at the heart of culture perpetuated by the media.[172] Her break from this role doubles the transgressive power and living on the cusp of the law in transgressive terms is still being defined by the law. In the history of drug literature, 'woman is passive or she does not exist'.[173] Paradoxically, through drugs or 'madness' there could be a level of resistance, as we saw with Charlotte Perkins Gillman's *The Yellow Wallpaper*. Clinical research on 160 users of early intervention for psychosis services found men experienced a greater number of symptoms in total and more delusions while women experienced a greater number of hallucinations including tactile ones.[174] Men were more likely to experience delusions of being attacked and possessing extraordinary powers; women experienced themes of people not being who they seem, hearing noises, and being touched and these gender differences are partially caused by different life experiences, including substance misuse and sexual abuse.[175]

[169] Ibid.

[170] Ibid., p. 182.

[171] Ibid., p. 187.

[172] Lee 2005.

[173] N. Prowse, 'Tracking Cixous's Medusa', in Lee (2012), op. cit, p. 8.

[174] Amy Jones, Gender Differences in the Experience of Psychosis', unpublished PhD, University of East London, 2018, p. 1.

[175] Ibid.

This chapter has traversed transrational trajectories concerning gender, class, sexuality, and 'madness', explicating seminal texts highlighting a failure in patriarchy revealing resistance as 'madness' and 'madness' as resistance. The importance of the transrational and the transgressive has been found and the problems of language in the West have been elaborated on further and how writing can be used subversively. In feminist theory that attempted to move away from Lacan to circumvent the view of woman as lack and the deficient mirror of man writing becomes the springboard for transgressive and transrational thought. We should not underestimate the power of this, but what happens when we attempt to go beyond the word? The converse side of integral reality is that perception has become the aesthetic abolishing the line between subject and object so, 'everything is verified by adherence to, by confusion with, its own image'.[176] Despite Warholian democratization of art via the power of reduplication the worship of the image epitomized by celebrity culture, including the self-image, is a regressive step.

Ownership of the performative self via an image that is self-constructed or performing on a reality television breaks divisions in a degenerative fashion offering false power. The operation of visibility can be equated with the banal, such as reality television where, 'everything is put on view and you realize there no longer is anything to see'.[177] But what exactly are we looking for? Exposing yourself in this fashion, or as an influencer on YouTube, or confessional star of a similar nature, means everything is put out there, so no secret is left. There is no inner world left, so no reality beyond the image. 'Is this self-expression the ultimate form of confession that Foucault spoke of?'.[178] This relates to being readable every second, to being fully exposed like the repetitive flasher, but could be a way to hide in plain sight.

'Madness' is at the heart of this ubiquity of semblance and while it would be inaccurate to condemn social media as an entirely alienating force the communities it creates can be dangerous. The liberation from when everyone becomes editors, critics, translators, and (co)authors of poor images is matched by the contradictions of the contemporary crowd.[179] The image here is the affective condition of the crowd: its neurosis, paranoia, and fear and this includes a flattening-out of visual content where economies of knowledge rip images out of context which is part of permanent capitalist deterritorialization.[180] To borrow Félix Guattari's phrase, this is capital's semiotic turn with flexible data-packages integrated into, 'ever-newer combinations and sequences'.[181] This means a prioritization of previews over screenings, compressed attention on impression rather than immersion, and a dispersal which optimistically leads to political global alliances amongst networks.[182]

---

[176] Baudrillard, op. cit., p. 60.

[177] Ibid., p. 73.

[178] Ibid.

[179] Hito Steyerl, *The Wretched of the Screen* (Berlin: Sternberg, 2012), p. 41.

[180] Ibid.

[181] Ibid.

[182] Ibid, p. 42.

Directors such as David Fincher in *Fight Club* (1999) built on the theme of mental breakdown in relation to capitalism's alienation and social breakdown, positioning this in a wider zone of conspiracy theory.

'Well-functioning people are able to accept individual differences and acknowledge the humanity of others'.[183] Accepting difference is key to human understanding, but many groups by definition deny difference. What in the past may have been thought of as paranoid and delusional has now become the new norm. According to the DMU a belief is not delusional when it is held by a person's 'culture or subculture'.[184] Those who the psychiatric establishment previously considered delusional can cure themselves, 'by seeking and joining an online community of like minds'.[185] No longer were you considered 'mad' to believe in an interconnected evil elite at the heart of all events, such as reptiles from another planet. Since 9/11 it was even more common to believe in these conspiracy myths. These were the new unifying narratives in a fragmenting world—'madness' in this guise was the new normal. Belief in these theories was a symptom and cause of wider fears which were embedded artistically in film and media narratives.

Discussing the murder of British television presenter Jill Dando in 1999 Sir Richard Henriques, who worked on the case in 2000 and 2007, argues that the process failed in instilling public confidence in the criminal justice system.[186] Barry George, who falsely claimed he was the cousin of lead singer of Queen Freddie Mercury among other aliases, served 7 years for Dando's murder then was exonerated and John Lennon, Gianni Versace and Rebecca Schaeffer were all shot dead outside their homes 'by dysfunctional obsessives' according to Henriques.[187] Behind the image is the notion that something has disappeared, hence the iconoclast denouncement of icons for making God disappear.[188] Due to endless reduplication on multiple platforms, celebrities' deaths become immortalized and God-like. Death is behind the image, any image but, 'digital, numerical production erases the image as *analogon*'.[189] The real is erased as something that can be imagined and the fetishization of images means things are never just objects. This is 'magical thought' where things are invested with 'supernatural powers' and is a materialist take with the commodity a, 'condensation of social forces'.[190]

Framing these celebrity narratives as the work of the 'mad' can dismiss them, as observed to define 'madness' or pathology in terms of functionality is inaccurate. As well as fan worship becoming pathological celebrities have often led troubled 'mad'

---

[183] Kolk, op. cit., p. 79.

[184] Bridle, op. cit., p 208.

[185] Ibid., p. 210.

[186] Richard Henriques, *From Crime to Crime. From Harold Shipman to Operation Midland. 17 cases that shocked the world* (London: Hodder & Stoughton, 2020), pp.171–186.

[187] Ibid., p. 183.

[188] Baudrillard, op. cit., p. 74.

[189] Ibid., p. 75.

[190] Steyerl, op. cit., p. 55.

existences. There is an increase in perceived insanity in certain creative fields, bipolar being a popular recent diagnosis for celebrities.

> Inspiration and madness have in common only the fact the ego is influenced by something emanating from a source beyond its ken, and what artists actually do is very far from being mad. Indeed, when artists become insane, they generally either cease production altogether, or else show a deterioration in their work.[191]

To be creative and original is a risk, stepping outside the status quo which involves danger and is part of the appeal. Albert Camus made a similar point but moves away from an either/or dualistic position—embrace the society of the sign and be utterly superficial or resist the audience and be utterly meaningless and negate life.[192] The media has this role of keeping such things in check and of defining the monstrous.

Are we now the machine's space, the human being the virtual reality, its mirror operator which is the essence of the screen? This is 'real time' with the nature of the virtual being to be empty and be, 'capable of being filled with anything whatever, it is left to you to enter, in real time, into interactivity with the void'.[193] Despite the rapid rise of reality television, along with online influencers via social media, this is not a recent phenomenon. Pierre Boaistuau published *Histoires Prodigieuses* in 1561 when monsters were viewed as omens and writes that of all things that can be contemplated nothing arouses the human spirit more, provoking both terror and admiration than, 'monsters, prodigies, and abominations through which we see the works of nature, inverted, mutilated, truncated'.[194] Today the press functions as a gate-keeper to what is deemed as normal or horrific and monstrous and 'mad'. Advocates for social media argue that it gives everyone a voice and is democratically getting rid of gatekeepers, but the antithesis is just as valid. On top of damaging democracy social media exacerbates constructs and destroys these new mythical monsters through shaming the perceived other. Marina Warner argues the more a work frightens the more it edifies, the more it humiliates the more it uplifts, the more it hides the more it gives the illusion of revealing. 'It is fear one *needs*: the price one pays for coming contentedly to terms with a social body based on irrationality and menace'.[195]

Media images define reality and identity usurping reality, becoming part of integral reality. The problem now is that finding a distance such as a critical, aesthetic, or ethical gaze is problematic, making even political reality difficult.[196] The media offers the framework for definitions of what is perceived to be appropriate, what is sane or insane, and celebrity culture puts a spotlight on this. This fluctuates with the political aspirations and beliefs of editors and is part of social control. Mental health is then defined via politics, driving what is perceived to be

---

[191] Anthony Storr, *The Dynamics of Creation* (London: Penguin, 1991), p. 263.

[192] Albert Camus, *Create Dangerously* (London: Penguin, 2018), p. 6.

[193] Baudrillard, op cit., p. 61.

[194] Bataille (2008), op. cit., p. 53.

[195] Warner (2000), op. cit., p. 184.

[196] Baudrillard, op. cit., p. 59.

normal for many purposes unconcerned with health. In Russia and China political psychiatry is more overt a subject we return to in Chap. 8, but should we be more concerned by covert practices?

In the theology and myths of monotheistic religions naming animals was a way the creator passed on power to the people with naming and language synonymous with power and ownership. 'Madness' contradicts this ownership being the gap in reason, the slip and the glitch in the system, the disruptor. There are numerous strands to 'madness', from the angry to the preposterous, to the endless medical definitions, classifications, and ruminations. Following the work of Darian Leader, we have seen medical definitions are primarily dictated by the pharmaceutical industry's need for profit. This observation does not condemn biomedical models outright, but the system within which it flourishes. Whether in the mental ward, or the maternity ward, woman's position is one of submission to predominantly male experts. 'Madness' could be an escape, a form of withholding compliance. Silence is a form of resistance to language. If language is hard-wired, as some linguists argue, then what is this resistance of? This stretches beyond the normal antagonisms concerning the obvious primal mother and father dynamics of psychoanalysis. In their dystopias George Orwell and Aldous Huxley explained this with social norms centralized. To step outside what is being dictated to by the centre is then insanity and in some cases criminal. Thinking and behaviour that is not 'group think' is anathema reflecting an ideology like Nazism where any form of otherness is relinquished. Here we get to the heart of the challenge of 'madness'; it is the othering of otherness in the extreme and to create a homotopia rather than heterotopia difference needs to be annihilated.

The route from typing to writing with feminist discourse has been examined, but what of the virtual machine and computer which results in hiding and disappearing. Chap. 1 concerned the happiness industry but, 'virtuality comes close to happiness only because it surreptitiously removes all reference from it'.[197] This virtual is not reality any more than science is theology. The course of traditionally perceived history terminated with the advent of the rolling recycled news media. This leads to a stage beyond the critical known as the ironic stage of technology which is followed by the ironic stage of value.[198] 'Madness' offers meaning within a gap of socially defined meaning, freeing us from the original illusion. Often this is without an externalised understanding. The phrase—they are 'mad'—refuses comprehension, positioning the other in a category outside the human which is difficult to reconcile with the view that all beings are as valid as each other. Problems concerning gender, class, sexuality, celebrity, and 'madness' in the context of transgression and the transrational have been examined to overcome binary discourse. Hagiographers, just as the contemporary media, love to document bad news; 'the difference between a saint's prediction of divine retribution and a witch's curse is to the victim merely academic'.[199] Positioning gender with class makes sense given, 'patriarchy is a

[197] Baudrillard, op. cit., p. 63.

[198] Ibid., pp. 63–65.

system where men control most of the money, and use that control to their own advantage'.[200] Under a century and a half ago women could not vote, own property, or control their fertility. There are numerous current outstanding inequalities.

Until October 2019 Northern Irish women were expected to bear their rapists' children. The UK parliament is still constructed so aristocrats pass titles and their seats through the male line. Dismantling patriarchy includes battling covert patriarchy fed by unconscious assumptions.[201] This chapter commenced acknowledging that the category of women materialized as a focus and object of study post-World War 2 along with those of youth and race. Research on the older woman is in its infancy.[202] Once women were set free from bondage to fathers, husbands, sons, and a 'lifetime of being told that they are unstable, unreliable, irrational creatures', they would make a principle out of 'instability and unreason', using superstition to subvert religious and secular authority.[203] This is addressed when examining witchcraft in Chap. 7, and was discussed in Chap. 2 where She believes women accepting witch status is actually empowering. The conclusions to Chap. 1 delineated the problems with language and terminology in a mental health context, and these have been examined further in this chapter. With its crude divisions, sociology sometimes is unhelpful as it tends towards structuralist simplistic divisions of humanity.[204] The danger is this draws us into a binary approach an emphasis on the transrational can avoid. Taking a blanket approach to patriarchy and evil, or patriarchy as oppressive evil, impacting on all in equal measure does have its draw backs. If, as Camilla Long maintains, the de facto position for feminists is 'being in pain', akin to Greer's position previously explained, then what of real pain? We might conclude with Long that all offices then become sexual harassment zones and all dates, in the words of FGM campaigner Nimco Ali, are 'life and death decisions'.[205] One study by psychologists at University College London observed 'victimhood' is spreading; from 100 students each one 'self-identified as having depression or anxiety disorder or both'.[206] A focus on mental health created a situation where everyone thought they were suffering when clinically they were not.[207]

Drawing together the themes of this chapter with the next, we can see that the worship of the 'English rose' ideal has been counter-productive to accessibility for roles, especially for black women in the film and television industries. There is the

[199] Greer (2019), op. cit., p. 404.

[200] Helen Lewis, *Difficult Women. A History of Feminism in 11 Fights* (London: Vintage, 2020), p. 315.

[201] Ibid.

[202] Greer (2019), op. cit.

[203] Ibid., p. 400.

[204] As previously discussed with regards to Rogers and Pilgrim, op. cit.

[205] Camilla Long (2021), 'It's not just rich for Samantha Cameron to claim she's a victim – it's genuinely harmful', *The Sunday Times*, May 9, p. 19.

[206] Ibid.

[207] Ibid.

double Otherness of being black and female, including a 'narrowly reiterative white middle-class femininity' feeding into a nostalgic vision of the past.[208] Cinema is only beginning to address deeply ingrained elements that discriminate doubly and, drawing on Richard Dyer and Cornel West, we can observe that there is an aesthetic assumption of cinematography that the subject is white, plus the film stock, lighting, and make up all privilege the white performer, especially the white women, as 'glowing' and 'angelic'. In truth, whiteness is politically constructed and parasitic on 'Blackness', that is, 'the Other upon which it depends and against which it defines itself'.[209]

Despite a desire for groupings to position identities there is no homogenous group or school of feminism making a genealogy of Black feminism, for example, within specific national cultures difficult.[210] After 1945, however, facing racism and sexism in employment, health, and education, plus endemic police violence still under-recognized today, there was a shared political identity and solidarity which included resistance to the far-right in the 1960s and 1970s in Britain, with significant industrial action by women workers such as that over unfair conditions at the Grunwick photo-processing factory, the Chix factory in Slough, and the Imperial Typewriters in Leicester.[211] In Marxist terms the media is a form of alienation but the mistake is to view the medium of media as merely a technique. We may prefer to base an approach on the imaginary that exceeds limits.[212] Such a move is more in tune with transrational approaches. This chapter's analysis exposed gender, class, and sexuality, as dictating methods for constructing and treating 'madness', deconstructing power by addressing narrative. This is supported by real world qualitative research in Chap. 5 but first 'madness' and the transrational in the context of another overt and covert power dynamic which has profound historical and contemporary resonances is addressed—race.

[208]Melanie Williams, *Female Stars of British Cinema. The Women in Question* (Edinburgh: Edinburgh University Press, 2017), p. 197.

[209]Ibid., p. 198.

[210]Brenna Bhandar and Rafeef Ziadhah, ed., *Revolutionary Feminisms – Conversations on Collective Action and Radical Thought* (London: Verso, 2020).

[211]Ibid.

[212]Baudrillard, op. cit., p. 63.

Chapter 4
Race

4.1 Introduction: Colonial Psychiatry

The conceptualization and division of darkness (as evil) and light (as good) in the West systemic in Christianity has had an inordinate impact on religion, culture, and society feeding racism. Chapter 2 analysed how evil, considered the antithesis of light and the totality of darkness, has been constructed philosophically and in art. Religious art depicts Satan as the quintessence of darkness, so it was only a small step to racial demonization in reality and this was carried out for political and economic purposes, including the protection of the slave trade.[1] If the 'mad' are predominantly constructed as the other then what of alterity and ethnicity? This chapter addresses this dynamic and its transnational dimensions along with the colonial history of psychiatry, engaging with key critical thinkers including Frantz Fanon. We shall understand how the pre-colonial era continued into the post-colonial era governed by racist psychiatric discourse.

The global treatment of the 'mad' has been constructed within a framework of imperialism and colonialism that has a damaging legacy with hegemonic power at its heart. National and imperial aims are pursued using the national culture which is mistakenly sanitized as, 'unchanging intellectual monuments, free from world affiliations'.[2] Psychiatry's development is part of this pattern of colonialism which still has a significant legacy. Postgraduate training in psychiatry has only been undertaken for the past 50 years in Asia, the most complex of continents. As of 2018 in China there were 15,000 psychiatrists for 1.2 billion people (approximately 1: 80,000); the UK has 12,000 for 70 million (approximately 1: 5800); India 1:

[1] Given Christianity's role for and against slavery, it is worth noting that Saint Anselm, who against his will was appointed Archbishop of Canterbury in 1093, obtained from the national council at Westminster the passage of resolution prohibiting the sale of human beings.

[2] Edward Said, *Culture and Imperialism* (London: Routledge, 1994) p. 12.

J. Lee, *Culture, Madness and Wellbeing*, https://doi.org/10.1007/978-3-031-37530-9_4

330,000; Indonesia 450 for 210 million people for over 13,000 islands.[3] In Nigeria in 2002 out of a population of 128 million there were seventy psychiatrists and fourteen psychologists.[4] The majority of the professionals live in the capitals and most senior psychiatrists are UK, France, Russia, Germany or USA trained. Political psychiatry is alive today used globally as a tool to silence protest, the transrational vanquished under the guise of racist scientific rationalism.

In 1916 John E. Lind presented a paper to the Washington Psychoanalytical Society where he noted that African Americans were just a short step from falling into the abyss of mental illness. He imbued mentally ill African Americans with, 'an ontological status that situated their mental disorders—their etiology, their pathology, and, ultimately, their management—within a larger transatlantic discourse'; this meant, 'maintaining particular social orders based on racial difference'.[5] There was a transatlantic dialogue with psychological research in America paralleling colonial research in an attempt to explain why the behaviour of colonial subjects did not meet with the preconceptions of 'primitives'. From the mid-nineteenth century to at least the 1950s this dialogue concerning race and insanity perpetuated. Challenging this hegemonic narrative went against the whole weight of white authority in the areas of medicine, psychiatry, and psychology.

Mental hospitals played a key role in international imperialistic projects and were fundamental in regulating local populations. Conceptions of black 'madness' were part of the larger transatlantic intellectual formation which had real impact on the way African Americans were treated in asylums. Martin Shaw highlights the work of Jonathan Sadowsky in Nigeria where the European system shaped medical treatment via what was perceived to be 'proper behaviour'.[6] The leading journals of the nineteenth century argued that insanity in the 'primitive races' was rare.[7] This included Africans, people of African descent in the Americas, and the indigenous peoples of the Americas, Australia, New Zealand, and the South Pacific. 'Evidence' also came from non-white sources; according to an article in an early issue of the *American Journal of Insanity*, Joseph Cinque, leader of the *Amistad* mutiny whose story was adapted for film (Steven Spielberg, 1997), claimed instances of insanity were rare in his native country.[8]

Whether this was accurate or not, this idea was spread on both sides of the Atlantic, so in the British *Journal of Mental Science* leading expert Daniel H. Tuke could write that mental disease was greater amongst, 'civilized and thinking

[3]R. Clay, 'Psychotherapy in China', *Monitor on Psychology*, Vol. 50, No. 9, 2019, p. 27.

[4]K. Aroyewun-Adekomaiya, Representation of Mental Illness: An Examination of Movies and Professional Perspectives in Nigeria, Unpublished PhD thesis, De Montfort University, 2017.

[5]M. Summers, 'Suitable Care of the African When Inflicted with Insanity': Race, Madness, and Social Order in Comparative Perspective. *Bulletin of the History of Medicine*, Vol. 84, No. 1, Spring 2010, p. 59.

[6]Shaw in Summers, ibid., p. 65.

[7]Ibid., p. 67.

[8]Ibid., p. 68.

people, than in nomadic tribes'.[9] Insanity was viewed as a breakdown of the higher functions plus modern developments were believed to exacerbate it. There was the notion that 'non-civilized' people were non-thinking and therefore had no stress, suffering none of the sense of fear, loss, anticipation, alienation, and regret of those in apparently civilized countries. Many of these theories stemmed from French alienist Dr. Mureau and his travels in Egypt in the mid-nineteenth century who summed up that the more people had to focus on the necessities of life the less insanity he found. Those in present day Sudan and Ethiopia, so the theory went, were supposedly immune to insanity. The same arguments are made today with reference to the American psychologist Abraham Maslow's hierarchy of needs.[10]

These pseudo-scientific anthropological conclusions that fed into mainstream myths were obviously not innocent with key economic, political, and social factors of the period feeding this accepted psychiatric discourse. Americans backing a pro-slavery agenda used these arguments to support their position, claiming the benevolence of the slave owner kept the slave from being vulnerable to mental illness.[11] When it came to freed slaves the position was reversed. Biological racism was employed to argue those freed had underdeveloped nervous systems and this made them more likely to go insane. The relationship between psychiatry and slave owning was clear and a common view amongst psychiatrists in the late nineteenth century was that emancipation had been more traumatic than enslavement.[12] The argument was that civilization drove Africans 'mad', so enslavement was benign. There was also the belief that there were different levels of susceptibility amongst different ethnic groups in the same colony. This view remained far into the mid-twentieth century and beyond.

Psychiatrists and British medical officers believed 'deculturation' or the 'cultural contact' (urbanization, Western education, and exposure to European culture generally), were responsible for rising rates of mental illness within the African population.[13] An argument was constructed that 'mad' Africans may have just become more noticeable and visible, but the consensus was that black 'madness' was fundamentally different to white 'madness'. A system of different disorders manufactured along racial lines was constructed supporting racist dogma. For example, mania was thought to be associated with the deterioration or abnormal development of the 'lower developed strata of the mental organism', and this was 'black madness'.[14] Melancholia was linked to 'higher and latest developed strata', and this was 'white madness'. Others pointed to the 'sexual madness' and

[9] Ibid.

[10] Richard Rohr, *Falling Upwards. A Spirituality for the Two Halves of Life* (London: SPCK, 2011), p. 6.

[11] Summers, op. cit., p. 69.

[12] Ibid., p. 70.

[13] Ibid., p. 72.

[14] Ibid.

'bloodthirstiness' of the 'emancipated negro'.[15] A diagnosis of mania was also found in the Malay Peninsula, but there was a consensus amongst European doctors regarding the differences with the black population across the Caribbean, Africa, and Australia. This construction within psychiatry of these differences had an inverse parallel with intellectual movements resulting in it being contradictory to the universalization found in Lukacs, Althusser, and Marx.[16]

We have previously seen how constructions of diagnoses change over time and place, being temporally and geographically specific and related to financial profit. Significantly, in the context of race by the 1900s psychiatrists were less likely to think of mania and melancholia as different. Following the clinical work of Emil Kraepelin these were now thought of as manic-depressive disorder. A study by Dr. Mary O'Malley of 800 black and white women admitted to Saint Elizabeth's hospital from 1909 to 1914 concluded that manic-depressive disorders were relatively rare among black people.[17] One other study of 3000 black men at Georgia State Sanitorium found the opposite, with black men having a higher incidence of manic-depressive disorder.[18]

While contradictions in this research proliferated, there was an agreement on both sides of the Atlantic using 'hereditarian' and 'civilizationist discourse' into the 1930s that suicide was a rare phenomenon in African American culture and colonial Africa.[19] Recent research has found suicide rates in black children to be twice as high as white children.[20] The accepted idea that those of African descent coped better with psychological turmoil by turning outward rather than inward meant psychiatric discourse added to constructions of black criminality. This had a significant bearing on what treatments were made available and were thought useful. A racialized approached has had a lasting impact to this day. Film and media have been immensely influential in this regard with films such as *Precious* (Lee Daniels, 2009) tackling these myths. Racial archetypes were embedded from this earlier discourse, including the black 'beast rapist', primitive insanity, and manic violence. These subjects are tackled, confronted, and complexified by black writers in the 1950s, such as James Baldwin.

Segregation was conducted within asylums, most superintendents believing mixing would hinder rather than help treatment. As we saw with gender in the previous chapter, asylums mirrored society, but the legacy of slavery within asylums went way beyond the period of emancipation. These asylums would mimic slave plantations in their structure with 'black lodges' in the stable areas. The containment of these black populations in the West was a continuation of the pre-colonial era with psychiatry and the discourse of mental illness enabling this. This mirrored

---

[15] Ibid., p. 75.

[16] Said, op. cit., p. 234.

[17] Summers, op. cit., p. 77.

[18] Ibid.

[19] Ibid.

[20] https://jamanetwork.com/journals/jamapediatrics/article-abstract/2680952?redirect=true

presuppositions in America and in the colonies, such as Nyasaland, Kenya, and Southern Rhodesia, with black inmates viewed as, 'the most dangerous class of people', 'demon-ridden', with, 'queer, almost mythical, cases of human abnormality'.[21]

Constructions of deviance, perversion, and transgression were at the heart of this. Black abnormality was linked to the white criminality along with the idea that white abnormality was akin to the black normal state of being. In colonial terms and in relation to mental illness this was a discourse of difference. 'When confronted with a "mad" African, Europeans had to figure out whether they were "observing the normal abnormality of the colonized or the abnormal abnormality of a sick African"'.[22] This legacy is still influential to constructions of otherness within the popular media today.

4.2 Social Theory

Edward Said's comparative analysis of the work and life of Frantz Fanon with Michel Foucault is germane in terms of social and political discourses in the field of 'madness' and alterity. Fanon was a French West Indian psychiatrist and political philosopher from Martinique whose works are influential beyond psychiatry, most notably in postcolonial studies, critical theory, and Marxism. Foucault from Poitiers, France, is a pre-eminent historian of ideas, theorist, and political activist whose ideas have entered most areas. Fanon treated colonial and metropolitan societies together, but Foucault's work moves away from a consideration of the social by focusing on the individual and the 'microphysics of power'.[23] In this comparison, Said argues convincingly that Foucault's theories became a colonising movement fortifying the individual in the containing system appealing to the individualism of the West; only Fanon ultimately is anti-authoritarian. Fanon encapsulates the non-binary approach advocated throughout this text and is part of a double constituency, 'native' and Western, held in high esteem within a certain paradigm of critical discourse and, taking Said further, it is not difficult to see why. Identity politics often triumphs over the politics of the collective and this had serious consequences for the politics of collective resistance with frequently the wrong enemy identified and attention levied in erroneous directions.

Fanon came to attack the distortions of psychoanalysis as presented by O. Mannoni, in works like *Prospero and Caliban*, where Mannoni maintains that the coming of Europeans was unconsciously expected by the future subjected peoples. 'According to Mannoni, colonization was made possible by an inherent

[21] Summers, op. cit., p. 85.

[22] Ibid., p. 88.

[23] Said, op. cit., p. 336.

dependency complex in the subject populations'.[24] This racism was matched by the further view that, conversely, Europeans were self-dependent and individual. For Fanon this view that colonization was somehow justified was not just anti-historical, but it skewered the objectives of psychoanalysis. Fanon contested the view that dependency complexes related to numbers, power being more important than numbers, pointing out that in Martinique there were 200 white people who considered themselves superior to 3000 members of the colonized population.[25] His reflections on the disciplines of psychiatry and on their inaccuracies led him to politics and in this he followed the inspiration of his mentor Professor Tosquelles who conceived the analyst to be responsible for the same world his patients knew; 'there was no all-pervasive identity of doctor and patient here, only a breaking down of the more rigid and artificial walls that some assumed to separate them'.[26] This is a radical departure, philosophically and politically, in the dynamics of mental health treatment and is still under-acknowledged in the wider mental health and wellbeing movement.

During the 1990s Fanon was condemned by American academics as a founder of terrorism.[27] Foucault was far more acceptable to the academy and filtered within most disciplines, even town planning. Drawing on Husserl, Heidegger, and Merleau-Ponty, and others, Fanon was the first black writer of his generation to use a phenomenological framework to understand the, 'man of colour in the dimension of his being-for-others [*pour-autrui*]'.[28] This was seen as a threat. For Fanon, the black man and white man are not realities; the 'negro' 'is' not (does not exist), and nor 'is' the 'white man'.[29] Trapped in their respective 'whiteness' and 'blackness' they 'are' only insofar as they create one another, but this does not imply reciprocity.[30] This profound point on being trapped resonates with recent discussions of institutional racism and the Black Lives Matter movement. Culture is key, as is media. An emphasis on shame, the veil of the look, is not unique to Fanon's work, from the 'veil of invisibility' of W.E.B. Du Bois's *Souls of Black Folk* (1903) to bell hooks' *Wounds of Passion* (1999).[31] Along with his psychiatric clinical experience, Fanon draws evidence from transrational fictional or semi-fictional texts of the period, such as Abdoulaye Sadji's novel *Nini* (1954), with their immediacy and emotional veracity which have more impact than sociological statistics.[32]

Fanon's work involves moving from the inauthenticity produced by the experience of being under the white gaze and the Martinican colonization that was so brutal

[24] I. Gendzier, *Frantz Fanon: A Critical Study* (New York: Pantheon 1979), p. 58.

[25] Ibid.

[26] Ibid, pp. 59–60.

[27] David Macey, *Frantz Fanon: A Life* (London: Granta, 2000), p. 21.

[28] Ibid., p. 164.

[29] I am aware of the use of the term 'man' being limiting, but I am quoting from sources that use this term.

[30] Macey, op. cit.

[31] Ibid, p. 165.

[32] Ibid., p. 168.

it traumatizes and annihilates. We can fathom how far Fanon was ahead of his time when we consider Islam which the Western media often still relates to 'madness' and evil which Fanon contested. Fanon practiced psychiatry in France and employed all the techniques of the period. He moved to Algeria in 1953 where there was a strong belief on the part of the French colonialists that Islam was pathological. Islam was termed a 'neuropathic state' and symptoms were framed as fatalism, an obsession with words (the repetition of 'Allah, Allah'), delusional sadness, perversion of the sexual instinct (masturbation and pederasty), 'auditory hallucinations that provoke sudden outbursts of violence'.[33] Fanon did not adhere to these views which over half a century are propounded by the nationalist and populist right-wing European press and by American broadcasters such as Fox News in 2020.

Research strategies were fed by a racist dynamic in psychiatry, psychology, and the related fields of mental health, psychotherapy, and sociology. Racial segregation defined research paradigms, strategies, and funding. Research was co-ordinated by a small group of individuals affiliated to the Carnegie Corporation, the Phelps-Stokes Fund, the Rockefeller Foundation, and specialists from the British Colonial Office.[34] Leading scholars, such as anthropologist Bronislaw Malinowski and Frederick Keppel, President of the Carnegie, held the desire to maintain racial boundaries. Philosophies from the American South fuelled apartheid backing thinkers in South Africa. While race mixing was condemned altruism towards 'the coloured races' was promoted, but paramount within all of this was the emphasis on the individual rather than group attainment.[35]

'Madness' and race were considered a tangible threat to social and political governance. The ruling classes were visibly concerned about miscegenation, especially race mixing with the working class, believing the latter would be mentally infected. The theory of the period did not see the problem as the impact of imperialism or racism, but failure to instil Westernization. This failure was deemed as being the cause of a high level of neurosis. Highlighting racism was deemed a mental illness. Race consciousness was thought to be an oversensitivity, a self-consciousness related to mental instability. We this is still highlighted today by those who condemn wokeness as insanity. The danger was also paramount if the white working classes were to be controlled, articles in the magazine *The Spectator* in the 1930s pointing this out.[36] The concern was that the lower classes would not be unable to maintain racial boundaries and this would result in the lowering of the white race to the level of the perceived inferior race. 'Madness' it was believed was spread by affinity. White people who mixed with blacks were considered pathological, 'immoral and weak'.[37]

---

[33] Ibid., p. 221.

[34] Frank Furedi, 'How Sociology Imagined 'Mixed Race'', in David Parker and Miri Song, eds., *Rethinking 'Mixed Race'* (London: Pluto, 2001), p. 23.

[35] This tallies with the predominance of Foucault's approach discussed.

[36] Furedi, op. cit.

[37] Ibid., p. 26.

To move beyond 'madness' would be to accept difference and otherness not as the same, but as valid in and of its own right. This step into transrationality for some is a step too far. The fear is the challenge of difference. Race is a good illustration, raising difficult questions for media and cultural studies. Is it important for people of colour to be represented in the media, for example, as the same proportionally as Caucasians, or is it just as important for people of colour to own the media? One argument is the mainstream media will always be the tool of the elite, in any form, so why enter this world when by doing so an inevitable stripping of identity will occur and a denial.[38] This argument has been partially backed by recent studies of new media which shall be returned to.

There are more people of colour locked up proportionally than white. Would a person of colour, trained in psychiatry by mainly white doctors, be looking for similar traits and thus become an administer of black oppression? Mental hospitals are often where damaged and aggrieved black men and women are contained, preventing them revolting against the power elite. In this sense, the mental hospital becomes the slave plantation feeding the mental health industry. The capitalist system allows for the expense of this containment because to not do so can be a conduit for its downfall. We might concur with Fanon that 'black' and 'white' do not exist as essential categories. They, 'are situational categories defined by the encounter with others'.[39] Fanon claimed that psychoanalysis could not provide an absolute explanation. The, 'theory of phylogeny and ontogeny must be complemented by one of sociogeny: the black man's alienation is not an individual question, and its causes are socially determined'.[40] Neither the history of the human species (phylogenesis), nor the history of the individual (ontogenesis), can explain what is a socio-political phenomenon.[41]

Written in the 1950s and first published in France in 1961, *The Wretched of the Earth* vividly reveals how colonialism through attempts at acculturation instigates mental illness.[42] For Freud, Adler, and Jung, 'primitives' were associated with the unconscious and drives.[43] For Mannoni, the black man is the white man's fear of himself; the unconscious.[44] Fanon argued the white world creates the black's neurosis. A normal black child growing up in a normal black family will be made abnormal by the slightest contact with the white world and the white gaze. This creates the black person as a 'phobogenic and anxiogenic object', so the black person becomes both the object of 'irrational fears' and 'source of anxiety' and the 'phobic object then becomes the screen on to which white fantasies, fear, and guilt, can be

[38] B. Chambers-Cooper, 'British Television Drama and Caribbean Families, unpublished PhD, De Montfort University, 2022.

[39] Macey, op. cit., p. 177.

[40] Ibid., p. 187.

[41] Ibid.

[42] Ibid.

[43] Ibid., p. 188.

[44] Ibid., p. 192.

projected in the form of perverted desires.[45] In today's world of global pandemics, war, and starvation, Fanon's *The Wretched of the Earth* is more relevant than ever. This is especially the case concerning his case studies, where he discusses the psychosis of pregnant refugees, mental disorders, and torture. Fanon confirms that the spread of African culture can only be realized when the practical support to create the conditions necessary for the existence of that culture are present, 'in other words, to the liberation of the whole continent'.[46]

During The Congress on the Dialectics of Liberation held in London at the Roundhouse from 15 July to 30 July 1967 Stokely Carmichael examined individual and institutional racism. He explained that in 10 years two thirds of the 20 million Black Americans living in America would be living in ghettoes in the cities, while white America would flee to the suburbs with Puerto Ricans, Mexican Americans, and Native Americans joining Black Americans. The resources would still be owned by the whites, creating a new order of colonization, capitalism by its nature unable to, 'create structures free from exploitation'.[47] The white population and economy had too much to lose by facing institutional racism, an issue still prevalent in Britain in 2021 with the Conservative government and Metropolitan Police refusing to admit its existence.

In the UK in 2019 it was reported up to the age of 11 the experiences of black and white children were similar, in terms of manifesting mental health symptoms and use of services, but after this point black men experience psychosis 10 times more frequently than white, and are four times more likely to be locked up in mental institutions than white.[48] This does not take into account the number of black people locked up in prisons who have mental health problems. By opposing external oppression and its internalization and moving beyond the tradition at the time what Carmichael attempted was revolutionary. The issue was those leading the field in psychiatry, such as Laing, remained locked in existential-phenomenological discourse and familial influences. Capitalism was seen to be an influence by Laing, but not to the extent that Carmichael framed it as white supremacy.[49] This was leading to fragmentation and psychosis within the black community.

In the 1960s America schizophrenia became less of a diagnosis for passive white females and more of a diagnosis for black Americans.[50] *The Diagnostic and Statistical Manual II* published in 1968 equated 'protest' with mental illness, so in

---

[45] Ibid., p. 193.

[46] Frantz Fanon, *Black Skin, White Mask* (London: Penguin, 1973), p.189. [check]

[47] Stokely Carmichael, David Cooper, R.D. Laing, Herbert Marcuse, *The Dialectics of Liberation* (London: Verso, 2015), p. 161.

[48] Anonymous, 'Discrimination in mental health services', 23 June, 2022, Discrimination in mental health services | Mind, the mental health charity - help for mental health problems (accessed 23 June, 2022).

[49] R. Roberts and Theodor Itten, 'Francis Huxley and the human condition', *The Psychologist*, May 2021, p. 69.

[50] J. Metzl, *The Protest Psychosis: How Schizophrenia Became a Black Disease* (Boston: Beacon Press, 2009).

an era of black protest it became easy to detain black people as 'mad'. The concept post traumatic slavery syndrome (PTSS) became popularized as a way of explaining how deeply slavery and its aftermath impacted on the current condition of black people.[51] The numerous YouTube videos addressing the subject make it sound convincing, but this itself has been condemned as a racist idea by leading black studies intellectuals.[52] The argument against PTSS is that it is premised on black behaviour being genetically predetermined. 'According to the historical record, Black people certainly had the physical scars from slavery, but mentally, they were not scarred'; they, 'as a group do not need to be healed from racist trauma. All Black people need is to be freed from racist trauma'.[53] The former position involving healing is from a psychology and a social work perspective, the latter is from the historical perspective. Again, a binary approach is unhelpful with an either-or position here is unfruitful, as this is defined by disciplinary boundaries.

There is a crisis concerning ethnicity and 'madness' with trauma caused from Central Americans moving north, seeking to escape gang violence and extreme poverty. Between October 2018 and February 2019, 260,000 people left the Northern Triangle (El Salvador, Guatemala, and Honduras), double the previous year.[54] Part of this migration is driven by climate change devastating crops and PTSD, drug problems, and suicidality is the norm. Following the liberation theology movement in the 1970s Jesuit priest Ignacio Martín-Baró developed liberation psychology, calling on psychologists to, 'redefine their role as socio-political and to support oppressed communities'.[55] While politics has been at the heart of some movements in the field, including aspects of a Laingian approach, this synergy between theological, psychological, and sociological political action is radical. Many in the established church condemned this as revolutionary Marxism. Because of isolation and limited resources often people cannot access treatment. Psychological awareness leads to work in areas such as human rights, especially to combat sex-based violence, public corruption, and income inequality. This includes restorative justice for past crimes, as with the Community Studies and Psychosocial Action Team in Guatemala. Other work includes psychotherapeutic treatment for Honduran survivors of torture and sexual violence.[56] Despite all the good work there are limitations. Honduras has a population of nearly nine million with just 185 mental health professionals. In countries with remote rural areas like Guatemala these parts of the country are under served. Across the region health care budgets allocated to mental health is 0.9 percent, mostly funding psychiatric hospitals. The United States

[51] J. DeGruy Leary, *Post Traumatic Slave Syndrome. America's Legacy of Enduring Injury and Healing* (New York: Uptone Press, 2005).

[52] I.X. Kendi, *Stamped From The Beginning. The Definitive History of Racist Ideas in America* (London: Bodley Head, 2017).

[53] Ibid.

[54] Anon., 'Support for Central Americans', *Monitor on Psychology*, Vol. 50, No. 9, 2019, p. 46–52.

[55] Ibid.

[56] Ibid.

spends 8 percent of its health-care budget on mental health.[57] In the UK it is roughly ten percent. Every individual is different and unique and understanding this is key, rather than generalisations, although indigenous groups can assist foreign psychologists in gaining some form of trust and cultural competency.[58]

Demonization works in numerous ways, as does the definition of alterity, and there is a further difficulty for those divided between cultures. For example, second-generation British-Barbadians (Bajan-Brits) returning to the land of their parents are accused by indigenous Barbadian nationals of being 'mad'.[59] Four factors have been found: (1) 'madness' as perceived behavioural and cultural differences; (2) elucidations that relate to the historical-clinical conditions of mental ill health among first-generation West Indian migrants to the United Kingdom; (3) 'madness' as a pathology of alienation from living in Barbados; and (4) 'madness' as 'othering', 'outing' and 'fixity'.[60] British second-generation people returning to the Caribbean raised in the colonial mother country exhibit hybridity and in betweenness so allegations of 'madness' fix the position of these young migrants outside the mainstream of indigenous Barbadian society.[61] Once again it becomes a method of controlling the perceived threat of difference.

4.3 Conclusions: History and Haunting

Historical and cultural trajectories of 'madness', colonialism, postcolonialism, and race, have been delineated, offering insight into versions of 'madness'. One argument proposes that in screen studies film's historical relationship with imperialism, colonialism and racism has been the least researched.[62] Chapter 1 confirmed how in cultural studies mental health has been overlooked when compared to areas such as gender and race, but the film medium since its invention in the late 1800s was powered by white patriarchal privilege and racist representations of Africans, Asians, indigenous communities and, in particular, Black people—still evident today in films and filmmaking practices.[63] A number of studies have examined differences across cultures in the way 'madness' is constructed.[64] Interestingly, there

57 Ibid.

58 Ibid.

59 J. Phillips and R. Potter, '"Black skins and white masks": Postcolonial reflections on 'race', gender and second generation migration to the Caribbean', *Singapore Journal of Tropical Geography*, Vol. 27, Issue 3, November 2006, pp. 309–325.

60 Ibid.

61 Ibid.

62 Robert Stam powerfully noted this in *Film Theory: An Introduction* (Oxford: Blackwell, 2000).

63 Joe Jackson, Call For Submissions, ScreenWorlds, April 26, 2021.

64 See N. Wig, 'Mental Health and Spiritual Values. A view from the East', *International Review of Psychiatry*, No. 11, Issue 2–3, August 1999, pp. 92–96.

is some evidence that there is less stigma regarding mental illness in Muslim and Arab communities.[65] However, interviews conducted for this volume and research in psychiatry confirm there is a poor understanding of mental health in Arab countries which lack services and professionals; mental health problems are framed as physical problems to avoid stigma, plus reliance on a deity and religious leaders can cause problems with women in Arab/Muslim countries at the most risk of mental health issues in politically volatile countries.[66] We have seen how in the West Islam has historically been demonized as 'mad' and when it comes to mediated acts of terror white terrorism is predominantly portrayed in the media as caused by a mentally ill person acting alone, not a terrorist. Not until 2020 did America brand acts of violence by far-right groups as terrorism. Perpetrators are often constructed as lone-wolves obfuscating links to wider terrorist organisations, as with the case with the far-right killer of pro-Remain UK member of parliament Jo Cox in 2016.[67]

Ethnicity is difficult to trace in some postmodern cinema, such as *Stranger than Paradise* (Jim Jarmusch, 1994) and *Blade Runner* (Ridley Scott, 1992), where there is a 'neutral mimicry' of forms of ethnic specificity.[68] The 'Japanese-ness' in *Blade Runner* is not a social code generating the effects of ethnic identification, but a 'global economic code'.[69] From a postmodern position there is a celebration of the non-person as Woody Allen's psychiatrist in *Zelig* (1983) puts it. Comedy here is multifunctional as it is elsewhere, for example *The Brother from Another Planet* (John Sales, 1984) asserts and subverts the concept of ethnicity and otherness.[70] The film is a parody of American history with the black alien standing out as a runaway slave tracked by white aliens lost in Harlem. Here blackness is not the issue; having only three toes on each foot is. 'Foregrounded here . . . are both the arbitrariness and power of the particular difference that makes a difference and thereby constitutes otherness'.[71]

Akin with the mental patient, the figure of the spectre is the figure of possibility politically enthused with heterogeneity and hauntology which is enabling, demanding justice. Exploring ethnicity and 'madness', *One Flew Over the Cuckoo's Nest* (Milos Forman, 1976) has an indigenous American watch the performativity of white patients and black orderlies as his very own theatre. Chief Bromden is considered so alien that he is believed to be mute, like a ghost, but through this he observes all, positioning him as the perfect narrator in the novel. His initial uncanny

---

[65] K. Aroyewun-Adekomaiya, 'Representations of Mental Illness: An Examination of Movies and Professional Perspectives in Nigeria', Unpublished PhD, De Montfort University, 2012.

[66] A. Al-Krenawi, 'Mental health practice in Arab countries', *Current Opinion in Psychiatry*, Vol. 18, Issue 5, September 2005, pp. 560–564.

[67] Jason Lee, *Nazism and Neo-Nazism in Film and Media* (Amsterdam: Amsterdam University Press, 2018).

[68] V. Sobchack, 'Postmodern Modes of Ethnicity', in Lester Friedman, ed., *Unspeakable Images: Ethnicity in American Cinema* (Urbana: University of Illinois Press, 1991), p. 338.

[69] Ibid., p. 339.

[70] Ibid., p. 346.

[71] Ibid., p. 348.

'madness' (fear) only exists in him not grasping freedom, which he also offers to others, should they choose to take it. The film *Beloved* (Jonathan Demme, 1998), based on Toni Morrison's novel, exposes the 'madness' of slavery and otherness, with the return of the repressed and again the focus on the ghost.

'Madness' like ghosts haunts every corner of rationality, embedding ambiguity via an ethically profound psychopathology of uncertainty and resistance which can be politically affirming. Outside race studies, uncanniness has been seen to be intrinsic to the nature of desire and significant relationships founded on acknowledgement of the 'strangeness' and 'differentness of another person'.[72] This is a step away from the hegemony of the same and, as explained throughout, what we find is that the central experiences of life and an understanding of life 'cannot be resolved by rational means alone'.[73]

Women of colour have been the subject of significant films concerning mental health, including: *Black Girl* (Ossie Davis, 1972); *Out of Darkness* (Larry Elikann, 1994), staring Diana Ross; *Call Me Crazy* (Bryce Dallas Howard, Ashley Judd, Bonnie Hunt, Laura Dern, Sharon Maguire, 2013), which includes one story about PTSD with Jennifer Hudson; and *Frankie and Alice* (Geoffrey Sax, 2010), where Halle Berry plays the true story of a woman with dissociative identity disorder; *Poppy Shakespeare* (Benjamin Ross, 2000), based on Clare Allan's 2006 novel concerning a day care mental patient; and *Precious* (Lee Daniels, 2009), based on the novel *Push* by Sapphire. Set in 1987, the film concerns Precious Jones (Gabourey Sidibe), a girl whose parents physically and emotionally abuse her. Precious gains a capacity for self-love and this film optimistically shows that even the most difficult of circumstances can be overcome. The above optimism does come of course with some major caveats.

For Kehinde Andrews there is an underpinning of attempts to rationalize processes of whiteness because they are rooted in the social structures inducing psychosis.[74] Critical Whiteness Studies emerged as an academic discipline that has gained attention in the last two decades. Central to this is the idea that if the processes of Whiteness can be uncovered then they can be reasoned with and overcome through rational dialogue. Andrews' argument is this is beyond rational argument. Through drawing on a critical discourse analysis of the two British big budget movies about transatlantic slavery, *Amazing Grace* (Michael Apted, 2007) and *Belle* (Amma Asante, 2014), Andrews states such films function as, 'celluloid hallucinations that reinforce the psychosis of Whiteness'. This then functions to distance Britain from the horrors of slavery, downplaying the role of racism. We saw in Chap. 2 how films can function as dreams and some could be considered psychotic within that framework. It is unclear whether Andrews is attempting to

---

[72] Roberts and Itten, op. cit., p. 70.

[73] Ibid.

[74] Kehinde Andrews, 'The Psychosis of Whiteness: The Celluloid Hallucinations of *Amazing Grace* and *Belle*', *Journal of Black Studies*, 2016, 47(5): 435–45, p. 435.

dismiss Whiteness as psychosis. If so, he obfuscates the notion that there is always meaning in psychosis.

There are resonances between cultural discourse and scientific discourse in this context. The media argued that the pioneer of cultural therapy Frederick Hickling claimed the occurrence of serious mental health problems is much higher in people of African-Caribbean origin than it is in the Caribbean due to European culture being psychotic.[75] Hickling claimed personality disorder in Jamaica was three to six times the global norm, meaning 40% of the population.[76] Again we have the problem with language and definitions of disorders as explained in Chap. 1. The problems with this binary discourse are blatant. The argument throughout this book is that transrational, non-binary knowledge, sometimes itself framed as psychotic, is useful. To deny this has caused mental health problems.

In 'The Cinematic Archive of Black Madness', an event in Toronto held on the 18 February 2020 with Ariella Tair, Trinity Square Video, the debates Fanon raised and explored in this chapter were investigated. 'Locating rage, incurable anger and Black protest on the axis of madness', this project works, 'from the shared understanding that global anti-blackness has produced the conditions of violence that preclude Black sanity'.[77] This statement is damning and Tair continues by explaining that mainstream films have negated characters of colour, and if they appear they are often in the service of the white protagonists. Black vernacular language is incorporated in this approach through reference to *Wayward Lives, Beautiful Experiments* by Saidiya Hartman (2019). This approach has a performative angle, placing the voice of the narrator and character in an inseparable relation, as she puts it, so that the vision and language of the wayward shape and arrange the text.

The genre could be termed 'critical fabulation', which enhances 'understanding of the ways that black women and girls have fought to make freedom a reality', those officially 'deemed unfit for history'.[78] *The Protest Psychosis: How Schizophrenia Became a Black Disease* by Jonathan Metzl is also used by this event. Previously, Metzl had cited drapetomania, the 'madness' that caused African American slaves to flee captivity, or the claim that they were unfit for freedom, arguments discussed in this chapter. Metzl shows how schizophrenia was shaped as a black disease, drawing on US medical journals, magazines, pharmaceutical advertisements, studies of popular opinion, music lyrics, oral histories, and films.[79] Other relevant texts for this event included *Medical Apartheid: The Dark History of Medical*

---

[75] Sathnam Sanghera, 'My Relatives, The Slave Owners', *The Times Magazine*, May 1, 2021 (54–61), p. 61.

[76] Ibid.

[77] Promotion for the Cinematic Archive.

[78] Isaiah Matthew Wooden, Review of *Wayways Lives, Beautiful Experiments: Intimate Histories of Social Upheaval* (New York: W. W. Norton, 2019), by Saidiya Hartman, in *Theatre Journal*, pp. 537–538.

[79] D. Wear, 'Review of *The Protest Psychosis: How Schizophrenia Became a Black Disease*', in *Jama – The Journal of the American Medical Association*, Vol. 303, Issue 19, 2010, p. 1984.

Experimentation on Black Americans from Colonial Times to the Present by Harriet Washington, and *Black Madness :: Mad Blackness* by Theri Alyce Pickens referenced here in Chap. 1. Washington explained how slaves were purchased specifically for the purpose of clinical experimentation, the use of black bodies for anatomical dissection, and the display of black subjects in fairs, museums, and zoos. He reveals how the father of American gynaecology, Dr. James Marion Sims, experimented on slave women without using any tranquilisers.[80] This is not something purely of the past, given Washington shows how recently African American prisoners underwent medical research using radiation and drug testing and how African American children were experimented upon. The author reveals that because African Americans were classified as inferior they were seen as exploitable and dispensable and today certain illnesses are constructed linguistically and morally as diseases of certain ethnic groups.[81] Ongoing aspects of biotechnology feed into this racial and racist discourse. This event offered an understanding into the ways in which 'madness' and Blackness exists in spaces between historical fact, archival abstention, and nationalist/white supremacist narrative.[82]

Much has been made of the 'madness' of social media and how it can stir racial hatred, but other research posits a colour-blindness and positive intersectional approach within social media discourse.[83] Within postcolonial theory, nationalism has been conceived as 'madness' and this chapter has addressed race, alterity, and 'madness', historically, culturally, and through social theory. The history of psychiatry within a colonial context along with the work of Fanon in relation to 'madness' have been examined. How black 'madness' and white 'madness' were configured has explained in the colonial and postcolonial era. How insanity was viewed as a breakdown of the higher functions only available to Caucasians, plus how modern developments were believed to exacerbate 'madness', was elucidated.

Amazingly in the mid-1980s comic books tackled the subject or racism and apartheid through humour, harking back to the past. *The New DNAAgents* is one example. 'It's so . . . so sixties! All you get out of it exercise, and Nautilus is so much more efficient . . . ,' says one character to a man of colour who is on an anti-racism march. While another taking a photograph comments, 'I need a souvenir of this . . . A genuine peace march!'[84] In this era there appeared to be a playing with nostalgia and retro culture, even in terms of activism, but 35 years later things had shifted. Following the murder of George Floyd by police officer Derek Chauvin in Minneapolis 2020 a global response re-invigorated the Black Lives Matter (BLM)

[80] Marius Turda, 'Review of Harriet A. Washington, *Medical Apartheid: The Dark History of Medical Experimentation on Black Americans from Colonial Times to the Present* (New York: Doubleday, 2006), in *Social History of Medicine*, October 2007, pp. 620–621.

[81] Ibid.

[82] Ibid.

[83] Devon W. Carbado, 'Colorblind Intersectionality', in *Signs*, Vo. 38, no. 4, 2013, pp. 811–845.

[84] M. Evanier, C. Patton and W. Blyberg, *The New DNAAgents* (California: Eclipse Comics, 1985), No. 4 (whole no. 28), December, p. 11.

movement. Unfortunately, racism gets, 'redefined as the product of black and anti-racist zeal that is both destructive of democracy and subversive of order'.[85] For Paul Gilroy there is an opposition to anti-racism, creating a version of the national past, challenging an emphasis on slavery.[86]

As with gender and sexuality examined in Chap. 3, we can mark the progress made, recognizing there is much more to be done, while in some areas there has been a backward step, corporate new media being one. Historically the Civil Rights leaders of the 1970s forced through enormous media reforms and major media companies dismantled 'pervasive practices of racial bias'.[87] They pressurize the federal government for a non-discriminatory media system, securing better access to news and information for non-white communities, but the problem was many of these leader then backed efforts by companies to, 'roll back those gains in communications policy'.[88] While new media systems diversify there was the need to examine, 'how power is challenged, reproduced and reformed'.[89] There was contestability with the view that the media does not merely mirror and reflect the population, given that assumes everyone relates to the media identically, and despite media activists adding a plurality to the debate black men especially are criminalized in the media and held up as deviant.[90] They embody the position the 'mad' have been situated in.

If race is an evolving idea created to legitimize inequality and protect white advantage, racism starts with ideology and the socio-political economic system.[91] A movement towards liberation, following critical race theory, entails counter-acting the normativity of cultural hegemony.[92] The transrational position here encompasses this movement away from cultural hegemony and combines with explorations concerning intersectionality where there is an examination of 'race, sex, class, national origin, and sexual orientation', as seen in Chap. 3.[93] Racial equality does not have a linear historical trajectory and this is especially true in terms of media history which involves economic and legal forces.[94]

The relationship between European psychiatry, racism, Africa, and the wider context has been explained with the controversial construction of 'black madness' and 'white madness' elaborated on. While being highly naive, Desdemona in

[85] Paul Gilroy, *There Ain't No Black in the Union Jack* (London: Routledge, 2002), p. 313.
[86] Ibid.
[87] J. González and J. Torres, *News For All the People. The Epic Story of Race and the American Media* (London: Verso, 2012), p. 371.
[88] Ibid.
[89] Gavin Titley, *Racism and Media* (London: Sage, 2019), p. 27.
[90] Ibid., p. 25.
[91] R. Delgado and J. Stefancic, *Critical Race Theory: An Introduction* (New York: New York University Press, 2017).
[92] Ibid.
[93] Ibid., p. 58.
[94] González and Torres, op. cit.

Othello asserts that, 'I think the sun where he was born/Drew all such humours from him' (Act 3 Scene 4, lines 30–31), arguing there is no way Othello can be jealous when her servant Emilia thinks otherwise. Shakespeare here encompasses the myth examined in this chapter concerning those who are non-white not feeling extreme emotions. Interestingly, we are more moved by those with intense desires as we identify with them and in this instance Othello's feelings can appear childish.[95] Critical work on culture relating to race has been analysed along with its relationship with 'madness'.

Colonialism and postcolonialism in America, Latin America and the Caribbean have been dissected. The construction of 'madness' is found to be at the heart of contemporary racism. How Islam has constantly been pathologized in the West has also been delineated. The media frame acts of political violence by white people as a lone wolf who is 'mad' while Islam is framed as violent ideology causing violence. Following Fanon, we examined how 'madness' is a construction as are constructions of 'whiteness' and 'blackness' within his paradigm. While not denying history and reality, this book's focus on transrationality concerns time being non-linear and haunted. This is how film operates, memory and time haunted, confirming a transrational approach transcending linearity is a more efficacious method for understanding the human and human understanding.

[95] Athony Storr, *The Dynamics of Creation* (London: Penguin, 1991), p. 229.

Part III
Politics and Economics

Chapter 5
Reality and Narration

5.1 Introduction: Lived Experience

Following the excavation of history, media, culture, and social theory in relation to 'madness', we now consider real-life accounts of 'madness'; 'people thought they just pressed 'rewind' on the little recorder installed in their heads, when in fact they constructed their memories. They 'developed their own narratives''.[1] The expressions of lived experiences are real and simultaneously narratives are devised with meaning and purpose illustrating in their own terms how culture creates 'madness' and vice versa. As explained in Chap. 2, we live in an overwhelmingly mediated world. This coheres with the view that the Lacanian Real is now the Simulacrum.[2] The following were interviewed: a retired medical doctor whose job was preparing patients for ECT; a psychologist working in the NHS and in academia; a psychotherapist working in the NHS and private practice; a mental health worker; an individual whose family had experienced 'madness'; and a person who had experienced mental health issues while working in communications involving managing the media. Methodologically there was an emphasis on an open and nuanced approach which is non-leading examining an individual's personal perceptions, rather than offering an objective statement of an event with the human at the heart of this process rather than data.[3]

In Chap. 1 it was explained how emotion involves the transrational. Blind faith in data which has been thought to be objective and rational has now paradoxically taken on a supernatural form that is unhelpful. The deification of numbers removes

---

[1] Liane Moriarty, *Truly Madly Guilty* (London: Penguin, 2016), p. 3.

[2] This is one interpretation of Jean Baudrillard. For a deeper analysis of Baudrillard in regards to fate see Jason Lee, *The Psychology of Screenwriting* (London: Bloomsbury, 2014).

[3] Interpretative phenomenological analysis (IPA) aims to fathom how people make sense of their personal and social world in a non-directive fashion. This method is loosely followed here.

J. Lee, *Culture, Madness and Wellbeing*, https://doi.org/10.1007/978-3-031-37530-9_5

the human.[4] It is important therefore to reinvigorate the human, but there are complications with trying to gain an insider's perspective. This will always have limitations, but during the interviews a level of empathy and relationship can be found.[5] Truncated examples are offered initially with four examples then given almost in their entirety. There is a two-stage process of interpretation, a double or even triple hermeneutic if you will: the participant is trying to make sense of their world, whilst the researcher is trying to make sense of the participant making sense of their world, and now you as the reader are making sense of this. Elements have been selected for relevance and appropriateness, but this was not carried out to fit a prescribed narrative.[6] There is an acknowledgement that relying on set questions can pose problems. For example, it is implying a consensus on what the meaning of the problem is, in terms of sociological categorises following Bourdieu, but this can be tackled by being reflexive, flexible, and the understanding ideological implications.[7] The richness of the responses here underscore how the method in these instances works.

ECT has been examined in fiction, especially in the research concerning gender presented and analysed in Chap. 3, and it is often thought of as barbaric in the current age.[8] The male perspective has left its presence on concepts such as immanence and transcendence. There is a paradox in the feminine ideal of transcendence and in the Hegelian sense women are relegated to outside the drama. The process of medicalization turns the women's body into an object for observation, but Simone de Beauvoir had the idea of making women 'lookers' rather than the 'looked-at'. With dominant male rationality conceived as the transcendence of the feminine it is then natural to affirm the positive in that which has been relegated.[9]

After qualifying as a doctor, A.2 had been an anaesthetist in mental hospitals delivering ECT over many years stating, 'I have witnessed absolute miracles, especially for those in a total stupor. One ECT brought them back'. The biological is stressed. They view mental illness purely as a disease seeing it as a chemical imbalance in the brain. 'Sometimes this is linked to enormous creativity, especially if you're bipolar', comments A.2. This is a popular view stressed in the media through celebrity cases, such as actor and writer Stephen Fry who has bi-polar disorder. It is also the focus here in Chap. 6, when we examine creativity and voices. This has been

---

[4] Iain Martin, 'Algorithmic Decision Making', *The Times*, 5 November 2020, p. 33.

[5] IPA assumes a chain of connections between the use of language, thinking, and emotional states.

[6] The format of each interview was the same consisting of the Freudian hour, recorded and transcribed by the author. Each participant was given an explanation in printed and oral form of this book, the interview purpose and content explaining this is qualitative research with an ideographic focus and invited to sign a consent form voluntarily. Questions were seen in advance and discussed along with areas such as data storage, anonymity, and what happens to the research. Participants were not paid.

[7] Jen Webb, *Researching Creative Writing* (Suffolk: Creative Writing Studies, 2015), pp. 138–150.

[8] Genevieve Lloyd, *The Man of Reason. 'Male' & 'Female' in Western Philosophy* (London: Routledge, 1995), p. 102.

[9] Ibid., p. 104.

the subject of psychiatric discourse, such as Anthony Storr's work on creativity and the 'schizoid character' and 'obsessional character, plus genius and 'madness' discussed in Chap. 1.[10]

There is the view that beyond a certain boundary a temporary shift in mood changes to a clinical problem. A.2 states the terms 'madness' and insanity are not helpful today, although it is acknowledged this might be a leading question. 'Environment, time and space,' to quote A.2, are a way for healing to happen. These three factors might not be in abundance, but this depends on the individual circumstance. 'There's a sort of grey area between sad, upset and depressed, and being depressed as an actual illness, where you've gone over a limit.' A.2 goes on:

> I can remember so clearly one person who was transgender, I remember her, she had transitioned so successfully that my team, all women, we felt about her as another woman. Whether the stress of the transition had caused her to break down, I don't know.

At the same time, A.2 concludes:

> I am glad that ECT is now only used for only the more acute patients, as it is crude. But in its time, it was the only thing you could do, and, of course, you can say psychiatric medications can only have side effects and can also do violence to people in a chemical way.

This is a valuable point and shows how progress does have downsides, bringing us back to Heidegger's view addressed in Chap. 1 on the problems with technological progress.

A.2 argues that many of these patients could not get support in the wider community in terms of treatment, but there were enormous institutions with thousands incarcerated who received real care from living in these large, regulated communities. The argument is the inner world of the institution was often more harmonious than the external world. Once these communities closed in A.2's view these people were lost exacerbating their mental health problems. As explained in Chap. 1, many historians of 'madness' make the same point. Feminist cultural historians examined in Chap. 3 argue that, while reflecting the hierarchy of the societies within which they existed, the 'mad' house offered a form of protection.

A.2 also mentions people with severe depression who had been in concentration camps. 'Some of these had ECT which helped a bit, but of course they were so damaged by the things that had happened to them they were never completely free of it.' These powerful observations show us how gradations of severity of mental health issues correlate with treatment and its impact. This is a salient point. The zeitgeist today is to promote the notion that everyone suffers from some form of mental health problem to a variety of degree and we can understand the logic to this, as it helps to destigmatize the subject. It can lead to people coming forward to get help. There is a clear danger with this argument, however, such as blurring severe mental health problems with, for example, normal anxiety creates problems can lead to neither end of the 'spectrum' being treated properly.

---

[10] See Anthony Storr, *The Dynamics of Creation* (London: Penguin, 1991), pp. 72–84; pp. 122–146.

For interviewee A.13, 'madness' 'goes against the grain' and is essentially 'non-conventional'. Someone 'mad' is holding a view outside the norm. This view equates with the work previously discussed where, due primarily to social media, even the most extreme views become the norm. What in the past would be termed delusional becomes accepted.[11] Because A.13 was originally diagnosed with bi-polar disorder they thought were misdiagnosed as being insane and, as they put it, 'they were scrabbling around, trying to find a definition for me'. Furthermore, 'I felt the medical profession let me down, I think I was experiencing post-traumatic stress disorder'. As explained, the media is our contemporary reality, and those who work intensely with the media can suffer PTSD which is explained in detail in Chap. 2. This also confirm Jung's view that a diagnosis of 'madness' causes 'madness' with the only truly 'mad' activity being accepting the diagnosis.[12]

There are also employment law ramifications in this case which relates to others. With a diagnosis of bi-polar for their employee organisations that might otherwise be culpable are exonerated, whereas if a diagnosis of PTSD was given then employees might be able to take their employer to court for damages. While media studies scholars have often steered clear of maintaining a direct relationship between media images and their impact, including attacking a hypodermic model of media influence, the severity and extent of involvement in media images needs to be kept in mind in this instance. A.13 experienced a constant bombardment of disturbing images in their media related profession. This included the most extreme end of images, including rape, murder, and suicide. In their opinion this was a direct cause of their mental health issues. The damaging impact of certain lines of work was felt by A.13 to be the cause of mental instability beyond than their own personal mental health.

> A friend of mine was talking about all the information he is dealing with lately, he is the gatekeeper, he looks at these images and decides whether they are suitable to go out to the media. It has had a massively traumatic impact on his mental health. I was dealing with similar issues. A.13

Discussing the causes, A.13 argues that the people in their own youth, 'had a tendency towards insanity caused by drug abuse, alcoholism, and alienation. There are a lot of people struggling to cope, and this is down to mental health problems'. They go on to suggest that people with PTSD should have time away from their jobs which are stressful. They continue that there are no counselling services until things get difficult. An earlier intervention strategy is a recommendation.[13] Why wait until things are too late and people are off with stress is A.13's key point. Unrealistic expectations are highlighted as a cause of the stress, plus bad management, and a dysfunctional culture, poorly structured.

---

[11] This has been highlighted when we consider how conspiracy theorists are now normalized and part of the free speech movement.

[12] C.G. Jung, *The Essential Jung* (London: Fontana, 1998).

[13] See Chap. 8. for recommendations.

> If you were failing it was felt you were failing by your own inadequacy, there was a huge macho culture. This was a really bad toxic environment. Here is the classic example. My boss who mentored me through six months off with mental illness is now off with stress. Rapes, murders, suicides—this is what we are dealing with. A.13

Personal treatments influenced professional outlook. With the affected role, the views on diagnostic assessment were more varied compared to the professionals. In A.4's case professionals had been arguing whether they clearly fitted into one diagnostic paradigm or not. A certain diagnosis may have then required long-term day-care. Once they entered short-term psychotherapy the participant decided this diagnosis was not useful. Perhaps the thought of long-term treatment made the short-term treatment more impactful in terms of wanting to avoid it. We might deduce from this that it depends on what experts in the mental health profession are seeing as the best tools. For example, borderline personality disorder (BPD) when it was developed was thought to be best treated by group therapy, but this often involves a long-term day-care setting.[14] This will have implications for career and life choices, possibly limiting prospects, and arguably when these day-care group therapy settings were established in the late 1980s there was an experimental edge to them.

Sometimes the initial diagnosis helped; it clearly does for A.28. A large amount of this interview is included to illustrate the background in establishing this viewpoint. The first two interviewees are professionals, the latter on psychiatric medication during the time of the interview. The third is a research scientist and the fourth is a psychotherapist. In all examples family issues arise. In the third the participant is trying to cope with their father's 'madness'. We find that the caring profession might be more female at the lower and middle ranking levels, but higher-level psychiatrists will often be white males.[15] This can cause problems when, as noted in Chap. 3, women are being treated by men or as explained in Chap. 4 cultural considerations concerning race are ignored with psychiatry a form of colonialization.

A.2 noted that when they worked in mental hospitals all the staff were female and A.22 also reflects on this.[16] A division concerning treatment was overt. In A.22's experience men of colour would get diagnosed as psychotic and then would not be referred for psychotherapy; women would be more likely to be diagnosed with personality disorders; and Asian women would have physical problems as a way of framing the issue when there was a psychological dimension not within their terms of reference; mainly middle class educated white men would receive treatment from a psychotherapist in the NHS. All of this exemplified the current barriers for treatment which are based on the predictable divisions we have previously examined

[14] Antony Bateman and Fonagy, 'Mentalisation-treatment training', NHS training the Anna Freud Centre, July/October 2019.

[15] See A.22.

[16] During my training as a counsellor and psychotherapist the staff and student body were over eighty-five percent female. The student body was 100% white, the staff eighty percent white, and none of the staff were people of colour.

in Chaps. 3 and 4 concerning gender, sexuality, race, and class and we could also include age in this.

Often interviewees had been both users of services at some point as well as mental health professionals. A drive to do care professionally for others came from a need to know about what it means to be human. There was a desire to learn how to help people based on direct personal experiences within the family. Some users of services were seeing multiple professionals which complicated matters, but this was not necessarily detrimental to treatment. This open approach to treatment could mean a more balanced set of treatments. Most of the participants who were in treatment recently were lower middle class without significant income. Two were still seeking a diagnosis that could be of use, believing this might be beneficial in the long run, in respect to gaining help. These service users were reliant on what provision was available on the NHS because individually they did not have private means for treatment. If they did go private, they were reliant on family members for financial backing. This was not ideal and caused further tensions, but this at least gave an urgency to the treatment and meant it was time-limited with certain goals. Participants were aware that many of the treatments felt like common sense. There can be a mystification where expertise is cloaked in language and exclusive norms that leads to reification.

A common drug noted by A.28 is sertraline, a serotonin reuptake inhibitor (SRI), prescribed for a broad number of symptoms, including anxiety and sometimes for borderline personality disorder (BPD). There was often a pattern in the interviews relating to a BPD diagnosis. Participants stated how there was violence in childhood and then aggression would be internalised against the self as a child leading to a high level of personal self-criticism. This often fed into an extreme sense of perfectionism which positively put was matched by success. This was an interesting observation concerning a popular diagnosis in terms of nature or nurture.

The work of Aaron Rosanoff and his researchers in the 1920s and 1930s is significant within this wider debate on nature or nurture. They gathered data on 1000 twins in California testing for the heritability of mental illness.[17] In 68% of identical twins when one had schizophrenia the other twin developed schizophrenia, but this was only the case in 15% of fraternal twins.[18] In the 1950s Franz Kallmann researched 691 twin schizophrenics in New York. His results were even higher with 86 per cent concordance for identical twins.[19] During this period American psychiatry was dominated by psychoanalytical writers, so some of this biological research

[17] For example, see, A. Rosanoff, L. Handy, I. Plesset, and S. Brush, 'The etiology of so-called schizophrenic psychoses, with special reference to their occurrence in twins', *The American Journal of Psychiatry*, No. 91, 1934, pp. 247–286.

[18] Matt Ridley, *Nature via Nurture: Genes, Experience, and What Makes us Human* (London: HarperCollins, 2003), p. 104.

[19] Ibid.

was silenced and even dismissed as akin to Nazism because of the use of twin studies, despite Rosanoff and Kallmann both being Jewish.[20]

The structure of interviews in this chapter allowed participants to reflect on their lives freely, away from a possibly more restrictive therapeutic model. Interviews were often linked to other personal goals, giving a purpose, plus non-directive reflection on careers and relationships which was suitably free flowing. Concerns around anger seemed clear with participants who had recent experience of mental health treatment. The belief that changes could come was raised by A.28 who had had a variety of treatments, including cognitive behavioural therapy (CBT), dialectical behavioural therapy (DBT), and gestalt therapy, as well as person-centred Rogerian counselling. Those participants in full-time employment and in treatment were forthright in setting goals having activities to occupy them, seeing this as a route for mental wellbeing. While it was recognised that these interviews were not primarily concerned with psychotherapeutic advancement, many stated they did benefit in a personal sense which was benign. The process was emotionally cathartic and fitting with this book's concern with the transrational and wellbeing and the importance of the emotional, as explained in the opening of Chap. 1 with reference to the work of Richard Rohr.[21]

5.2 Interviews

5.2.1 Example One

Interview A.3 is with a mental health professional with a fifth of the interview included. As explained in Chap. 1's conclusions, language is central to how we conceptualise disorders and A.3 states it is important to reflect on the historical development of terminology. The questions are directive to a degree, but the direction the discourse flows is open with the researcher and participant trained in person-centred counselling. What resonates is the deep personal struggle with initial treatment and diagnosis—autism and connected disorders. A tremendous amount of adversity has been overcome and while the retelling is emotional there is hope. The participant would not have made a successful career in the field without these early experiences. Towards the end of the transcript A.3 claims little has changed in 40 years which is damning. This is in the context of patients being moved across the country away from their families. Their conclusions marry those of Chap. 3; often men are in control and this is a major part of the problem, both within the mental health system and externally in politics and internationally leading to war. This informs an area around expectations.

[20] Ibid.

[21] Richard Rohr, *Falling Upward: A Spirituality of the Two Halves of Life* (London: SPCK, 2011).

> I think we need to stop thinking about separating the social model from the medical model and start thinking about how can we actually integrate these ideas, to get a more holistic idea about what it means to be human, and what it means to be a human with a mental health condition. And what a mental health condition actually is, and how we cope with that, and how we manage it in society so we can live the best quality life we are able to live. There are always going to be restrictions. So, going back to your first bit of the question, class, race, gender. Those things are always going to set limits. A.3

What is noticeable about this participant is how their family had to fight so hard to get help and how professionals took over the family. This had an impact on each family member, in some cases detrimentally. A battle gives impetus to the participant to help others via their job. There is the acknowledgement of areas that appear fixed and the political implications of this.

I: What is your understanding of the terms insanity and 'madness'? What do you think these things mean?

A.3: I think they are very interesting slightly outdated concepts, and I think that reflects the evolution of language and the ways it shifts and changes in terms of how we conceptualize mental health. And I think insanity is one of those concepts in lay discourses that unfortunately bought a range of negative associations with it, which is not how it was necessarily originally intended to be used. But I think like a lot of concepts in mental health the shifts in meaning and semantics around a particular concept and the way in which society uses that concept changes its core meaning. And unfortunately, I think the meanings around 'madness' and insanity now have got very negative associations with them, and I think you know Foucault's work around 'madness' and the asylum and the power of psychiatry has helped to shift those terms. But ultimately you can change the word but the ascription of meaning remains constant to some extent. So, while we might not necessarily use those particular words anymore, we just have other words to mean what we mean, if that makes sense, so we now, even things like mental health disorder versus mental health condition which are quite contested concepts. So, we wouldn't say someone was insane we would say they have a mental health condition, if you were kind of socially minded. If you were clinically minded you would say mental health disorder. But the sociology scholars would take issue with the word disorder, but the clinical medical scholars still see that as part of their framework of understanding mental health. And as someone who sits in the middle of those two disciplines, I tend to use them interchangeably, depending on which context I am working in and who I am working with.

I: OK thanks, are these terms valuable, you've said that they are outdated, but do you still think they are valuable, these terms insane and mad, or is it too ambiguous, as you've said we've got other words now anyway?

A.3: I think as singular concepts they've still got some value. Not in terms of value of how we treat people today, but in terms of our understanding of language and how it's shaped what mental health means. So, you can never completely disregard terms because they are all part of rich history of language and they will always have some meaning and although that meaning has shifted and changed understanding how that has shifted and changed is actually relevant to how we treat people in practice today. So, if we didn't have the history of our terminology, we wouldn't be able to move forward and be more progressive in our understanding. Does that make sense?

I: So, we have to refer back to it anyway.

A.3: Absolutely, so our understanding of the asylum and how people were very badly treated, and then there were more humane treatments, and then they were very badly treated again, and then we moved into more community care, that kind of shifting cycle of attitudes of terms, of language, of people, we need to be able to understand that, so that we can do better today. We can't do better today without looking back at yesterday.

I: So, what are your personal experiences of insanity? This can be coming from causes, impacts, treatments, and so on.

A.3: I guess my motivations for starting the charity work when so young and going into psychology as a career, at least the foundation of my career, was my own personal experiences, because my relative was diagnosed with autism. But interestingly the process of that diagnosis was a long painful process. And you read the literature around autism and parental experience and family experience of the diagnostic process these metaphors of it being a battle and terrible and hard work and struggling to access services. Unfortunately, they are still the narratives today. My mother said to the nurse there's something wrong with this baby, because in her words she said he went very stiff in her arms and she'd already had me by that point, I'm older than my brother, and so she was making the contrast between the two babies.

I: And so, she knew what a so-called normal baby was like and they told her what, that she was just paranoid or something?

A.3: Absolutely, they told her stop being so stupid women, you know just hold on to him.

I: Do you think that was not conscious denial on their part, just lack of understanding?

A.3: I have a horrible suspicion that nurses today would still say something like that.

I: Because they can't be bothered to deal with the problem?

A.3: I guess there's this kind of idea that you can't know there is something wrong with a child when it's only two hours old. I don't know. I'm not sure where that comes from. But I suspect the same experiences are being re-lived by mothers today. And I doubt that attitude has changed much. The idea that you can't possibly know with a 2-h old child, but she did, which is really interesting really. But as he grew slightly older as toddler, she really knew there was something wrong because he wasn't meeting his developmental milestones, he wasn't talking, he wasn't walking. All the things that children typically do he wasn't doing and she kept going back to the health visitors then and then the doctors and as he grew older more and more signs were developing that he had issues and she still kept getting told that there was nothing wrong with him, stop being so silly woman you know and she was also told this common thing parents of autism children are told, you need to love him more.

I: Often, it's the woman who is blamed, the cold mother.

A.3: Yes, which goes back to Bettelheim's idea of the refrigerator mother. He was sent to a special educational needs school and it was at that point that our family became flooded with professionals.

I: So, what was that like?

A.3: Well, that was fascinating in one sense for me I guess as a kind of curious inquisitive child anyway, and quite academically driven even at that age. To suddenly start meeting social workers, clinical psychologists, the lot, speech and language therapists, educational psychologists, the head teacher at the special educational school, and I guess it made me really curious to know more about my brother in the first instance, but other children like him. Because he was a very violent, so we encountered as a family a significant amount of violence from him, and he was only young, when he was diagnosed. But I've still got quite a few scars from things he did when I was young, he threw a Rubik's cube at my head and it hit me point on and I've got a scar here on my forehead, that was a Rubik's cube, it bloody hurt. But there were lots of instances. He broke my sister's wrist. They were watching fireworks, they'd climbed up onto a dressing table to watch fireworks and he just pushed her off, randomly. He was very unpredictable; it was that instantaneous shift.

I: So, it was more than just autism then, it was lots of different things you think?

A.3: Yes, he's been diagnosed with additional co-morbid conditions, as time goes on. He has co-morbid anxiety disorder which is treated with medication. He's on two for anxiety, one for depression, an anti-psychotic, he's on about 5, PRN as required.

I: What did you do as individuals or as a family to cope, because you began by saying about systems?

A.3: People cope in different ways. It certainly had a profound impact on my family, I guess for me interestingly I developed quite strong coping mechanisms, I was quite resilient. And what I did was make sure my time was filled with sensible stuff. I used to stay back at school and do extra homework. I did all that charity work.

I: That began around the time he was diagnosed?

A.3: Absolutely, and that was partly the influence of those professionals telling me stuff and talking to me about him and what they did for a living, made me curious you know I started doing all the voluntary work, and I stayed behind at school.

I: I don't want to stereotype you as a woman, but would you say before you found that out about your brother you were also a helpful person, wanting to understand other people and help them have a better life, was that in your nature do you think?

A.3: Yes, I think it was to some extent. I was always a bit of a people person, if you can be in primary, a people person. So, I guess it was always in my nature to be organized and driven and do stuff for others.

I: So, this was when there was starting to be an early understanding of autism, how were the professionals relating to your family, were they good, bad, a mixture, did they see him as a guinea pig?

A.3: It was a real mixture, I guess. The clinical psychologist and the head teacher at the special school were brilliant, without a doubt we owe them a lot because they really helped. So, it was a really turbulent few years after his diagnoses. Because of his violence. That violence became sexual. Inappropriately sexual, towards my mother and my sister. And so social services stepped in. We had a crisis point. I can't remember how old I exactly was, I would have been about 14. But memory plays tricks, it was about that, and social services stepped in and they took him away. So, they decided he couldn't be part of the family home anymore, because he was too much of a risk. Because they said, his sleep was terrible, he would wake up on the hour every hour and go and wake my dad up so my dad was awake on the hour every hour but getting up at 6 am to go to work to do a full day's work. And so, the medics said all that sleep deprivation, all that turbulence probably contributed to the stroke. So, then that left my dad disabled. Yes, I can guess that's a reflection on how badly mental health is treated in this country that there's nowhere available anywhere near where we lived.

I: Because we hear those stories now, don't we?

A.3: Nothing's changed in all that time. So, they whisked him off to Liverpool, and he didn't cope with all that change, massive change. To be ripped away from your family, he was only about 12 at the time, and he thought it was because he'd been bad, and it was. So how do you, you know, managing that was tricky, but they had him sedated for about 6 months. They had to keep him under sedation for quite a long time. So, my poor mother, she struggled. Her husband had had a stroke and was recovering from the stroke. Her son has been ripped away from the family and sent up north and her youngest daughter was struggling at this point because of all the impact of her brother and I just carried on, removed myself to some extent, with my own coping mechanisms and got on with my homework. But I guess it really took its toll on me when I went on to do my A levels, that's when I noticed it, and that was another 2 years later, so it was like I was so focused on getting my GCSEs and working through and being successful and doing something. So, I went to college to do my A levels, and I met my personal tutor at college, and interestingly was the first person to really talk to me. And even though that was 2 years later he was the first person to notice that there might be actually something wrong. And so, I went through two really difficult years of suffering really badly with headaches, which reflecting back I realize was just the release of all that pressure and stress that I had stored for so long was finally coming out physically, as it does when you suffer from stress and anxiety. And I really struggled through my A levels and this guy really helped me. And I've stayed in touch with him and I still write to him every Christmas.

I: Looking at your own perceptions of human psychology then, summing all of that up, what do you think, how these things have shaped your view of human psychology? If you could sort of synthesize your experiences of your brother, plus also of others when you did the voluntary work and your career working as a practitioner and as an academic and your experiences of your own mental health and your sister's, how's that shaped your view of human psychology?

A.3: Well, it's been hugely influential, I guess. But it's left me constantly questioning things. It's left me more curious and inquisitive. I don't think that anyone's got the answers. It's a bit like religion, it's kind of like there must be an answer, but we've spent centuries trying to find it, and we still haven't found it. And

I think mental health is a similar, a similar theoretical object in that sense. That we are constantly seeking answers, but we've yet to find them. And I think part of the difficulty of mental health is that people tend to treat it in a homogenous way, mental health as a singular object. When actually even one condition isn't a singular object, when you start to really look at it. So, when you use autism as the example, a brilliant example of a mental health object, you can't even say that autism is a singular mental health condition when you define it label it and say you've got autism that's the end of the journey, we now know what the problem is. Because autism means so many different things. It's a spectrum condition anyway, we know that. You can have ten autistic people in a room, and every single one of them will be different from one another. And they might have some similar characteristics that mean they are autistic, but the differences across that group is so vast, that you can't narrow it to something homogenous. Does that make sense, can I ask you questions?

I: Yes, it does. So, you're saying actually because of these things you're not locked down into a black and white thinking over it. And I suppose, because you're an academic you're still diving into these things, you haven't latched on to, like you said before with religion, latched on similarly to say this is the answer, this is it. You know, psychosis equals this, or autism equals this, or because of that I can cure it using that. So that's good in a sense, I'm not morally judging that, I'm just saying that means you're open for more discoveries in a way, which is great. This is a bit locked down this question, but can you think about issues concerning gender, sexuality, class and race? And I will say the next question as well, just so you know, is a sociological approach relevant in the context of mental health psychology. I know you teach sociology. And if it's relevant, how relevant, you see what I mean? Because part of this book I'm writing is actually called beyond sociology, so you know there's this whole period where we went from a kind of biological model to a sociological model. It's kind of gone back again. So where do you think all these things fit together, I suppose?

A.3: Well, I think you just nailed the problem in a nutshell there. Because this idea that we are shifting from a medical to a social model to a medical model as if they are completely separate insular ideas that are disconnected from another. And I think going back to my earlier point and the object of mental health and the solution to it isn't ever going to be a singular domain, it's never going to be singular discipline that manages to find a solution either. I think we need to stop thinking about separating the social model from the medical model and start thinking about how can we actually integrate these ideas, to get a more holistic idea about what it means to be human, and what it means to be a human with a mental health condition. And what a mental health condition actually is, and how we cope with that, and how we manage it in society so we can live the best quality life we are able to live. There are always going to be restrictions. So, going back to your first bit of the question, class, race, gender. Those things are always going to set limits to what the best you can live is.

I: So, something behind it all. What do you mean by human nature then?

A.3: It's a range of different things isn't it. So human nature is your temperament, your personality, it's your drives, your motivations, your ambitions, your personal make up, your own mental health, your attitudes, your ability to cognitively process, your intellect. It's an entire, a lot of things, but there's certain things the human species has been doing for centuries and continues to do. The mistakes it continues to make over and over. That's got to be down to something more than, you know, that's got to be down to human nature. I don't know how else to describe that.

I: Do you believe then, the cliché is the more civilized we get or more humanized, the more conscious we get and therefore the more choices we can make. But do you believe that because there is such a thing as human nature that's sort of deeper than our consciousness, that sometimes we don't have a choice in that sense, because human nature will get played out. And we are kind of like puppets of human nature.

A.3: I think that we kind of make the same choices, that we've always made, but we do them in a different framework. So, for example, bullying, kids have bullied one another for centuries. The mechanisms through which they do it have changed. But their behaviour is still fundamental to human nature, it's still kids doing kid things. And some of that is quite cruel and some of that is quite extreme, but most of it is just kids being kids. It's just that now they don't, you know the names they call each other have changed over centuries, and now we are doing it online instead of in the playground. But the behaviour is the same. So, I think humans are making the same mistakes over and over again. They are still making the same choices, to use that word. Over and over again. But we are not learning any lessons. We say we learn lessons from history, but we don't. We do the same thing, but we do it in a different package. Politically, if you look at the politics of Britain, we are doing the same thing. We are not learning; we don't learn lessons. And the fact we still have all this political conflict and war is down to the fundamental issue that there is down to certain people, predominantly men, who are seeking powerful positions, and they don't care what they do to get it.

5.2.2 Example Two

Our next interview is transcribed in full. The participant is a more junior mental health professional than A.3, trained in counselling, youth work and drug prevention, and undertaking academic work in psychology and criminology. What is striking is that the participant had to find their own way and that in childhood there was no one there in the family to listen or help. This then led to their own difficulties with anxiety and depression, including minor levels of psychosis with the underlying issue being anxiety. Of course, saying minor we should not underestimate the depth of feeling and its impact. There is a view that extent of the trauma is not as important in terms of its long-term impact on wellbeing as having someone empathic at the time, plus there is evidence that the more severe childhood trauma the greater the level of adult empathy.[22] They are a former client of mental health services and now a professional.

Once they found a job in mental health and moved out of their earlier environment the past resurfaced which they then had to deal with. This relates to the analysis in Chap. 2 concerning PTSD, plus Derrida's concept of hauntology.[23] In the introduction to this chapter it was also explained how, in the main, those working in the mental health profession have their own mental health issues from the past they had to deal with and become reconciled to. This might not be a linear process and depends on the individual, but often this is a driving force for those entering the helping professions. In some professions, such as psychotherapy, there is often still a need to publicly deny a personal traumatic past for professional reasons indicating there is still stigma attached to mental health. Through their own resilience and work on personal wellbeing people were more effective in helping others.

I: OK, so what's your background in the field of mental health?

A.28: Mine stems back to childhood, now I am medicated for anxiety, putting the pieces together of how that developed and progressed throughout my life.

I wrestled with it for a long long time, I didn't know where to go, what the answers might be, I was trying to find myself for a long time, and it wasn't until I broke away from the confines of where I lived, which was a very community-based place, so moved, that it gave me a bit of scope to search for answers really.

And so, when I applied for the job I am in now, dealing with kids with challenging behaviours and a lot of mental health issues, a lot pops up, and some of it we are trained to deal with, some of it we are not. Some of it is a bit beyond our remit. It helps you develop knowledge, and with that I think came me wanting to sort my mental health problems. Because I would find myself in situations, family situations, where I would be absolutely petrified from saying a word, as my mind would recoil in horror. And in them situations you feel you should have a sense of being comfortable and trust, and all that stuff. And it didn't pan out like that for me, because of anxiety. It's an absolute minefield.

So, as I say, that's my experience from an early, early, age, from being that rebellious teenager full of hormones, testosterone, going through the change, I didn't have parents that really wanted to try and understand, it was just a lot of behaviour projected and—what is wrong with this boy, is he delinquent—it was very black and white, there was no scope for—well, shall we sit down, do you want to speak, and let's find out what the problem is? There was never any of that, never any of that.

And I think, looking back, it was me lashing out, trying to make them understand, to the effect of let's sit down, and it never came, that talk never came. And it was difficult, it was really, really, difficult. And I believe in my mind since I was 15, to probably 3 years ago I was suffering in my mental health, and it was never addressed. And I think with the family going back, looking at relatives in the past,

---

[22] DM Greenberg; Baron-Cohen, S.; Rosenberg, N.; Fonagy, P.; Rentfrow, PJ (2018), 'Elevated empathy in adults following childhood trauma'. PLoS ONE 13(10): e0203886.

[23] See Chap. 8.

my granddad's brother and nana's sister suffered from mental health problems, so I think, I think a lot of it stemmed from that as well, maybe, but like I say it was a journey I had to go through myself. And I've sort of cracked my own code, with regards to it, because I felt there was something wrong, I went to see a counsellor and she said I believe you might have this, and the next step was to try and get medicated for it, which I have been now. So that's helped immensely, it has changed everything, in regards to having a bit of confidence, doing things that you thought were never ever possible, which was, as I say, over the years a struggle.

That's my personal journey, and it was anxiety, maybe a little bit of depression because there were dark times, it was like I was doing this on my own, not anybody knew anything about it, not even to this day, I haven't expressed how low it got, to family, or friends, just a counsellor I spoke to for 12 sessions. She knew everything about me, because she had to deconstruct it, there was a lot of—did you feel suicidal, did you attempt it—and I think possibly there were two times I did think right I have had enough.

So, you are now the second person I have told about that, and they were two very isolated incidents. As suicide attempts are, because you don't want to tell anyone how you are feeling, because that's the way my life was going, it was hard, but it was also determination to go hang on a minute this isn't right, there's got to be an answer, and luckily, making that transition from north to south and finding out that there's a bigger world outside those four walls that you are bought up in, and there was a lot of scope for change, meeting different people, so yes it was a struggle, I feel now I've sort of conquered it a bit, and now I am, with the job I am in, you've got to promote, you've got to promote mental health, you've got to promote the child, and believe in that, and if you feel like that, again, going back to cracking the code, you have to crack your own code, because if you feel if you've got this, you need to go to a doctor, you need to tell your symptoms, because if you don't you're going to suffer, and you're going to suffer a long time without any help, so you've got to reach out, you've definitely got to reach out, but with my childhood there was no real chance of that, it was just looked as if I was just a naughty boy who was lashing out, rebelling against parents, father son relationship, that struggle a lot of boys have. So that was the catalyst.

My parents were singing off different hymn sheets bringing me up. There was a lot of tension in the house. A lot of violence with my dad. And so, me mam was the go-to person. My dad was just, I think he was just doing his own thing, you know, there was lot of awkward silences for not just an hour, not for days, but for weeks.

I: That sounds difficult, the silences, painful.

A.28: It was two parents sitting in different rooms not speaking to each other, with a child thinking what on earth is going on here, with me trying to gravitate between the two, and until then something happened, then, it was a horrible horrible atmosphere, just talking about it then made me go back. It was terrible, and I think that's where the anxiety sprang from: these are my parents, why are they sitting in separate rooms for this amount of time and not speaking with each other? So, yeah, that's where the anxiety came from, it all depends on your upbringing I think, which is highly important, so I carried it a while, I'm repeating myself, so that's my personal journey with it.

I: Well thanks for being so open, you mentioned hereditary elements as well, which is interesting, and I like the way you said about cracking the code and helping others. So, through helping others, you then realised you've got to help yourself. And you also mentioned the medication and how that is helping you. So that's really positive, as far as I can see it. There's one thing you said about not saying a word in a family situation and there was a sort of nightmare around that, do you remember saying that, what did you mean by that?

A.28: Well every time there was a family gathering, everyone sat around a table, conversations were going, I had to muster up a courage to get involved in that conversation, and now there is a second generation of kids coming through the family, and they're learning, and everything like that, and you can never gauge what kids are going to say, so there was that element, and there was a comment around the table, I remember it as if it was as clear as day, it was family, but someone said something to me, and I panicked, someone said something to me, and I wanted to get out of that situation, and you shouldn't feel like that, it's family, it's unconditional, and that was kind of a defining point for me. It was just a young child, going well, pointing the finger around family, and me disappearing under the table really, do you know what I mean, the horror, the horror. And so, that again made me realise there is a problem, that it is difficult not just in communities but within the family structure as well, so that made me think there is a massive problem, and I need to deal with it. That's when I reached out and went to the doctors and said there is something wrong here, and that I have either got this or this or this. So, I went down that road.

I: It's great the medication has been so useful there, so moving on to an understanding of the area of the professional area, as a professional mental health worker, but also the personal, because as you say they correlate, they sort of bleed into each other. What do you understand then by insanity and what do you understand insanity or madness to mean? I know it is a very difficult or complicated question, but what do you understand these terms to mean, if anything? You know, I mean are they useful?

A.28: To me when you mention insanity or 'madness' to me the majority of that term in my mind conjures up evil. But in regard to it being useful it kind of is because I am all for trying to put a label on something. I know a lot of people aren't, I know a lot of people disagree with that. But I think if you put a label on you know what you are working with. And probably from an early age I have read a lot about criminals, across a whole genre, from tricksters, to crime organizations, to serial killers, as you know, and they dress that up a lot as madness and insanity. So, when these people are charged and assessed they get these labels which is associated with them and that to me like I say conjures up evil acts, insane acts. So yeah, I do think it is.

I: Do you believe in evil? Just thinking about those labels. So, you've got those labels, so you've got madness, could be classified as criminally insane, or whatever you want to put it, but you mentioned immediately conjures up evil, because the two go together if you've got people committing horrendous crimes. So, what about evil then, because I'm thinking about possession and evil and all the rest of it, so in the past someone might be called possessed or even today we might say possessed by an evil spirit. So, is evil a useful term?

A.28: Like I say, evil to me is a useful term, and it is relevant, it's all about finding out the psyche of a person or an event, I mean look at the holocaust, is that the act of an evil man? A lot of people say Hitler was a genius and that's a fair point as well, he was great at oratory, and a great speaker, but running parallel to that was the holocaust, where all these people suffered. So, I think evil has a place on the planet, it exists, and a percentage of the population are just doing their daily business, getting on with things, and then you have the element that is criminally insane. I don't know, look at the Rachel Nickell murder, on Wimbledon common, where she was stabbed to death in front of her 2-year-old son. I think that was an act of sheer evil, unnecessary. And the guy now who did it is in Broadmoor. And again, you look at Sutcliffe, he was deemed probably to have a mental psychotic disorder, murdered 13 women, and I think that was some sort of act or revenge, but you've got to equate that with some sort of act of evil, how he went back to visit the victims and did whatever he did to them. I would say they were acts of evil men, so it does have a place.

I: So, they are valuable terms?

A.28: Absolutely, they are valuable terms.

I: So, what's your experience of insanity, personally or professionally? So how does this relate to environment, so causes, or treatments. You mentioned treatments to do with anxiety. So, all those different elements, again it's very complicated, and an open question. And is there a difference between insanity and madness?

A.28: I think the environment is very important. Going back to see my environment, that had the power to affect me mentally. And I think having a stable environment to develop in to a young adult is very much important. And I know it's difficult for parents because it's a coming together isn't it, because they've got backgrounds, their ancestors have got background, and they come together to create this being, and it's whether that person has a good start in life, or are they subject to neglect or abuse, or parents that don't fully comprehend the magnitude of bringing a defenceless being into the world. I think a lot of it is important, it's kind of nature versus nurture isn't it and all that debate.

I mean there was a case up in Newcastle in the 40 s and 50 s, she was a child killer, her mother was a prostitute, and her father was a gambler and an abuser, and a substance misuser, drank a lot. So, she had this very unstable environment in which to exist. She then went out to commit two murders with two boys, which inevitably she thought she would get away with. The job I am in at the moment when we do our introductory work we are told about the story of Mary Bell, how this girl did not have the right environment to be bought up in, to know the rights and wrongs, killing or not killing. So that's interesting, when you going into this type of work, so you are always given a chronological history of a person when they come into our environment, and it's always interesting to look at the background because ultimately these are children who have been damaged by adults. And it's, you look at it and you think should they be responsible, and quite frankly yes, they should be, because that child is just learning from patterns and imprints of your behaviour.

I grew up with a very violent dad who was very violent towards my mother, which I witnessed on a number of occasions. That was instilled in me, and I admit that I went out and committed acts of domestic abuse, until I was arrested for that, I was taken to court, I pleaded guilty, I was given a sentence. It wasn't custodial, it was a fine, community service, counselling, for a year. And what I learnt in that counselling through probation was seeing the signs. You've got to read the signs in any situation, because if you don't you are going to go down a road. A lot of it was me not reading the signs. I felt it was instilled in me. It was hard-wired into me, growing up, and it shouldn't be because I know a lot of parents who don't do drugs or domestic violence, or abuse or anything like that, and their kids are trying to live the best lives they can. But when that is put to you as a child, how to treat a woman, then I took that. I took that behaviour from my dad, and I projected it onto other women, I knew it wasn't right. But it was hard to disassociate, how do you end a violent argument, well you make that person shut up, and that's what my dad did, that's what I did, until the age of 30 when I realized that this wasn't the right road to go down and it was my environment, and it was the abuse of drugs, it was the abuse of alcohol, the place where I was, combined.

I remember I stood in that prison cell thinking this is the lowest of low, this is the bottom rung, and there is only one way out of here, one way up even, and it was a struggle, but at that moment in that room, 12 by 6, or whatever it is, there was a lot of me walking around in a circle thinking I have reached the bottom, this is it, have I gone completely, have I lost the plot, had a breakdown, gone mental, or whatever. So yes, with growing up to that point there in my life it was, I was brought up, I mean initially I was brought up with what I thought were two great parents. But as you grow older you see their faults. But within that environment I was witnessing domestic abuse, and like I say it was hard-wired into us.

And, so, I took that experience, I took it and found out that it doesn't get you anywhere. I mean, I was in a prison cell. So, I totally believe, absolutely that it is lineage, hereditary, parenting, environment and behaviour. They all add up, abuse, they all add up to how you are created. You witness these things then it is time served, go and live your life, and then that's it, go live your life. That's it, go live your life, if that's the way to do it? Is that the way to do it? So, I am 16 years old. I'm sure it's not, but that's what I have learnt for the last 10 years off this man, who has beaten my mother, so that's why I wanted to leave that environment, that's why I got out early because I thought it was my fault that these people were having these absolutely monumental arguments. So, I left, thinking things would be better, and they weren't, so I left and a year later my parents split up.

So, thinking that for all those years those arguments were my fault to find out hang on it wasn't your fault, that took a bit of a toll. I remember the day it happened and my mam telling me it isn't your fault it is the man in that environment who was controlling what we did. He is to blame for that. He is to blame for that. So, yeah, I went on this path, to escape, to find something meaningful, get married, let's do that, let's see what that brings. Again, I found it claustrophobic, I thought I was going mad, hated it, anxiety attacks just flooded over me. I remember being invited to parties, going there and just running out, running home. My wife going, "what is wrong?" and going, "I don't know, I'm going mad, something is going on."

I: But you literally thought you were going 'mad' maybe?

A.28: Yes, absolutely yes, thinking I should be safe in this environment because I've got a wife, a child, all the trappings that a marriage could bring, so this is my sanctuary, surely, surely. No, no it wasn't, it was just pushing down. I remember running home from that party and a car pulling up and it was my mate in there, and they were like what are you doing? I said, oh yes, just nipping home for something. Oh yes, you going to the party? Yes, I am going to the party. No problem, I carried on running home, it was about two miles, got there, walked through the door, what you doing here? I've got to come home. I've got to come up. I was just freaking out, freaking out. What's happened? Nothing's happened, I just needed to leave.

Faces were just speaking to me and I could feel it, I could feel my heart was beating, the sweats were coming, the negative thoughts, yeah, I felt absolutely, it was traumatic, that was the height of it I think, being in that situation of the marriage, thinking well this is what I want, surely? Looking back, it wasn't what I wanted. But it was that sense of escape from another horrible violent environment to go to an environment that was, had domestic violence in it, but was carried out by me this time. How's that, how's that worked? Well, you've learnt that from that environment and taken that to that environment. That's what you've been taught, surely. So, get out of that environment. Had to leave. Had to leave. And then.

I: How long were you married for, I mean you say got out of that environment, how long were you in that environment for?

A.28: Four years, and so I left that was sort of bouncing around from one disaster to another, and then got into another violent relationship with a woman who was a drug dealer. Unbeknownst to me at the time, learnt that further down the line, was told numerous times to leave by friends, all that sort of thing. Ignored every warning possible. Until I was in that prison cell, stood thinking, that's it man, what do you do? You've lost everything.

You've lost the relationship, you've lost respect, you've lost, you've lost a bit of pride, you've lost probably your job, how you going to live, wage, you know, I'd lost everything. There was only one way up, surely. So yes, that was the decision there, and I think it was a year later I did leave, and so, got out of that paranoid claustrophobic environment.

I remember moving, walking down the street one day in my new town, and I remember lifting my head up, man, thinking you can walk with a bit of confidence surely, so that made me kind of believe in myself again. Nobody knew who I was, so I could put a stamp on anything, I could reinvent myself. So yes, that was a good period.

I went to live on my own in a single room. It was me on my own with a bottle of whiskey every night. For however long it took. Hallucinating. No contact with friends. I think it was the alcohol, a closed environment.

I: What did you see when you were hallucinating?

A.28: I saw a lot of dark figures, they weren't fully formed, so spiders, spiders' legs, my greatest fear, was my greatest fear. I thought oh my god, so when the opportunity was right, I left and moved into a flat with a guy who was pretty cool, and that was the end of it. I put all that behind me. All that negative behaviour behind me, it just wasn't allowing me to grow and develop. So, that was me 30 s, and I went through job, job, job, until I am where I am now, realizing, having an epiphany that's what I wanted to do. It was a tough old journey, a lot of thinking in strange places, thinking this is your life! Thinking, how do I make a life for myself. I'd bowed down to other people—my father, my wife, but to do something for yourself, you know?

I: You must feel, because you've been there, you can be there for these people you now work with?

A.28: Absolutely, yes.

I: And in that context then, in a professional context, what's your experience there of insanity and its causes. You've mentioned it briefly, and some of the treatments, you've come across a lot of adolescents, have you got anyone there you feel it's OK to talk about?

A.28: Yes, in the environment I am now in there is a lot of mental health issues with young people. And it's down to them whether they address it or not. And I am there as a facilitator.

I: You say down to them. I mean you can't intervene?

A.28: Well, I can advise, I can say I knew somebody, a friend of mine . . . it's like a person who takes substances, it's up to them at the end of the day, no one else can help them. So, I think again with mental health, with young people, they do come through the door, and they are bouncing off the walls. I remember one case study, a young lad, he was getting dragged out every week, tied up, and in hand cuffs, he was just lashing out, lashing out. I got on quite well with him, and he was doing things, it was like he had OCD or ADHD, something like that, but he'd not been diagnosed. It was just him, being carried out, by the police, in a full body wrap, every weekend. And I noticed one day, when he was making a cup of tea, he put his spoon in the same place, not in the sink, but on top of the sugar jar, every time. I used to purposefully say, make me a cup of tea, just to watch what he did, and I went back to a couple of colleagues of mine and said this young fella has got more than we think and this environment isn't working for him, and he needs to be assessed by a professional because he needs structure. We are not helping him by seeing him get carried out, we might see what he is doing in the home, but that's not a sight you want to see every weekend. So, it was determined that he should move to a different environment, see a doctor, get medicated, and he did. And this boy transformed so much, his behaviour stopped, his outbursts stopped, he never ever got arrested once he was moved, it was another house in our company, he just thrived. He absolutely thrived; he went to college. So, looking at the boy that got dragged out, that came to us initially, and seeing the boy that left us was, was, team work. Hang on a minute, need to address it, so it went through a chain, being in that environment, which is very observational, and trying to see people's behavioural patterns, trying to see how they react. Because every situation is a communication tool, whether someone is punching you in the face or whether someone is crying in the corner, it's a way of communicating. And some kids you can break down the barrier, and some you can't.

And again, with another girl, I worked with on a daily basis, she was massive, massive, she was non-verbal when she came in. And she met me, I am not saying I changed her world, but she was very non-verbal, she started doing a lot of self-harm, a lot of self-harm, she said to one of my colleagues I can't sleep at night in my bedroom because I see figures, I see dark figures. She didn't tell me, my colleague told me, and I said to my colleague at the time, I said that is a sign of anxiety, that is sleep anxiety, I suffer from it myself, I've had two really bad experiences of it, and now I can learn, I can see it when it comes in the night. It is a black figure; it is a black shadow in the corner. It is hallucinations which you see, which you can't do anything about, you can't scream, your eyes are up, but you are in a state of rigidity, I said you've got anxiety, sleep paralysis, I give her all this information, I said you need to go and see, we call them CAMHS, Children and Adolescent Mental Health Services, and she was treated ultimately for anxiety, put on sertraline, it's difficult because they try and find out which is the best medication for her. They've put her on sertraline, they've put her on fluoxetine, which is Prozac, but now they've put her back on the sertraline because her behaviour on this different drug had changed a bit.

I: What when she went back on Prozac?

A.28: Yes, on the Prozac she was self-harming, it's sort of a minefield, experimenting with young people's minds. Once you stick with, once you focus on, communication is key, you need to go back, and get the medication that feels right, and like I say it's about cracking your own code. And she did comment, because we were talking one day, on the holiday I have just been on with the kids, she did comment in the group session, she turned around and said I was the only one that understands her. And I didn't say anything at the time, but I took that to be a sort of badge of merit. You know what I mean, because I have worked with this girl since she's come in the house, she didn't know what was wrong with her, she was hearing voices, black visions, and that's not 'madness' that's anxiety, it might seem like you're going into a world of . . . but let's address it, let's drive on with it, let's see what we can do with it, here's a load of information that you probably didn't even know existed, about what you've suffered. And this girl, hopefully, I've not seen her for a week or so, hopefully she is back on the right track.

And it's just seeing these kids come through, I know one kid who is very aggressive, but he's not medicated, not diagnosed, it's just aggression, it's just him acting out behaviours he's grown up with. His background I think was his mother was passing him around, and now he's got an interest in young girls. He's 16, but you've got to be careful, you can be arrested as an adult, but if he was medicated and he was counselled, which he is not having anything to do with, then we could see a different child there, he wouldn't be doing all that, he maybe would take a different route, but he's not. But this other kid who is, is a completely different child.

Maybe every time a kid comes in, he should be assessed by a mental health professional, and let's move forward from there, but these kids are scared, they've been in environments where they don't know, they don't know us, but we are there to help, advise, support, encourage, so I have seen a lot of scared kids come through who think they are on the brink of going down a really dark path but it's just grabbing them and going, listen, I know someone who suffered from that, this is this,

this is that, this is the other, this is what you need to do, and it has worked on occasions. And the kids probably think they are a bit 'mad' until someone with knowledge comes in and says this is going on.

I: Have you ever had to bring in social workers and doctors to section someone?

A.28: We . . . yes, we have. Again, I experienced a young girl, self-harmer, she'd been raped by her dad, chasing her one night through the town centre, ended up on the railway tracks, of all places—I want to kill myself, I want to kill myself—with me going—don't kill yourself.

I: Just you and her on a level crossing?

A.28: She stood on the tracks and I thought, this was before the old procedure came in, because I thought if I am there with you, you might have a second thought if you're going to take your life, you're going to take someone else's with you, you know what I mean?

I: Sorry, I don't know, what do you mean there?

A.28: Well, she went to commit suicide that night, she wouldn't take any notice of me. I phoned a colleague, I said she's heading towards the train track, she's stood on the line, so I have sort of encroached where she's stood, and so thought well if she's going to take one, she's going to take two. I didn't want that to happen, of course I didn't, and I said look we are stood in the middle of train tracks here, can we talk somewhere else? And eventually she came around to my sort of thinking, but after the police were called and cars turned up then they did section her, they did put her in and she went to the hospital.

So yes, I have had to do that, it was a real drastic situation, but when the police turned up, I was like listen she's got mental health issues, she's on medication, I've just been in a situation which I didn't want to be in, and I think I believe she did try and commit suicide, and unfortunately that girl is now dead because of her mental health, because of her incapacity to try and fathom out why her father raped her, probably. All that self-harm just gradually built up.

I: What, so she committed suicide, in the hospital?

A.28: A lot of colleagues of mine went to the funeral. I didn't, because of the background. She put me through quite a lot that girl, like stealing cars. I tried to prevent two girls stealing a car, wrestling them on the forecourt, thinking it was my fault, I just completely broke down. That girl came back the next day without any feelings of, of remorse, she was then arrested for that, and then she eventually did leave, but with regards that episode it was three girls going down the same track, being groomed.

I: Sorry, say that again, there were three girls?

A.28: There were three girls portraying the same behaviours and they were together constantly. And they were going out the house, self-harming, self-medicating, being abused, doing sexual acts for older men, for gangs, that sort of thing, coming back, smoking spice, being hospitalized, that went on for months, it was a horrible, horrible period for everybody that worked there. We were trying to reach out to them, but you can't, the lure, the pull factor, the gangs, the drugs, the sex, it was too much for them. So, in that respect I think ultimately there was an intervention and that shut the placement down. I had to go to a meeting with all the directors and staff involved and express what we went through and I was the only one that went in depth in front of all these people, it was very emotional.

I: Did they appreciate that?

A.28: Well, the directors did, because a lot of people were very tight lipped about it, like they could have done more but didn't. Well, when you are wrestling with a car at three in the morning you are trying your best, you know what I mean.

I: And so, we've just passed the Freudian hour, a question a lot of people in your position must get, how do you separate work and play, your personal and your professional? Because that is intense, it is difficult to get more intense than that, at work. And obviously it has an impact on you, so what stops you getting so worked up. You've mentioned some areas, is there anything else you would do, or you would advise people to do in your position?

A.28: I've been doing what I am doing now for just over 7 years, and I remember in the beginning, because with a job like that there's a lot of information to take in, I remember in the initial stages of it being curled up on a couch, in the foetal position, going I can't do this, it is too much, like rocking back and forwards. Back in the womb! Thinking it was too overwhelming, dealing with the children and learning a new job running parallel it felt to me like too much. At first, I struggled, I took this job everywhere with us, and that's all I ever talked about. And I still do in a way, I wear it as a badge of honour really, but it's quite a tough job to do, not everybody can do it, so yes, I thought this is going to change my life. And I mean it has, in a good way. But with the initial getting the job it was integrated because I lived only a couple of minutes from work, and then I was in another environment with a partner and her child and it was like a steamer ready to go off. Working there and living there something had to give, because I was just going home thinking about everything that went on, did I do this, did I do that. And eventually I wanted the job more than the relationship, so the relationship went. Now, because I am in a caring environment, it sounds a bit harsh but I don't take it as personal any more. I don't take it personally one bit. I know that might seem a bit steely cored, but I think if you took every story home and dwelt on it you would be an absolute wreck. Like I say, the beginnings were eventually like that, but after years of being in every given situation you can possibly be in, restraints, people leaving, people coming.

I: You say restraints?

A.28: Yes, if you put someone in restraints then you are a paedophile and a rapist, you know, I am just doing my job, just trying to prevent you hurting yourself and other people. And I've been called every name under the sun, and I will probably get it when I go back. I have become hardened to it, and although it is a, like I say a sort of inspiration moment, this is what I need to do, this is what I have got to do, and so I went out to do it. I made sure I went to the right places and got the right qualifications, and so I have chosen to be in that environment, I want to be in that environment, and separating it now which is a lot easier, because I am 7 years down the line, and I don't live near there anymore, I have got that separation. I have got that environment where I can just go and switch off totally, and that is what I do. I will go to work now that the anxiety is not there anymore, again sounds a bit cold, I am just going through the motions. I know what to do, I know when to do it, I know how to do it, and I know what to say to this person, to that person, so yes, I have found it over the years very therapeutic to be in that situation because I have learnt a lot about myself.

In another job you probably wouldn't learn so much about yourself. So that job now it's part of my DNA. And I am glad for it, because it has helped me to become who I am today, not just through all the mental health areas, but regard to helping other people, being honest, being empathic, being congruent, being allowed into people's lives, trying to fix it I suppose. It's made me who I am today. And I wouldn't have it any other way, it's given me lots of relationships, but it's also helped me get rid of loads of relationships I didn't need. So, in that sense I have become quite strong, so again in being able to address my own personal problems it's just proved that things can be done. Like I say, I was never one to become very ambitious, but now I do want to achieve, I do want people to know that I am doing things not just for me but for others. And I am trying to learn other things. So, I find it now easier, but I don't want to sound too cold blooded.

5.2.3 Example Three

The final section of the interview above shows how professionals can achieve a healthy distance from their work and relates to what psychotherapists call bracketing, enabling clients to compartmentalise aspects of their lives in a healthy fashion. The term bracketing has also been used in counselling research to overcome prejudices and expectations to focus on the actual research. Interestingly, this was the double movement of reflecting on pre-understandings and consciously being open to new information and demonstrated the success of bracketing, such as revealing the actual findings differed from expectations.[24] Overall, this is also good for wellbeing.

In this next example an individual encounters their father experiencing 'madness'. The participant questions the whole process of finding meaning. Derrida was referred to with regards to Example Two, but in this case, this is more akin to the poststructuralist thinking of Jean Baudrillard as previously discussed where a desire to find meaning is 'madness'.[25] Class is raised as a major issue, as it is in the other interviews. This next interview offers insight into how 'madness' manifests itself. Unlike the previous example, 'madness' is not thought to be a valuable term. As with the first two interviews there is a sense of loss and frustration, but there is again

[24] R. Elliott, D. Shapiro, J. Firth-Cozens, W. Stiles, G. Hardy, S. Llewelyn, and F. Margison, 'Comprehensive process analysis of insight events in cognitive-behavioral and psychodynamic-interpersonal therapies', in *Journal of Counseling Psychology,* No. 41, 1994, pp. 449–463.

[25] J. Baudrillard, *Fatal Strategies,* trans. Philip Beitchman and W.G.J. Niesluchowski, ed. Jim Fleming (New York: Semiotext(e), 1990), p. 176.

gratitude for how things are currently all showing a journey where obstacles have been overcome.

I: So, what is your background in the field of mental health, how do you see mental health, where do you situate yourself?

A.6: Well nowhere really, mental health is how I think about the world, no expert, just a person who sees it.

I: OK, what do you understand insanity or 'madness' to mean?

A.6: It's a bit of a label isn't it, to be honest, everyone is a bit crazy. Who is OK and who isn't, it is a matter of opinion. I would say some people are acting in a way where they are not looking after themselves, that's for sure. I would say insanity and 'madness' is almost like you have to look after the event, and look back on it, and then look—is that a sensible thing? It's a matter of opinion, it's hard to define.

I: Do you think you can't, do you think they are bogus terms, insanity and 'madness'? Or do you think psychosis is an actual thing? When you are getting into clinical psychiatry, things like that.

A.6: 'Madness' or insanity, it depends where you are coming from. To the person who is being 'mad', to them it is very OK, it is exactly what I should be doing, so it depends on which direction, exactly in what moment you talk about it. We call it 'mad', but it is a matter of how you look at it. So, I would say the whole process of existing is 'mad', it doesn't make any sense. And that's 'madness'.

I: What, to make sense of it is 'madness' or the fact that existence exists, is 'madness'?

A.6: Trying to conceptualise what it is to exist is maddening, so if you can't define what it is, to kind of exist, you know, what it is we are here to do, how do you define when we go outside the boundaries.

I: So, you can't define normality so you can't define abnormality, is that what you mean?

A.6: No, you can define socially acceptable, that's alright, someone doing that is OK, someone doing this is OK, someone doing that is actually crazy—so 'madness' is a funny concept.

I: It's interesting, one definition might be repeating the same thing—that is 'madness', one definition is it's not being able to see any other point of view, but another definition of that is just being self-willed, so you're focused. Do you think they are valuable terms?

A.6: There are definitely people you look at and they are outside the norm . . . my mum called up and said, "your dad's gone mad".

I: Your mum actually said that, she used those words, "he's gone mad"?

A.6: Obviously some threshold had happened, been crossed.

I: So, she used that word did she, "mad"? She'd didn't say he's psychotic, or he's lost it?

A.6: Yes, I think so, she's very precise. She didn't want to say anything, she was desperate, it was dramatic enough, and it might be sort of 'mad', and it made me go there, so there was some limit that we'd gone over that mum then labelled it differently.

I: What is that limit then, what makes that 'mad', what is he doing?

A.6: Well, when we got there, he didn't make sense, you couldn't have a conversation with him, he was like there was something happening in his mind, it was about his school, he lived opposite a school, asbestos involved, and he was paranoid or something, but whatever it was, he was talking in little snippets that didn't make sense.

I: Didn't make sense to you, but they made sense to him?

A.6: Without a doubt.

I: He was convinced, about some form of conspiracy or what, what was going on?

A.6: He looked nervous, but he didn't look confused.

I: He was convinced.

A.6: Yes, he was convinced his house had poisoned the school opposite.

I: He was worried he had infected the children?

A.6: Yes, and as the children were leaving the school, he was going, "oh no you have to protect them," so he was in a . . .

I: And what's the rational explanation for that then, is there one?

A.6: No, there isn't one, there's a limit he's gone over, and we don't understand that.

I: Is there something in there about influence, I don't want to get psychoanalytical about it, but was there a repressed notion of wanting to connect but can't? So, the paranoia makes him connect. What is the reason; you must have thought of that?

A.6: I just thought he'd been on his own too long. He's a little bit reserved, he wants a quiet life that kind of makes sense to himself. And you know, peaceful, maybe he's respected, intelligent, how he thinks, he thinks "I think things are good", and wants everyone else to think he thinks things are good, and maybe that didn't happen in his life.

Yes, so he's kind of angered, and he retreated into his own world and without external stimulation, feedback, he kind of got anxiety about anything. Depends; how dark you want it?

I: So how has this shaped your view on human psychology?

A.6: I am scared. How it's shaped my philosophy of human psychology is how fragile that mind of yours is, that is really scary, it is unbelievably fragile.

We think we have an idea of what is real, and we are OK, and that's OK, but if you look around you, you could moan at everyone, everyone is 'mad', they are 'mad' for doing that, and that and that. Katie Price is 'mad'. Sometimes you use schadenfreude about it, oh she's 'mad', but she's made ten million pounds. So, you think she's not 'mad', but maybe she loses it all, and you think oh maybe she was really, and the schadenfreude, there's always this feeling for me, there's always this weird limit. Am I actually alright or not?

I: So, it makes you question your own sanity.

A.6: For me, I've withdrawn yes.

I: Have you? What do you mean?

A.6: I think it's a really delicate moment. My dad was always a bully, boss, patriarch. Not as in anything weird. He's the most scared individual, so he gets what he wants, so with society and everything, mum married him, and she's been in his shadow, barked at a lot. So, what happens is when dad actually loses his mind, what I think is he can't make decisions about what to do. The house is worth this, for example, let's move here or there. There's no sensible decision, or any kind of cooperation, such as that's a good idea and let's all do that. All that goes out the window.

I: Do you think, just thinking about rationality and 'madness', so because he had depression and then he had dementia, this thing about being stuck like that, do you think this is almost deliberate, or is this part of the so-called illness? Do you see it as an illness, he can't make decisions, or do you think he doesn't want to, and that's comfortable? Do you think it's deliberate or not? Is there free will or not here?

A.6: He never helped himself. When depression kicked in there are things he could have done to avoid it, I'm not sure about the dementia or whatever, or whether it's a physical thing.

I: Can you elaborate a bit more on that, your experience of that in terms of treatments, causes, environments. You know, where's that at with him, or in a wider context?

A.6: Causes: if you isolate yourself, you will go crazy, yes.

You will develop an idea of the world, and if you isolate yourself from the world, you will just continue to develop that model of the world. If no one is around to change that model, you will just keep building it and reinforcing it. So, if you just keep building that model, without any influence, you will just go off in a direction.

I: So, he had no influence at all, no groups.

A.6: No, I don't think he was seeking influence, I think he was very opinionated, he wasn't easy on people, he didn't take their point of view and try to understand it.

It was a very difficult one for me. I think my dad accepted he was right, I don't know where it came from, maybe his childhood or something, but he put an iron wall around himself.

I: Really, at what point?

A.6: I have no idea, but it was always there. For me. I felt his guidance all along, but I didn't feel bullied. It's a story of a man who came from the shit into a world in which he finds shit.

I: So why become fixated on your own sense of what's right, and everyone else is wrong, what's the need for that?

A.6: He's born and he became aware—his mum's sixteen, his stepdad is a useless git.

I: What happened to his dad?

A.6: We don't know anything about his life.

I: Do you want to?

A.6: To be honest, as he drifts into his worries, I feel really sad, but in my life, I've asked him to write about it, to write a book about it; he's maintained that isolation forever.

I: I don't think he ever will. He's incredibly yearnful, he understands, he cries, in a way he's kind of lost, because he can't share it with anyone.

What do you think the issues are here in terms of class? Are there any, doesn't have to be, in relation to his 'madness', or your understanding of 'madness'.

A.6: In a way it's the key. I think my dad is a really smart guy, and so he's born into this environment surrounded by arseholes, and he wanted to go to the naval college, and they couldn't afford it. So, my dad built up some stuff, got out of there, and at the same moment there's some princess being bored, who has none of that shit. Then his 'madness' comes from class, because he can see around himself, that's what I said at my wedding, thanks for getting us out of this shit.

Yes, because he comes from such a working-class background, we stand on him, but he's paid a massive price, because I can understand. I can understand you asking all these poncey questions, but I don't think he could understand it.

I: Is sociology relevant when talking about 'madness'?

A.6: I tell you what's 'mad', the person who wrote that question. I mean, what are you trying to understand? I mean even science is gone, it had its tail up 200 hundred years ago, we've dealt with religion and, as science goes on, we understand quantum mechanics. The people who really understand, understand the least, the physicists. The absolute physicists don't understand. What's real or not, they can't tell you. Fundamentally, what's happening, there isn't a reality. The more you look at something it goes crazy. You can follow rabbit holes; physics has done that. What is real?

You open up things that go wrong. What is happening when an electron goes through a slit. Many worlds interpretation. The universe splits. For me, if people understand me and I understand them, then I'm not crazy, but if you go into the real world and dig deep you find nothing but craziness. You don't find sanity anywhere and it is ridiculous to look for it. The best you can do is to be polite to your friend, that's about it, in terms of being sane there is nothing else, and that's what I think.

I: So, on a very detailed level, it is insane, reality? Meaning you cannot comprehend it, so why try and comprehend it, it gives you feedback that there is an insanity at the quantum detailed level?[26] Is that what you mean?

A.6: Yes, there is nothing there. It's difficult for us, because we are trying to develop a society where we want to be in control. But when you try to look for the fundamentals, is there something that's fundamental, something good, or some fundamental truth? If you try and do this at any level, you find it just goes all over the place. Physicists try and say we will ignore the human race and any opinion, and we just look at the dots around us, and even they have got into a rabbit hole, going - my god it's all probability - there's nothing here that's real. This is very difficult, from the fundamental to the biggest level; very difficult to say this is real, this is right. So, I think when the 'mad' guy goes 'mad', he's only in his own world, it doesn't matter to us he's 'mad' but as long as he's happy.

Example 4

I: What is your background in the field of mental health?

A.22: I am a trained as an existential psychotherapist. I used to be a volunteer counsellor with child-line and bereavement care (Cruse Care), and I also used to work as a stop-smoking counsellor, and then about 10 or 12 years ago I trained to be

[26] See A.3.

a psychotherapist, and I specialise in existential psychotherapy. I work with individuals of working age, and I run one group.

I: OK, thanks a lot. So, what do you understand 'madness'/insanity to mean, are they valuable terms?

A.22: They are not particularly valuable terms in a professional context. They are romantic terms in a way that sort of sound like they are in a film or a book or poetry or something. So, in a professional context they are not helpful, although sometimes in a team meeting one or other, either me or a fellow clinician, I work in the NHS, might describe something as really 'mad'. By which we mean it just really did not fit any other context in which we could explain it. Something about it just really is not adding up. If somebody is presenting with OCD, or a personality disorder, or depression or anxiety or depersonalisation, we might expect certain things to be present in their presentation, a way of communicating. But sometimes people will just veer off, and then it will be a bit like that is quite 'mad', just to describe it I suppose as beyond our own personal and clinical experience.

So, insanity, I don't even know if that is a medically recognised term, and I'm not a doctor, and I'm not a trained medical professional at all. In terms of understanding mental health, I guess it would mean, it would equate with something like psychotic which is a term I might use and that would mean really out of touch with a sort of shared understood reality. So that's the term I would use instead, professionally.

I: So, what are you experiences of insanity personally and professionally?

A.22: So professionally, I have worked with people who . . . I guess I don't work with people who are psychotic or in an insane state, as it were. The work I do requires people to be and to have demonstrated a reflective capacity and reflective function and be able to engage in something in that way. I don't tend to see those sorts of people, or people presenting in that state professionally, although I hear of them, and I hear some ideas that seem quite strange.

I would tend to think of people perhaps veering into something we might ordinarily describe as 'mad' when people have got very fixed states of thinking, or just start telling a story that doesn't actually, really couldn't make sense. I suppose my experience of those sorts of people is that their stories are really quite plausible, and it is only sort of often afterwards that you sort of step back and think hang on, how the hell could that have happened, and hang on that's not true. But often when you're with them there is something quite plausible about their presentation. I don't know, for some reason I am thinking Jekyll and Hyde, you know, people running around with their hair all over the place isn't really the case. Although, you know, it has been known! So, I don't tend to see those people presenting with those sorts of symptoms so much.

My own personal experience, I suppose I feel that you know that there is, I don't think that I have ever been psychotic, but I know certainly that I am quite prone really, quite like obsessive sort of thinking about not being able to stop thinking about something, and becoming quite consumed by it, and you know so that in a way I might then, then like a friend might say something to me like you know that's not real, or how do you know that, or calm down, or something like that. I mean 'madness' seems like such a highfaluting phrase. I mean my experience of mental ill heath, of which I think there has been many over the years, I get quite depressed, I mean really depressed actually, and, and, can stay quite depressed for long time. I see myself and I sort of prefer in a way being depressed, so things like Melanie Klein, the depressive position to actually being anxious.

There is something quite safe about being depressed. It is horrible, it is horrible, but it doesn't feel quite as dangerous in a way, because I suppose I know that I'm not going to kill myself. Whereas when I'm anxious, and think someone is going to kill me, I don't know quite if they are not going to kill me in some ways.

So, I think I probably started to show signs of a sort of, you know, a pathology. Well, probably, probably, when I was about 14 and had a sort of eating disorder actually, and then got very depressed when I was 17, and 18, and 19. During those years I was sort out of control in some ways, and during those years I exhibited behaviour that probably I would now call 'mad', because I feel they were very out of character for me. But then I was also young, very young, and before I had loads of therapy, so I guess I don't know that. And then when was 22 or 23 I was sort of diagnosed with a borderline personality disorder which you know isn't 'mad', but you know as an existential psychotherapist, pure existential psychotherapists don't work with medical diagnoses and don't believe in medicalisation, so I don't diagnose people. And in a way when people come and say I've well, you know, I've got depression or something, the first thing is like, what the hell do you mean by that? But in some ways, having that diagnosis for me personally is quite helpful, because I guess it sort of contains those aspects of myself that might become a bit 'mad' or out of control, as in, you know, perhaps something like a life event has happened I might be able to think OK so I know there are some things which I find perhaps are more difficult to deal with than other people, such as being abandoned, for instance. It's going to, like, you know, can be quite difficult sort of thing, so in some ways it's quite helpful. And I guess for my patients sometimes their diagnoses are quite helpful, because it's a way of them checking in with themselves, actually, you know, is what I am feeling understanding what is actually happening or is it objectively there, and maybe 'madness' is an over concentration on the sort of subjective nature of things.

I: OK, thanks a lot, so how has this shaped your understanding of human psychology.

A.22: See, when I hear that question it's funny because I work with a lot of psychologists. I actually feel like I don't know what you mean. What is human psychology? You know, seriously, it's like one of those things I don't know what that means.

I: Well, I suppose you've already explained that in terms of your practice, but I suppose in terms of human psychology, psychology one sometimes thinks psychology is more related to constructions of the mind, and personality, both personally and professionally, I suppose this is more a disciplinary question.

A.22: It seems to me that I might not understand it particularly because as I say you know those highly trained in existential psychotherapy they don't really have like a model of the mind, my discipline would not use that language at all. Which actually puts me quite at odds working with the culture where I work often, because people do use terms that I don't necessarily know what actually they mean. But in my own opinion about models of minds and how people form relationships I guess funnily enough I suppose what I see happening actually is people who are fucked up as children nearly always grow to be fucked up as adults, and that is quite depressing in a way. You know, I would say that about myself, and sometimes I think I'm quite high functioning in some ways, but actually the damage that's done to us as children never ever goes away. And I then guess our challenge is to try and understand it, and to tolerate it, bear it, you know that how people are when they are quite small children and throughout their childhood and their teenage years does set a pattern that is actually very diff . . . I don't know whether it is that difficult to deviate from, you deviate from it, but it's always there. So, you know, perhaps in times of distress you go back to. Like those early attachment patterns, ways of behaving or defences. You know, like some people shut down, some people act out, and I see that sort of time and again with the people I work with that often people, you know I have to sort of class myself with this, and I do when I talk to my patients. You know, often people who have been quite hurt as children grow up to become helpers in one way or another, as a way of getting control. So, I think actually that's probably my view of human psychology. It's always about trying to get control in a way to stop yourself being hurt again.

I: Can you think about gender, sexuality, class and race in this context?

A.22: Yes definitely, you know speaking as someone who is on the bi-sexual end of the spectrum. You know you grow up knowing what the mainstream is, so you know that most people in this society are white, and you know that men have power, and you know most people are straight, and you know if you're rich you have more choices, and therefore all of those people tend to have more control. And so, if you know you're in one of those groups that isn't in the ruling classes and the elite, then you have to find other ways of subverting that control and getting it another way. It's just there is a lot of discrimination, you know. I guess now the big thing we are seeing is young people who identified as trans or non-binary who meet with, you know, in my experience they either meet with people who are a bit like, "hang on though this is a question of identity and meaning," and think it means something other than just gendered identity. And I guess I would put myself in that sort of camp. If they come and see me that's probably that's what they would be facing, consciously or consciously. Or they meet someone who is like "yeah all genders matter, it's all cool, be whatever gender and all that," which in a way you might argue is another way of avoiding the reality of what it might feel like to be a non-binary. I don't know if I'm going off on one actually, it's all discrimination, if you are black in our service, out of a team of say seven clinicians two are non-white that's in our team, you know everyone in our team, it's quite an elite team, because everyone who is there has had quite a lot of training. Then in the mental health team, which is sort of lower down the pecking order that's a much bigger team, and there's much more diversity of black and Asian people in that team, because you don't have to spend loads of money on training so it's more accessible to work at that level than work at our level, so that's the first level of the hierarchy in terms of race and class and culture. And you know you're much more likely to get you know if you see a psychiatrist who will assess you and put you through to our team, you're much more likely to come through if you are an educated middle-class white man even if you are not that ill.

But in terms of whether it makes you 'mad' I think it does, because I think you are always aware of being somehow other, or somehow having to apologise for yourself, or more scared of losing status or knowing other people ... and you're carrying a sort of duality ... and again speaking from my own experience of knowing what the norm, you know the heterosexual norm is and sort of carrying that, and having that as sort of one filter of how the world is viewed, but then also having that other filter which is a sort of you know as sort of lesbian or bi-sexual sexuality. So, I'm always looking at things from two angles, which is a strain sometimes.

5.3 Conclusions: Psychic Reality

This chapter studied 'madness' through the eyes of mental health professionals and those impacted by mental health problems. This included someone who worked closely with extreme media images and believed the work gave them PTSD. The chapter began by recognizing perceived reality is a narrative of selected meaning. As frameworks for understanding, A.22 mentioned that 'mad' was used in meetings in the NHS to describe when something was beyond clinical and personal understanding. Most mental health professionals interviewed found specific diagnostic tools useful. The more academic the participants the more nuanced their approach to diagnostic terminology and these tools. Binary approaches were found to be unhelpful when it came to approaches to mental health with biomedical and sociological models combined being the best way forward.

For those being paid to help those with mental health issues the personal was evidently driving the professional with early childhood experiences linked to emotional experiences and the transrational central to world outlooks. A vivid account was given in interview A.28 of what it is like to experience mental health issues and what happens when professionals deal with the end process. Medication was seen as part of a solution, as was a clear diagnosis and 'cracking your code'. This positive account shows how much an individual can grow in a complex and challenging work environment. To speak of reality is contentious with analytical psychology downgrading our reliance on external reality making the human internal world more important. All is a construction and a narrative with storytelling the key. How we create the narrative around the incidents of our lives results in the myths we rely on and our depth of transrational knowledge, our emotional awareness, informs this. Personal storytelling is sanity or 'madness' if we want to situate these as binary and broadening this binary opposition in a transrational sense leads to mental health.

As A.28 shows, clients enter a mental health facility believing they are 'mad'. They are then educated, and a specific diagnosis is found making them feel less desperate and different. Rather than being 'mad' they are then positioned into a wider medicalized narrative that may offer hope, as they come to understand they are not alone, and that there is specific help for their diagnosis. For A.3 'mental health condition' is more appropriate language. They still find misogyny and sexism such as blaming the 'cold mother' is at the heart of treatment. For A.6 physics disproves reality, so this makes analysis all the harder when it comes to ascertaining what we are dealing with both on a personal and on a social level. If we cannot get to grips with the foundations of matter, if the micro-story is unfathomable, how are we supposed to understand the more complex macro-elements of abnormality? Such questions are useful but suggest a desire for singular answers which are unforthcoming and which we have seen in Chap. 3 is the nature of epistomophilia. As we have seen throughout this is the beauty of seeing life as an open quest and a narrative in a transrational fashion with the films and culture examined making this same point. As Stanley Kubrick put it, to say anything truthful about life a movie or play must avoid conclusions, the point of view must be intertwined with life as it is through, 'subtle injection into the audience's consciousness. Ideas which are valid and truthful don't yield themselves to frontal assault'.[27]

A.28 believed their own diagnosis of anxiety helped them come to terms with their issues. They also believed they were going 'mad' and had mild psychosis so any support was of use. PTSD might also be an appropriate diagnosis, given some of their reactions. This confirms Nassir Ghaemi's thesis regarding mental illness and empathy and leadership, elaborated on in Chap. 7 with Gandhi being a complex example.[28] Not all accounts are so positive when it comes to diagnoses. A.13 believed they were misdiagnosed with bi-polar disorder and PTSD would have been more appropriate. These differences are notable; personality types respond differently to diagnosis, making a bespoke approach more fruitful. This needs to be the future of mental health and wellbeing work in terms of treatment and policy.[29] Some appreciate being told where they fit in, diagnostically, desiring a clear-cut treatment, offering safety with the certainty of the parameters that diagnosis gives. Others find it offensive. A.28's account explains clearly how young people might be so isolated they believe that are the 'mad' and a diagnosis helps them understand this is an issue that can be treated, rather than indigenous to them alone. As they explained you, 'don't need a history of trauma to feel self-conscious and even panicked at a party with strangers—but trauma can turn the whole world into a gathering of aliens'.

Our philosophical outlook and belief systems are central to our ontological sense of self and our culture's (haunt) ontology, how we collectively feel about illness, and how we feel about diagnosis, treatment, and further help. Psychiatrists describe a normal personality as one which is, 'never too sad, too angry, or too excited',

---

[27] Stanley Kubrick, 'Words and Movies', *Sight and Sound 90 Years Anniversary Special*, Summer 2022, Vol. 32, Issue 6, p. 67.

[28] Nassir Ghaemi, *A First-Rate Madness. Uncovering the Links Between Leadership and Mental Illness* (London: Penguin, 2011), p. 86.

[29] See Chap. 8.

problematically branding people as ‘neurotic’ and ‘infantile’ for example.[30] There is a cultural assumption here of a set perfect norm, that never expresses more emotion than is appropriate and, as we discover through further acknowledging transrational knowledge, the problem is that science has often relegated and even deleted emotion.[31] This is to remove the transrational and in Chap. 1 we saw how this position developed historically and how difficulties branded as mental health problems are emotional difficulties. The mental health profession developed a system for treatment to verify views on ‘madness’, to systematise the industry, and in their own view better process people to achieve data-driven results to fit targets, ignoring the human. Patients may not understand the severity of their illness unless this is addressed by an expert, this possibly being part of their ‘madness’. Work of this nature is in its infancy; to presume otherwise inflates capabilities within the mental health profession leading to accusations of narcissism.[32] This is partly why the anti-psychiatry movement expounded upon in Chap. 1 gained such traction during a period when many areas of power were contested. This can be termed the psychopathology of psychiatry; group institutionalised self-belief being over-blown and delusional. As we saw in Chap. 1, and A.22 explains here, psychiatrists are those believed to have pre-eminent insight which means other professionals lower-down the hierarchy are not as heard. But, as Dr. Glyn Lewis of the Royal College of Psychiatrist put it, we still do not understand how the brain works and there is no way of predicting who can improve or not on medication.[33] Traditional psychiatric drugs are convenient and can work for anxiety. Because of the ubiquity and long-term harm of depression, individually and to economies, there is a return to earlier treatments such as that involving LSD. In March 2021 Britain opened its first clinic combining talking therapy with controlled sessions of taking ketamine used to break down repetitive thinking common in depression.[34] In 2021 Imperial College was researching the benefits of DMT, a drug related to that used by traditional shamans and again the idea is to break the repetitive negative thinking of those with depression to develop new neural pathways for healing.[35]

Interviewee A.6 makes the direct point about class. People who are rich still feel pain and have mental health problems and some argue even more so.[36] A.6 outlines, those without wealth may have made certain sacrifices for the next generation that

[30] Erich Fromm, *The Fear of Freedom* (London: Routledge, 1989), p. 212.

[31] Ibid.

[32] This point is made by various contemporary psychologists.

[33] Glyn Lewis has made this point in a number of interviews, see Dr Natalie Ashburner interviews Professor Glyn Lewis: Antidepressants (rcpsych.ac.uk) (accessed 22 December, 2021).

[34] Rhys Blakely, ‘Ketamine on prescription at first psychedelic psychotherapy clinic’, *The Times*, 27 February 2021, p. 19.

[35] Linda Geddes, ‘Psychedelic Drug DMT to be trialled in UK to treat depression’, *The Guardian*, 9 December 2020, Psychedelic drug DMT to be trialled in UK to treat depression | Drugs | The Guardian (accessed 24 January, 2022).

[36] *Ecclesiastes* makes this point about the dangers of riches. See *The Bible*, Revised Standard Version (London: Collins, 1977), pp. 529–535.

can then lead to the deterioration of their own mental health, so it seems endemic to an unequal class system which ongoing mental ill-health perpetuates. When it comes to suggesting treatments being with others to certain personality types is hell, but community may heal. We saw how group therapy has been promoted for certain diagnoses like borderline personality disorder. How isolation can lead to 'madness' is underscored in these interviews. While genetics may play a part, any single causality theory is too simplistic and what is needed is the openness of the transrational which is often rare within health services with drama and art therapists on the lowest salaries.

Not even the deepest preliminary knowledge could lead to a true understanding if it were not accompanied both by an attentiveness to others and a self-abnegation and openness rarely encountered in everyday life.[37]

Real experience examined in this chapter includes the imagination and the transrational. As observed in Chap. 1, types of diagnoses change over periods due to cultural and social changes and can merge. As well as the lived experiences in this chapter, we have examined media and culture, including photographic history and theatre, illustrating a two-way relationship, the development of 'madness' with art creating conceptions of 'madness, including what it is and how it is understood. I was explained how the rational is not objective. An incessant desire for limited rationalism, the 'madness' of the real, is part of the problem not the cure, creating a need for reinscribing transrational knowledge which concerns the imagination. Instead of cutting off the imagination there is a need to explore its uses which is the subject focused on next. Derrida maintained the belief that spoken language has more integrity than writing.[38] While we can question his form of logocentrism there is a truth within the interviews in this chapter. Creativity is a fruitful way 'madness' is explored and tackled, counteracting the fear mentioned in these interviews. Having methodology drawn from personal experiences along with that drawing on analysis of media and culture is beneficial due its multidimensionality. In some sense there is no divide with the interview process a form of media, a mediated process, but reflecting on Derrida's point again there is a deeper truth, an integrity in these interviews. Emphasising the human as an individual is imperative, against the encroachment of data worship. For the outside world the 'mad' person has changed,

---

[37] Pierre Bourdieu, ed., *The Weight of the World: Social Suffering in Contemporary Society* (Stanford: Stanford University Press, 1999), p. 641.

[38] Mark Fortier, *Theory/Theatre: An Introduction* (London: Routledge, 2004), p. 63.

but for the 'mad' person change has taken place in the world.[39] But binary non-transrational divisions between these worlds are problematic.[40] Categorisations can lead to an unhelpful binary approach.[41] This returns us to the significance of empathy and the transrational, along with the importance of expanding what it means to be human fuelled by creativity and imagination, the subject of Chap. 6.

[39] Wouter Kusters, *A Philosophy of Madness – The Experience of Psychotic Thinking*, trans. Nancy Forest-Flier (Massachusetts: MIT, 2020), p. xx.

[40] Lucid dreaming is one practice that confirm this.

[41] For example, we cannot say science is outside culture/s.

Chapter 6
Creative Voices

6.1 Introduction: Voices and The Other

Over 20 years ago I went for a job interview at an Australian university. I say went; I was standing semi-naked in a rented semi-detached in Lancaster on the telephone at one in the morning. 'I'm a philosopher, I don't have a creative bone in my body, how would you teach me to be creative?' Good question, you might think. Based in empiricism, the analytical philosophy of the Anglosphere is often held up as of a higher level than what has followed in that discipline. Previous chapters explained how the rational and reason are just as full of prejudice as the irrational. I understand what this philosopher meant, and why they asked this; but it misses a major point concerning the relationship between creativity and philosophy. 'Culture and artistic creation are part of the ontological order itself . . . they make the understanding of being possible'.[1]

Chapter 1 examined the history of the prioritization of the rational and the problems that followed. We have seen how mental health issues are primarily emotional issues which are part of the transrational, but the emotions and the transrational have been overlooked leading to an increase in mental health problems. This chapter appraises 'madness' in the context of hearing voices and creativity, addressing questions concerning mental health, wellbeing, creativity and the transrational. This is an area that some have found dangerous, and yet creativity has long been equated with a visionary form of 'madness'. We shall see in Chap. 7 how successful visionary leadership in a crisis and 'madness' are synchronous.[2] We should not romanticise 'madness', including hearing voices. But we shall see there is

---

[1]Emmanuel Levinas, *Basic Philosophical Writings*, eds., A.T. Peperzak, S. Critchley, and R. Bernasconi (Bloomington: Indiana University Press, 1996), p 41.

[2]Nassir Ghaeni, *A First-Rate Madness: Uncovering the Links Between Leadership and Mental Illness* (London: Penguin, 2011).

J. Lee, *Culture, Madness and Wellbeing*, https://doi.org/10.1007/978-3-031-37530-9_6

an essential component to this form of transnationality that is part of the creative process and that guides.

Prolific film music composer Thomas Newman receives his music from outside of him not from within him and he sees the film business as the emotion business.[3] Similarly, for poet Paul Muldoon writing works like a radar, picking up signals and transcending the self. In his author's note to his collected poetry, he states that, other than correcting factual errors, he has made few changes given, 'the person through whom a poem was written is no more entitled to make revisions than any other reader'.[4] The interesting word here is 'through', as opposed to 'by', negating the capitalist idea of ownership. This conjures up the image of a shaman who is channelling a voice, rather than speaking from their own individual voice. This may sound 'mad' but is part of the depth of the transrational and the emotional.

The Bakhtinian literary theory term heteroglossia is relevant when discussing the multiplicity of 'voices' in writing.[5] Understanding and pursuing excellence with regards to voice in the context of narrator and character, for example, is an area covered by books on writing craft.[6] Using a layered approach, a diversity of voices, this chapter employs pedagogic theory, psychology and anthropology, as well as literary and cultural theory, to tackle voice in the context of 'madness' and transrationality. For Jung, what is not made conscious appears like fate.[7] There is a need to access this unconscious mind, this transrational world, and to subvert the conscious mind that might be repressing more imaginative work, more original voices. A relationship exists between the transrational and what is often demonised and dismissed as 'mad' and creativity. Why creativity is seen as such a threat is partly down to fear which relates to the fear of 'madness'. Creativity always begins by stepping into the unknown. Acknowledging the power of the 'imaginary self' means we can begin to subvert it.[8] Some writers get overly concerned developing what they hope is their own style and voice. Ultimately it is not about finding your own voice, but the story's voice.[9] This is a form of liberation and takes us beyond the obsession with the individual and is helpful in the writing and editing processes and in other activities, including the process to wellbeing. Overall, it leads to a more profound understanding of what we mean by the complex terms voice and 'madness'.

In practice this includes relinquishing the search for our own voice; working with and for the reader; welcoming the competing voices of characters; 'to find our voice

[3]Mathew Sweet, 'Thomas Newman in conversation', BBC Radio 3, Sound of Cinema, 16 April, 2022.

[4]Paul Muldoon, *Poems 1968–1998* (London: Faber & Faber, 2001), p. xv.

[5]M.M. Bakhtin, *The Dialogic Imagination: Four Essays*, ed. Michael Holquist, trans. Caryl Emerson and Michael Holquist (Texas: University of Texas Press, 1982).

[6]Jason Lee, *The Pschology of Screenwriting* (London: Bloomsbury, 2014).

[7]See Roger Brooke, *Jung and Phenomenology* (London: Routledge, 2015).

[8]A. Boulter, *Writing Fiction: Creative and Critical Approaches* (London: Palgrave, 2007), p. 62.

[9]Ibid.

we must lose it . . . in the voices of others'.[10] This has a *New Testament* resonance, ontologically, as well as a Buddhist character. To find yourself you must lose yourself; 'to find their voice the writer must know, at whatever level of conscious or unconscious imagining, their own intentions as an artist'.[11] What, then, is our intention as an artist and human being, and is this focus inhibiting? Boulter is writing about fiction when she comments that every word is caught between the conventions of the literary, the languages of the world, and our own 'voice', but this is relevant for other forms such as screenwriting. The reader in this instance is the co-conspirator.

This view is in some ways antithetical to the Amherst Artists & Writers (AAW) Group manifesto that begins with—'1. The teacher believes that the student possesses at least one unique, powerful voice that is appropriate for expressing his or her own lived experience, memory, and imagination'.[12] The AAW manifesto, following an order of priorities, goes on to command the tutor to tease out the primary voice of the student through teaching craft, convincing the student of the, 'value, beauty, and power' of their own voice.[13] These are guidelines, but the style they are written in suggests a form of pedagogic dogmatism implying if the teacher does not do so they are failing the student. It is important to question whether the complexities of the voice concerning the context, story, character, or social structures, are made as paramount as the stated utopia of coaxing the 'real', 'primary', 'authentic' voice from the writer. There is within this assertion the debatable implication that this 'voice' truly exists and is something outside the text.

Philosopher Emmanuel Levinas claims it is via the Other and from our responsibility to the Other that we have our subjectivity.[14] This can be equated with finding subjectivity through the plethora of voices emanating often from non-physical sources, as many non-fiction and fictional texts have revealed. I would add this might also come from the image, but Levinas would not concur given his Judaic belief that art, 'does not belong to the order of revelation'.[15] Jung maintained we do not create these voices, but the voices create us, seeing the unconscious as something beyond the individual.[16] This reversal has profound implications in our understanding of 'madness' and transrational knowledge. For theologian Karen Armstrong in all cultures artistic and religious inspiration has been conceived of as 'benign possession' in both artistic and religious terms.[17] But it has also be conceived as evil. What is profound is the notion that this is not the rejection of reason, but it is

---

[10] Ibid.

[11] Ibid., p. 68.

[12] Pat Schneider, *Writing Alone and With Others* (Oxford: Oxford University Press, 2003), p. 320.

[13] Ibid., p. 321.

[14] Emmanuel Levinas, *Totality and Infinity*, trans. Alphonso Lingis (London: Kluwer Academic Publishers, 1991).

[15] Sean Hand, *Emmanuel Levinas* (London: Routledge, 2009), p. 68.

[16] C.G. Jung, *Memories, Dreams, Reflections: An Autobiography* (London: Fontana, 1995).

[17] Karen Armstrong, *Islam: A Short History* (London: Penguin, 2000), p. 85.

more akin to reason advanced, speeded up, where the seer enters most fully into the moment equivalent of the 'event', as discussed by Deleuze. As we have seen, drawing on Spinoza and Nietzsche this becomes the purpose of philosophy or, to put it another way, of the experience itself: 'Philosophy's sole aim is to become worthy of the event.'[18]

Restrictive linear time ceases with a deeper result. There is a direct equivalent between religious revelation, artistic inspiration, and creation. In this sense solutions appear to enter the mind independent of their source. Armstrong explains clearly how religion was never supposed to supply answers within human reason and like art is concerned with the symbolic and mythic and enables us to live creatively when there are no easy answers to areas such as pain.[19] This is the same point I have argued throughout this book concerning the importance of the transrational for dealing with areas that are no black and white, such as emotions. There is the added problem when reason collapses in the modern world into mere instrumental rationality separated from the values intrinsic to daily life.[20]

For Muhammad, for example, hearing voices was not felt to be a benign experience initially, and the scepticism and fear is good proof as to the level of healthy doubting and analysis that occurred. In Sira 153 by Ibn Ishaq we learn, 'When I was midway on the mountain, I heard a voice from heaven saying: "O Muhammad! thou art the apostle of God and I am Gabriel"'.[21] Karen Armstrong explains that up until Muhammad's revelation the tradition in the region had been overwhelmingly poetic rather than religious and throughout his life Muhammad was careful to distinguish the Qur'an from ordinary Arabic poetry. He considered ending his life because he did not want to be seen as someone possessed by a jinni.[22] Others began to reassure him over the authenticity of his experience. Here there is an overwhelming by the numinous and a kinship to the 'terrifying otherness of God'.[23] This is an allowing of the transrational, prevalent in all main religions, often mistaken as 'madness'.

Looked at historically and culturally there is an equivalence with the existential thinking that fed into modernism and current philosophy and literary culture. Only through this entering into the otherness can depth occur. Virtually every account of prolonged silence mentions hearing voices coming in the form of divine intervention, or the tongues of 'madness'.[24] In the eyes of contemporary diagnosticians these are labelled visionary or pathological, although classic psychology calls elements of

[18] Paul Patton, *Deleuze: A Critical Reader* (London: Routledge, 1996), p. 15.

[19] Karen Armstrong, *The Case for God* (New York: Knopf, 2009), p. 318.

[20] Martin Jay, *Reason After Its Eclipse. On Late Critical Theory* (Madison: University of Wisconsin, 2017).

[21] Karen Armstrong, *Islam: A Short History* (London: Penguin, 2000), p. 83.

[22] Ibid.

[23] Ibid.

[24] Sara Maitland, *A Book of Silence* (London: Granta, 2008).

mysticism 'cosmic consciousness'.[25] It is interesting to compare this to the inner critic that writers can engage with, subvert, or ignore. Part of the self disassociates from the pain and the voice appears outside of the pain in a bullying way which can enable the individual to move through the pain, a good example being the memoir *Touching the Void* by Joe Simpson, which covers the true story of two travellers traversing the west face of Siula Grande in the Peruvian Andes, adapted for film by Kevin McDonald in 2003.[26]

Psychologist Steven Pinker thought he was going 'mad' because he heard human voices emerging from what he knew to be a randomized synthesizer.[27] This is sine-wave speech that can be deliberately manipulated to represent human sentences. Combinations of two or three bands of sound waves create noises that can be heard as human or quasi-human voices. Similarly, Sara Maitland queries whether the choir voices she hears in the wind might be formed from a combination of waves.[28] Hearing voices can easily be romanticised, but for balance it is important to consider their benign elements, given hearing voices is commonly associated with mental breakdown and the lack of creativity. For musician John Cage there is no such thing as real silence for there is always some sound, even if it just the human body sound.[29] The brain is always looking to interpret. Even in anechoic chambers, designed to stop the reflections of sound or electromagnetic waves, sound can always be heard, such as the heartbeat or pulse of the human involved.

There is a culture clash between an acceptance of the importance of transrational knowledge and dismissing it as 'madness'. Space is supposed to be the ultimate silent zone where voice does not travel, and yet the media frenzy around the space traveller, especially those involved in the moon landings, meant silence on earth at least was impossible. Furthermore, there is then the voice of those that filter into us in our interpretations of voice. As Andrew Smith explains in *Moon Dust*, his brilliant analysis of what happened to those who went to the moon, after reading J.G. Ballard's *Memories of the Space Age* he felt Ballard was whispering into his ear as he entered Kennedy Space Center doing his research.[30]

While this might be dismissed as a metaphor for the power of Ballard's writing, returning to earth in Apollo 15, Jim Irwin is purported to have heard God whispering to him at the foothills of the majestic Apennine Mountains. Irwin left NASA for the church upon his return. The shamanic tradition equates healing with channelling the voices of the dead but is sometimes viewed in the West as 'madness'. Stu Roosa, an

[25] William James, *The Varieties of Religious Experience: A Study in Human Nature* (London: Penguin, 1982), p. 398.

[26] Joe Simpson, *Touching the Void* (London: Vintage, 1998).

[27] Stephen Pinker, *The Language Instinct: How the Mind Creates Language* (London: Penguin, 1995)

[28] Maitland, op. cit.

[29] Ibid.

[30] Andrew Smith, *Moon Dust. In Search of the Men Who Fell to Earth* (London: Bloomsbury, 2009).

astronaut on Apollo 14, became exasperated when visiting Nepal because he was forever being asked the question, 'so, did you see my grandmother on the moon?' as the Nepalese believe their dead reside there.[31] Here silence does not reign on the moon but a cacophony of voices, be they the souls of the dead or the broadcasts of the living.

Dr. Edgar Mitchell, the sixth astronaut to walk on the moon, also underwent a mystical experience, returning to earth and founding of the Institute of Noetic Sciences. Similarly, the writing of pioneering travellers is revelatory concerning their engagement with the preternatural. For example, the pilot Charles Lindberg heard voices while flying the Spirit of St Louis in 1927 on the first solo nonstop transatlantic flight: 'First one and then another presses forward to my shoulder ... conversing and advising me on my flight ... giving me messages of importance unattainable in ordinary life'.[32] Every day reason cannot comprehend this transrational knowledge so dismisses it. So, during these breakthrough moments in human discovery there has been assistance and revelation from the transrational.

Whatever voices that come to us, some are the voices of others we have picked up and internalised until there is no differentiation. Issues of authenticity, uniqueness, and essence, so highly valued in creativity, become questionable. This relates to the examination of PTSD in Chap. 2 and queer theory in Chap. 3 on identity. In this respect the writing becomes a form of regurgitation, after the absorption, however we should not dismiss this as a mere parody, plagiarism, or postmodern bricolage. Shamans, for example, attempt to access the voices of spirits who are often from a world more connected to the dead, a world where theoretically all knowledge is possible and transmit this to the living.

In the novel *Unholy Days*, for example, the mayor of Tenerife hears voices deliberately courting them as they move him from the twenty-first century back to 1797 when Nelson invaded the capital Santa Cruz and stole his ancestor's wealth. 'With these few gestures and a lowering of his breathing he was transported in space and time'.[33] Here Jorge plays with 'madness', as does the title character in the novel *Dr Cipriano's Cell* where voices taunt him, rather than guide him, and push him over the edge.[34] In *Unholy Days* they function more like self-induced mediums. This can be read as too black and white and binary, as in one interpretation of a psychoanalytic view that the inner world is equivalent to that of the child and nature with the outer world that of the adult and intrinsically inauthentic. Everyone has an ability to channel this voice if they try, as it is innate and this inner voice will bring them back to what some term God, a prelapsarian state. 'Our judgement of the inner voice varies between two extremes: it is regarded either as merest nonsense or else as the

[31] Ibid., p. 3.

[32] Maitland, op. cit., p. 61.

[33] Jason Lee, *Unholy Days* (London: Roman, 2011), p. 9.

[34] Jason Lee, *Dr Cipriano's Cell* (London: Chipmunka, 2010).

voice of God.'[35] Jung continues that there might be a middle-point worth considering, but no one normally does.

In nineteenth-century literature this voice is shown to be accessible as a form of channel to a purer world. After World War 1 there was an upsurge in interest in the paranormal, especially seances, so much so that the Archbishop of Canterbury started a commission to find out why church attendance was falling, but seances were crowded.[36] Similarly, but more overtly, twenty-first century fictions address this need for multifarious voices. Hilary Mantel's 2005 novel *Beyond Black* depicts a professional medium Alison Hart with humour and in specific detail.[37] Alison may be able to communicate with the dead, but she has problems with the living and must team up with a financial guru Colette to sort her life out. We are immersed not only in the living character's narrative voice that is sharply alive and believable, but also with the non-living voices until we come to question the idea of who is speaking and whether such divisions are necessary at all. This confirms the non-binary view and the need for deeper transrational knowledge propounded in this volume. We are placed in the position of the living dead who themselves may not know they are dead. Instead of making profound statements about the nature of the universe they are often more concerned with types of cakes and kitchen fittings.

As well as the comedy there is a dark edge to the novel that subtly reveals the often-tragic underbelly of British life and mores, but it is not a postmodern tract claiming there is no individual self or soul and mere constructs of culture and society. In the transrational sense it confirms we are more than this. The medium Alison remembers more of her past which was like being brought up in the home of serial killer Fred West. *Beyond Black* functions as social commentary and by questioning the concept of voice it invites us to look profoundly at whom or what it is that is driving us, personally. This then enters transgressive and transrational knowledge asking what voices have we got inside and outside our head that makes us feel, think, and behave in the way we do? When Alison is in a state of trauma as a child these voices arrive as aids, but not all are helpful. What can heal us can harm us; a real danger and limitation is when we believe these voices are all we have.

David Peace's novel *The Damned Utd* (sic), (film directed by Tom Hooper, 2009) concerning Brian Clough's 44 days as manager of Leeds United in 1974, dexterously uses multiple voices to reveal how harsh Clough's inner critics were.[38] There is an unsettling quality to the prose with the reader, along with Clough, never being sure these voices are just a projection of his paranoia. Historically many writers

[35] C.G. Jung, *Psychological Reflections. An Anthology of the Writings of C.G. Jung*, ed. Jolande Jacobi (London: Routledge & Kegan Paul Ltd.), p. 271.

[36] Various authors have examined this. See Alex Owen, *The Place of Enchantment: British Occultism of the Modern* (Chicago: University of Chicago Press, 2004).

[37] It is interesting to note that in real life the author Hilary Mantel claimed she had seen a spirit when she was a child which influenced her entire life and fed her writing practice. When she died in 2022 the press focused on the claim ghosts infiltrated her fiction, literally and metaphorically. This included the ghosts of her Irish Catholic ancestors and her unborn children.

[38] See Chap. 7.

heard voices and this is well documented; St Ignatius of Loyola, who was known to be addicted to letter writing, heard voices and had visions.[39] Today a psychiatrist would drug the saint and have him locked up, the voices a threat to rational order. R.D. Laing revealed how the voices schizophrenics tell us hidden truths about society.[40] This is why those in the establishment want them to be silenced, especially when it comes to accounts of child sexual abuse one of the primary causes of mental illness.[41]

Can accessing these voices lead to a profounder originality in the way characters come alive, the writer stepping outside the text? Dr. John Dee, known as the counsellor to Queen Elizabeth I, and the subject of an opera by Blur and Gorillaz frontman Damon Albarn, conversed with spirits to gain mystical knowledge. These conversations appeared to enhance his creativity although they had their dangers as Benjamin Woolley shows in his biography of Dee, *The Queen's Conjuror.*[42] Stepping outside the text we step in creating objectivity through a knowing fluidity. This might seem like a call for writers to divorce themselves from their writing and eliminate emotion, but the antithesis is proposed here with a move towards the transrational. An interviewer may ask a writer if this or that character was the author or were they using them to expound their philosophy. In a world obsessed with celebrity culture this might be superficially interesting, but it takes us away from the story, an entity outside the author. This also could appear to be stating in laypersons' terms the New Critical mantra that there is nothing outside the text, but in New Criticism the structure and unity of a text contains, 'subterranean connections with its author', such as a verbal icon that corresponds to an author's intuition.[43] Despite this theory believing there is nothing beyond the text things are not this simple as was shown in Chap. 3. The known and yet unknown zone in a non-binary transrational sense cannot be escaped.

Characters encompass poststructuralist openness, such as the photographic model in Dennis Potter's miniseries *Blackeyes* (1989) who is there for the mark of the observer's gaze.[44] There are also well-known earlier characters, such as Tess in Hardy's novel first serialised in *The Graphic* in 1891 with numerous adaptations set up by the male gaze, and Sarah Woodruff in John Fowles's 1969 novel *The French Lieutenant's Woman* who is considered by the author to be the enigma who cannot be known.[45] Fowles follows the dictum to know your intention as an author and by

---

[39] W.W Meissner, *Ignatius of Loyola: The Psychology of a Saint* (New Haven: Yale University Press, 2009).

[40] See Chap. 1.

[41] Jason Lee, *Pervasive Perversions* (London: Free Association Books, 2005).

[42] B. Woolley, *The Queen's Conjuror: The Life and Magic of Dr Dee* (London: HarperCollins, 2002).

[43] R. Selden, P. Widdowson, and P. Brooker, *A Reader's Guide to Contemporary Literary Theory* (Harlow: Pearson Longman, 2013), p. 157.

[44] Ibid.

[45] Ibid.

this very process he allows his characters to become more enigmatic, more entrancing to the reader.[46] This dictum appears more important than finding an original voice. In this context and in the world of the story the apparently unknowable is engaged with, a sly metaphor for the creative process itself immersed in the world of the transrational.

6.2 Conclusions: Outside Conformity

The importance of voice has been explained in the context of 'madness', creativity, and the transrational. Discussing theories of affect and creativity, Sandra W. Russ referred to comedian Robin Williams who claimed that characters came through him, he just piped them, which has clear shamanic connotations.[47] This we saw was also true for poet Paul Muldoon. Many performers, such as rock star Mick Jagger, profess a shamanic quality to their art, where they appear to move or be moved into and by another being and become possessed, to truly take possession of their art. Interestingly, Harold Pinter begins his play *The Homecoming* with, 'What have you done with the scissors?'. Initially Pinter did not know who was saying this, and even whom they were talking to, which brings a level of openness to the concept of voice that transcends convention. This is refreshingly antithetical to the dictum 'find your voice', or even the more open 'find the voice of your story'. 'I sit back and get passive, and something is given to me .... When I have a subject, the subject tells me the style that he needs .... The whole world comes to me'.[48]

Numerous psychologists have related children's pretend play with creative writing and primary processes.[49] For Deacon (2006), 'aesthetic cognition may involve representational manipulation of emotional experiences', and what distinguishes humans from other primates is this feature.[50] Here we see that it is emotion, part of the transrational, that is the distinguishing feature of humans. It has been clinically proven that children who use play well can maintain more emotional memories to begin with and then have better access to these memories than those who cannot use play to deal with emotions.[51] This confirms the argument here concerning the importance of transrational knowledge for wellbeing as explained in Chap. 1.

Emotional awareness, transrational knowledge, advances us as individuals and as a species. Research in this context found that expressing negative affect was

---

[46] Ibid.

[47] S. Russ in A. Kaufman and J. Kaufman, eds., *Animal Creativity and Innovation* (New York: Academic Press, 2015), p. 251.

[48] Ibid.

[49] Ibid., p. 252.

[50] Ibid., p. 254.

[51] Ibid.

important.[52] Taking this childhood paradigm into adulthood the shaman, or creative writer that is any good, has a greater ability to play and to access these memories in play, ritualistically and artistically, translating them to the wider community. As Ingmar Bergman put it with regards to his screenplays, he had maintained an open channel with his childhood and at night between sleeping and waking he entered the door of his childhood where everything is as it was.[53] This is the root of transrational wellbeing which leads to creativity, rather than anxiety. How do we resurrect the past or tap into the eternal which includes the past, present and future? We have seen how through a focus on the transrational these false time boundaries become immaterial.

Bergman is most renowned for *The Seventh Seal* (1957) in which medieval knight Antonius Block (Max von Sydow) challenges Death (Bengt Ekerot) to a chess game to save himself and his friends. The film *Meet Joe Black* (Martin Brest, 1999) similarly concerns Death (Brad Pitt) who arrives on earth for basically a look around before taking the soul of media tycoon William Parish (Anthony Hopkins). Pertinently, the voice of Death is initially that of Parish (Hopkins), the soul Death is taken, as if he is talking to himself. At one point Parish says to his daughter Susan (Claire Forlani) that he is talking to himself when he responds to Death talking. Talking to oneself is assumed to be saner than to be talking to Death, but it can be argued every action and inaction is a response to Death whether we are conscious of this or not. By accepting Death can appear like this, accepting the transrational, this is part of the healing of William Parish, part of his sanity.

In the days leading up to his sixty fifth birthday before his soul is taken by Death William Parish learns from Death and vice versa. William Parish has a passion for life, that is why Death has chosen him to show him around earth, and yet he appears stuck in grieving over his dead wife which may have traumatised his two girls. How creativity deals with early childhood trauma is an interesting area, full of many voices, the theory being those constricted by unresolved mourning use this unresolved grief and identity issues in their transformative creative work.[54] For Morrison and Morrison (2006) early intense memories serve as motivation for later creative expression, as in the work of Emily Bronte, J.M. Barrie, Isak Dinesen, and Jack Kerouac.[55] The voices of writers and their characters and stories are tied up uniquely with this bond and with that of death, the voice with the strongest echo.

One argument is that when there is no physical external other, as with the experiences of the sailor or pilot or explorer, these become invented often for the purpose of high functioning, such as navigation as we have seen, so multi-layered personal discourse that is benign can continue. But this theory could be limiting, because those who experience these voices do not state they are invented. They might hear them, but to them they did not instigate them. Creativity that engages with the variety of voices explored here creates a higher resonance and impact.

---

[52] Ibid., p. 256.

[53] Ibid., p. 257.

[54] Ibid.

[55] Ibid.

Those grappling with the unknown were thought to be ‘mad’ or possessed by spirit, and these voices may or may not have been their own. Leaders who deal with the unknown are more able to do so in a crisis if they are affected by ‘madness’ and this is part of leaders engaging with the transrational, a subject to which we now turn.

Chapter 7
Cults, Leaders, Groups

7.1 Introduction: Cults

Media, communication, and cultural studies in the main has focused ideology and power. When it came down to the human on a personal level psychologist Alfred Adler believed everything was about power.[1] Along with an analysis of real-life narratives and creativity, so far, we have examined power dynamics concerning the context of 'madness', gender, sexuality, class, and race. The significance of the transrational has explained and it has been argued that the transrational has been ignored leading to poor mental health. This chapter analyses cults, leaders, and groups, where power dynamics are also primary and draws on films and popular culture to illustrate this.

Chapter 1 explained how leaders in the happiness industry created an ideology from the notion that the world is merely how we perceive it to be. We know from Bergson that internal experiences, which he contentiously called intuition, are just as important as the real world. Such an argument then gets dominated by accusations of irrationalism. What is more interesting about Bergson is that he believed novelists, such as Virginia Woolf mentioned in Chap. 1, were able to convey a more accurate depiction of experience. Here is where the transrational and imagination are important and it is this argument that has been made throughout this book. Ironically, something beyond reason cannot be accepted by reason. This ought to flag up to us the limitations of just relying on reason which is not as objective as we might think.

'Madness' can be a trait of leadership producing better results in a crisis.[2] Popular films about famous leaders, such as politicians like the trilogy by Oliver Stone, including the banal *W.* (2008), humanize flawed or dangerous leaders, some verging

---

[1] Alfred Adler, *Understanding Life. An Introduction to the Psychology of Alfred Adler* (London: Oneworld, 2009).

[2] Nassir Ghaemi, *A First-Rate Madness: Uncovering the Links Between Leadership and Mental Illness* (London: Penguin, 2011).

J. Lee, *Culture, Madness and Wellbeing*, https://doi.org/10.1007/978-3-031-37530-9_7

on 'madness'. Unfortunately, as Stone found with his George W. Bush film, the problem is this approach makes for dreary drama. The humorous and zany part of W.'s character was deleted, and he was sanitized, making the film excruciatingly dull.[3] Like Donald Trump, Bush was often dismissed for being stupid and crazy. Paradoxically, when it came to crisis leadership decisions like 9/11 and the Iraq War like Tony Blair US President Bush was too mentally well to be a good leader, although during the twentieth-anniversary of 9/11 attempts were made to reconstruct him as a great leader. That was not difficult when we compare him to Donald Trump.

Unlike J.F. Kennedy and many other renowned leaders such as Winston Churchill, there is no evidence that Blair or Bush suffered from mania, psychosis, depression. This is a complex factor concerning leadership that psychiatrist Nassir Ghaemi makes clear; however, there appears to be a contradiction in his argument when he claims Bush and Blair were not realistic enough to not invade Iraq. That single act, with no evidence of weapons of mass destruction, seems like 'mad' behaviour of sorts. Unfortunately, being able to construct lies (a psychopathic trait) is also felt by psychologists to be a sign of maturity and mental health.[4]

Donald Trump's White House rule was in part a backlash against the first black president 'no drama Obama', but it is interesting to note how the perceived stability of Obama may have been viewed as a weakness.[5] When it comes to leadership the media are hell bent in creating a dramatic 'mad' narrative every day pushing the drama that comes through conflict creating click bait online and bigger audiences. Even when there is no crisis the veneer of crisis is promoted.[6] Each Tweet sent by Trump was poured over and often seen as a sign of his unhinged mind and constructed as such by parts of the media. If we cannot predict someone's next move, their entertainment value increases. Due to Trump not being a good leader in a crisis, such as the COVID-19 pandemic, following Ghaemi's argument does this then prove his sanity?[7] According to the narrator of *Enduring Love* there is not a human society, 'that did not have its leaders and the led; and no emergency was ever dealt with effectively by democratic process'.[8]

Whether we call it 'madness' or mental illness, the oddity of the leader can be their strength. Genetically and/or epigenetically it has been argued leadership is rooted in our biology with paranoia a key trait for leadership.[9] There is a spectrum of course: Winston Churchill had the correct level of paranoia; Adolph Hitler's was psychotically destructive. Other forms of psychopathology are not as useful for a

[3]P. Bradshaw, '*W* Review – Dubya presidential biopic without dramatic fizz', *The Guardian*, 7 November, 2008, p. 42.

[4]See the television series *Lie to Me* (2009–2011), based on the work of psychologist Paul Ekman.

[5]Ghaemi, op. cit.

[6]S. Price, *Worst-Case Scenario? Governance, Mediation, and the Security Regime* (London: Bloomsbury, 2013).

[7]Ghaemi, op. cit.

[8]Ian McEwan, *Enduring Love* (London: Jonathan Cape, 1997), p. 11.

[9]Ghaemi, op. cit.

leader. The narcissist is tuned into their own wants and needs rather than that of their followers, using lying and deceit with their lack of conscience bringing ruin to their followers. Threatening times lead to charismatic and messianic leaders which explains the unexpected success of Brexit and Trump.[10] One criticism of this approach is that this is confirmation bias; just because leaders show these traits it does not mean that genetics has made this so. Introversion rather than extroversion could just as easily be a trait of great leaders, as with Mahatma Gandhi and Barack Obama.[11]

David Peace's novel *The Damned United* and the film (Tom Hopper, 2009), discussed in the previous chapter, concerns the trials and tribulations of the best manager the England football team never had, Brian Clough (Michael Sheen), during his brief tenure at Leeds United in 1974. Clough, renowned for being outspoken which was media gold, wrestled with many inner demons and paranoia. The fact he possessed a genius, despite or due to these demons, makes him a heroic leader, 'madness' or not. His extraversion, charisma, clear and direct communication, entertaining use of language, sensitivity to his men's wishes, and his paranoia enabled him to know his enemies. All of this positioned him as the perfect leader. But this is only up to a point. What Peace does so superbly is explore that mental health issues behind Clough's cock-of-the-north mask exterior. In all respects, his strengths were his weaknesses—he could never be wrong, and was brilliant in instilling confidence in others, but this can lead to hubris and a fall. In Peace's version of the man, paranoia runs rampant and at times it is in control of him. If Peace had written a traditional biography, the depth of Clough's internal 'madness' would never have been illustrated so vividly.

The follower projects notions of perfection onto their leader, seeking a superhuman messiah figure encapsulating their utopian desires. The imperfections of a leader, including their 'madness', can be spun by their public relations team as the trait that makes them more human, more authentic, more like one of 'us' despite their weirdness, with Donald Trump again a great example of this. The whole idea of authenticity took on a whole new meaning under Trump, given the way he thrived on dichotomies, such as condemning the mainstream media as 'fake news'.

Like 'madness' and leadership, 'madness' and wisdom have also been equated, but not without controversy. Writers such as George Feuerstein have popularized the term 'crazy wisdom' in works like *Holy Madness* (2006).[12] The immediate nature of this wisdom infuriates some, given this wisdom appears to not have to be worked for contradicting all the Puritan position stands for. The parallels between the 'mad' and leaders are blatant: the 'madman' is convinced of their delusion more than anything

---

[10] Savvas Pappacostas, *Madness and Leadership: From Antiquity to the New Common Era* (Cheltenham: Edward Elgar Publishing, 2015).

[11] It is a truism that our strengths are our weaknesses.

[12] Georg Feuerstein, *Holy Madness: The Shock Tactics and Radical Teachings of Crazy-wise Adepts, Holy Fools, and Rascal Gurus* (London: Penguin, 2006).

else; the leader can be obsessed with their vision more than anything else. The leader then can deny reality in the process.

Here we are at the heart of why a certain level of mental ill-health is paradoxically a good thing. This is partly why depression is a healthy trait in leader, as is well-known with Churchill; it offers a realism, given people without mental health issues are naturally over-optimistic.[13] *Darkest Hour* (Joe Wright, 2018) portrays how Churchill (Gary Oldman) had to overcome the over-optimism of those in his war cabinet who wanted to appease the Nazis. Leaders are often psychopathological and in popular culture this difference can be laced with aspects of evil which audiences find attractive and glamourous. For example, they can cross a line not many of us would—including murder. This is framed as being for the greater good given, 'leadership and followership are evolutionary adaptations that developed in order to enhance group cohesion, to maximise chances for survival and reproduction'.[14] We might find the inordinate number of pages of print media devoted to leaders tedious, or how their every movement is broadcast banal, but this biological understanding offers a further reason why this is. Simply, if our leaders are not functioning well our survival is threatened.

Following the death of American president Frank Underwood (Kevin Spacey) in the hit TV show *House of Cards* (2013–2018), in Season 6 the president's chief-of-staff, recovering alcoholic Doug Stamper (Michael Kelly), has a breakdown. Only in Episode 8 is it revealed Doug killed his former president because Frank was about to kill his own wife, sitting President Claire (Robin Wright), 'protecting the legacy from the man'. The extremes everyone goes to gain, keep, and protect power appears 'mad' here, but also totally necessary, with this narrative's fictional world mirroring reality.

The president has previously killed his journalist-lover. Doug sees a psychiatrist confessing to this murder, one he has not committed, again protecting the legacy of his boss. The 'madness' of loyalty is dissected and the group psychosis of belief in a corrupt leader unveiled. Political parties, executive boards, and large police forces, often try to mimic this level of loyalty and paranoia which is akin to the mafia and reflects on both the Clinton and Trump presidencies. For Claire this therapy is to gain information, Doug's therapist feeding her every detail. The therapist jumps to the conclusion Doug is psychotic and truly 'mad' because he has confessed to a murder.

Aware of the bigger picture, as the audience we know the patient's way of thinking is more strategic than this. Speaking is of course often equated with wellness but, paradoxically, expressing our thoughts and feelings can be a way of avoiding experiencing them. One other danger of psychotherapy is that it can add to hopelessness. Stories are repeated, emphasizing an inability to change. Despite a recent surge in narrative-therapy, telling a story is not enough for healing. A patient

---

[13] Ghaemi, op. cit.

[14] Savvas Pappacostas, London School of Economics *Business Review*, 'A bit of madness is good for leadership potential', https://blogs.lse.ac.uk/businessreview/2017/09/04/a-bit-of-madness-is-good-for-leadership-potential (accessed 18 November, 2020).

must be prepared to change the narrative, to move beyond the framework of the previous narrative, otherwise they are in danger of being continually re-traumatized. If not, this enables 'madness' to perpetuate, keeping the real trauma at bay.

Cult-like behaviour occurs in many organizations including those considered mainstream, such as governments, corporations, universities, and schools, as well as religious groups. Indeed, it might be in organisations where the ideologies are not as overt where the power dynamics and hold over people is stronger because it is less opaque. What we may have considered to be on the fringes is part of the mainstream and understanding this enables us to realise that 'mad' behaviour is often normalized. Political cults create extreme behaviour, such as the storming of Capitol Hill in January 2021 when six people died.

Knowledge of cults is popularized and glamourized through documentaries, such as the Netflix series *Wild, Wild, Country* (Maclain and Chapman Way, 2018) about Bhagwan Shree Rajneesh (Osho). Frequently these figures are demonized as charlatans in the media, and yet evidence as to their transrational healing powers comes from all quarters, including the psychiatric profession: 'the greatest successes of all have not belonged to psychiatrists but to the shamans, priests, leaders of sects, wonder-workers, confessors and spiritual guides of earlier times'.[15]

Figures like Bhagwan, who promoted a communal alternative lifestyle in the 1970s and 1980s, are perceived by the political and social establishment as a threat to the status quo. On the surface they often challenge the propaganda of individualism and materialistic consumption at the heart of Western society's capitalist ideology. Bhagwan's cult blended capitalism well with spiritualism. The Western world is termed sick and 'mad', and it becomes again a matter of one group with its defined ways of being and behaving asserting its identity and difference through condemning the other.

For American transcendentalist Ralph Waldo Emerson believing in your own thoughts and knowing these are true is a sign of genius, but this is also a sign of narcissism veering on 'madness'.[16] In various interviews the documentary filmmaker Michael Moore termed Trump an 'evil genius' but we need to be careful with the term evil in case in glamourises deviant behaviour and places it on a supernatural level beyond human intelligence. The need to prove an almost supernatural level of power is innate in many humans, not just psychopathic cult leaders.

Freudians argue there is the primary narcissism of children and then the secondary narcissism of schizophrenics. Adults who remain narcissistic in adult life, 'retain this need to be loved and to be the centre of attention together with the grandiosity which accompanies it'.[17] But many actors, extroverts, and leaders could be described in this way, making it very difficult to distinguish what exactly is a mental illness.

---

[15] K. Jaspers in Anthony Clare, *Psychiatry in Dissent – Controversial Issues in Thought and Practice* (London: Routledge, 1989), pp. 38.

[16] Anthony Storr, *Feet of Clay – A Study of Gurus* (London: HarperCollins, 1997), p. 208.

[17] Ibid., p. 211.

Unfortunately, those seeking transcendence and oneness are sometimes led by those creating divisions to assert their power and absolute authority, such as David Koresh.

Cults were part of the foundation of America which was concerned with freedom of religion and America is most popularly associated with cult behaviour for good reasons. What was known as the Burned-Out District in New York State became an epicentre in the nineteenth century for all manner of movements.[18] Some of these, such as the Quakers, are known as mainstream today. Others moved towards spiritualism and the belief in the supernatural.

The common denominator here can be summed up in three words: power, profit, and paranoia. Again, the separation between the mainstream and the marginal is not as overt as might at first be believed. The People's Temple is an especially salient example of this. Founded by the Reverend Jim Jones, at first Jones was a mainstream ordained minister. He established a church in San Francisco in the 1970s which had the support of political figures, but those deeper within the cult knew the healings they claimed were fake. After moving the cult to Latin America, Jones advocated revolutionary suicide and 918 followers died. Overall, the American constitution, including the Bill of Rights, makes it easy for groups to establish a religion which is tax free.

Again, when we consider the main attributes of a cult—behavioural control, informational control, thought control, emotional control—we see overlaps with other, more normalized, organisations, such as corporations and political groups. Whether it is a belief in salvation through alien forms, as in the cult Heaven's Gate which carried out mass suicide, or promoting the end times Biblically, as in David Koresh's Brand Davidian cult where eventually 75 followers died, the actual belief is immaterial. What is more important is the control of vulnerable people seeking answers from a charismatic leader which is big business. From the 1960s to the 1980s cults attracted young people fighting the system, dismayed by war and seeking a new way of life. Since the 1980s members tend to be in the middle age bracket, highly educated and having a solid income. As with the Witch Craze, we see the pre-eminence of finance.

Chapter 1 examined the contradictions of the happiness industry. In some sense the cult industry and religion business are part of this, promising true happiness here or in the here-after. The tax-free religion business in America alone is estimated to be $4.8 trillion annually, so we should not underestimate the financial incentives for establishing cults.[19] As with the Witch Craze, some researchers tend to over-emphasize psychological and/or religious elements, but economics is key. The Kabbalah Centre linked to celebrities such as Demi Moore and Madonna, exemplifies this. It has drawn controversy due to its selling practices, despite being a non-profit organisation. Like some forms of 'madness', if you are in a cult, you often do not know you are. You refuse to believe it, trusting you are consenting and

[18] P. Knight, *Conspiracy Theories in American History* (New York: ABC Clio, 2003).

[19] B. Grim and M. Grim, 'The Socio-economic Contribution of Religion to American Society: An Empirical Analysis', *Interdisciplinary Journal of Research on Religion*, Vol. 12, 2016, pp. 1–31.

ignoring areas such as the coercion and control. Video footage with believers from cults like Heaven's Gate where 39 died of suicide confirms that these believers sincerely thought they had never been happier. We might doubt this as outsiders, seeing this as staged for the cameras, but who are we to judge?

It would be wrong to call all these leaders and followers 'mad'. While openness is one of the five main traits that psychologists use to measure human personality (along with conscientiousness, agreeableness, neuroticism, and extraversion), paradoxically having a closed mind is in part essential for living, an open mind leading to an increased risk of mental illness.[20] This openness is largely determined by genetics and environment.[21] Followers lose their ability to be individuals. Individualism may have caused them angst and unhappiness, so they deny their individuality and separateness for a new sense of all consuming belonging. This might bring some happiness, but for society this has meant mass suicides, bio-chemical attacks as with the Osho cult, and terrorist bombings.

There are an estimated 5000 different cults in America alone with approximately 200,000 members.[22] Those in cults believe the mainstream's concern about them is further evidence of their truth and conspiracy theories have been enhanced by this paranoia. For example, a question that still concerns some is who started the fire in 1993 on the Branch Davidian compound led by David Koresh which led to over 75 deaths? We return to economic and the financial incentives, not religious motivations; Koresh was buying and selling guns without paying taxes. This was why the cult was flagged to the authorities. It had been operating peacefully in various forms since 1935, Koresh not moving to the cult until 1981. If greed had not consumed the cult leader with Koresh making money from selling weapons plus stockpiling them the government would have left them in peace.

Film and media often remove the complexity concerning why people follow leaders. An analysis of Italian fascism and the media reveals economics is more relevant than the 'mad' charisma of the leader.[23] Via a plethora of popular documentaries, the media often situates the main danger of a cult as being the leader's mental health, condemning figures such as Koresh and Osho as psychopaths. This is just one-way explanations that dwell on personality usurp analysis drawn from socio-economic factors that seeks to establish why people may be drawn to cults in the first place. Our culture of narcissism thrives on such a focus. A more nuanced approach comes from interviews with survivors of cults such as those in *Wild Wild Country* who often still maintain their cult offered a level of freedom that was unavailable in 'straight society' burdened by conformity and the rigidity of a rational normality. This is confirmation of our wider argument concerning mental health problems being created by society's prioritisation of repressive rationality and a non-engagement with transrationality.

---

[20] James Marriott, 'Why a closed mind is key to a happy life', *The Times*, September 3, 2020, p. 27.

[21] Ibid.

[22] Stephen Hassan, *The Cult of Trump* (New York: Free Press, 2019).

[23] John Dickie, *Cosa Nostra: A History of the Sicilian Mafia* (London: Hodder & Stoughton, 2007).

Unfortunately, when people move into cults, they discover that far from being open explorations of transrational knowledge they falsely use so-called secret knowledge, with truth being literally purchased at a cost. Membership involves an obligatory transfer of financial resources to indicate commitment, or a staggered increase of financial commitment as you go higher up within the cult system as with Scientology. In some respects, there is little difference between groups like Scientology and the Freemasons, although the latter seems more benign. Despite murders connected to it, the Freemason have dominated the foundation of the modern world with many prominent leaders being members, including Winston Churchill, King George VI, and one third of all American presidents.[24] People thrive within secret societies.

Celebrity culture and new media have exponentially advanced desires to gain public approval, turning more people into overt followers giving rise to cultish leaders and life-style gurus, such as Russell Brand mentioned in Chap. 1. Globally, the rise of nationalism and celebrity worship has normalised this further, on top of the mainstreaming of New Age beliefs. This is tied to an exponential rise in belief in conspiracy theories that grew further when governments took measures to combat COVID-19 in 2020 which to some looked to draconian and dictatorial. Interestingly, older humans are better at learning than other animals who age because we preserve a level of flexibility and adaptation depends, 'principally upon learning rather than upon those built-in behaviour patterns which govern the lives of creatures lower down the evolutionary scale'.[25] Our infancy and childhood are prolonged relatively to our total lifespan differentiating us from most animals. Just because some retain the childlike willingness to learn this can be counterbalanced by a deliberate sense of knowing-it-all. Teenagers are frequently cited here, but it is fallacious to stigmatize any stage of development as less open to knowledge and learning and development.[26] Maturity can be associated with doubt which is healthy if we compare this with the absolute belief in authority figures as exemplified with belief in gurus or certain leaders.[27]

The opposite of faith is not doubt but control, and it is control that exemplifies cults. Although it cannot be healthy to blindly follow any human being, the temptation to relinquish power over oneself with the deluded sense of freedom this can bring is strong. The success of fascism in the twentieth century shows this. To the insider in a cult this is pure liberation despite the cult enslaving the follower. In tough times people seek fixed answers and cult leaders are more than willing to provide them. As conspiracy theorist David Icke states in one of his advertisements which have been banned from Facebook but still appear under other names, 'I have the

[24] John Dickie, *The Craft: How the Freemasons Made the Modern World* (London: Hodder & Stoughton, 2020).

[25] Storr, op. cit., p. 215.

[26] Sarah-Jayne Blakemore, *Inventing Ourselves: The Secret Life of the Teenage Brain* (London: Doubleday, 2018).

[27] Storr, op. cit., p. 221.

power!'. These figures sell themselves as uniquely gifted and possessing a secret, the ultimate secret that they have been especially chosen to reveal. And all for a fee, of course, possibly everything you own.

One leading thinker and practitioner on psychological wellbeing, psychiatrist, and founder of analytical psychology Carl Jung, was termed 'mad', indicating a correlation between 'madness' and health and wisdom. Jung's movement has also been termed a cult.[28] Some concluded Jung was schizophrenic at one point in his life, or at least suffered forms of psychosis.[29] We have seen how great leaders had a mental illness. Paediatrician and child analyst D.W. Winnicott, previously mentioned due to his BBC role bringing health to the nation, believed Jung was a child schizophrenic and a recovered psychotic.[30] This is placing his experiences within a medical framework. Another way of looking at this is Jung was engaging with different parts of himself on purpose.

Between 1913 and 1918 Jung underwent several experiences, including hearing voices, which he said were psychotic, but he also saw this as an experiment being performed on him. We saw in Chap. 6 how hearing voices is far from abnormal and is related to creativity. Jung worked with these experiences leading to his influential form of transrational knowledge. The Jungian engagement with the mythopoetic imagination which vanished from our rational age could then be once more used to understand the human psyche.[31] Jung's personal experiments with the unconscious confirmed what he had observed in his Burghölzli psychiatric patients, namely, 'that there exists a collective substratum to the human psyche on which the personal psyche is based.'[32] An increase in mental illness is caused by the denigration and lack of integration of the mythopoetic imagination, that is, attempts at deletion of the transrational. To gain mental health means to re-invigorate the transrational.

Issues such as class are notably untouched in many examinations of Freud and Jung and in their own work. This is despite the work of influential figures such as Wilhelm Reich, Geza Roheim, and Herbert Marcuse, known as the Freudian left.[33] Overly concerned about what he thought was the boredom and conformity of Marxism, Jung read texts as warnings against communism, rather than warnings against the conformity of capitalism.[34] The immense emphasis on the individual in systems that work to cure a patient fosters the idea that the individual is permanently at battle with the group, or the individual is solely at fault. An essential belief of Jung is that the psyche mirrors the universe. This takes us outside what is thought of as nature and is expansive, but some may consider it 'mad' that Jung insisted that his

---

[28] Richard Noll, *The Jung Cult: Origins of a Charismatic Movement* (Londone: Touchstone, 1994).

[29] Storr, op. cit., p. 89.

[30] Ibid., p. 90.

[31] Anthony Stevens, *Private Myths. Dreams and Dreaming* (London: Penguin, 1996), p. 125.

[32] Ibid.

[33] Paul Robinson, *The Freudian Left. Wilhelm Reich, Gerza Roheim, Herbert Marcuse* (New York: Harper and Row, 1969).

[34] C.G. Jung, *Psychology and the Occult* (1977), p. 177.

most esoteric discoveries were more than metaphysical assumptions. For him they were provable scientific facts.[35]

In the sublime film *My Summer of Love* (Pawel Pawlikowski, 2004), adapted from the novel by Helen Cross, Paddy Considine plays released prisoner Phil. He is now a born-again Christian leader with followers. Phil and his sister Lisa (Natalie Press), known as Mona to Phil, live in their dead mum's pub which Phil converts into a spiritual centre. With resonances of cult-like behaviour, this is more a free-church house group manifesting gifts of the Holy Spirit as described in *Acts*, including speaking in tongues, and being slain in the Spirit. As the leader, Phil is initially humble. 'If I can be saved, anybody can be saved,' he preaches on the hillside, arguing that evil dominates their Yorkshire valley. 'The Devil wants you to do bad things, if he's got a grip of you,' Phil says to Tamsin (Emily Blunt), Mona's upper-class new friend, then saying God is more powerful than the Devil.

'Is he totally mad?' asks Tamsin. Eventually Tamsin reveals how divided Phil still is, including his propensity for physical violence not being fully vanquished. Tamsin is apparently mourning her sister Sade death from anorexia, but this we learn late on in the film is utter fabrication, giving Tamsin an opportunity to perform the role of grieving romantic for Mona, one-upping the latter's real story of her mother dying from cancer. Along with Tamsin's father's infidelity, this story presents the familial problems of the moneyed upper-class in comparison to the working-class, despite part of this being a sham.

Phil and his band of Christians dream of taking their Yorkshire valley back for Christ, so he builds a giant cross to mount on the hillside. Some members, like Phil, who was incarcerated for stealing and fighting, seem damaged and needy. Mona does not want to believe what is happening to her brother and their pub, declaring she wants her old pre-Christian brother back, and she now has nobody. The film momentarily breaks class and sexual taboos, and as with all transgression by doing so reinforces them.[36] Importantly, Phil sees his new life as the authentic one, an issue addressed further in Chap. 8. Meanwhile, Tamsin feeds Mona lines from cod Nietzsche about God being dead, which Mona repeats to her brother and his Christian friends.

Despite all his public display of godliness, Tamsin easily seduces Phil. By proving he is a fake, not possessed by Christ, following Tamsin's argument Phil is sane. 'If you leave me, I will kill you,' says Tamsin. 'If you leave me, I will kill you, then I will kill myself,' replies Mona. Then Mona fakes her suicide. When Phil finds Mona, he attacks her, throwing his gang out of his Christian centre, accusing them of being 'fakers'. Who is fooling who is the major theme, because Tamsin is lying about her sister Sade's mental illness and death. This is played out when Lisa and Tamsin use a Ouija board and Sade's spirit apparently moves the glass. 'You're too easy, you fucking fraud,' mocks Tamsin to Phil, who gets violent again, not having dealt with his demons. 'Madness' is explored via religious belief, leadership, and

[35] Ibid, p. 133.

[36] Chris Jenks, *Transgression* (London: Routledge, 2003).

cult-like behaviour, with grief, adolescent yearning, and romance, plus the art of imagination and storytelling, and family breakdown across the classes.

Gurus, such as the founders of cults, are often condemned for emphasising a world beyond the everyday. Paradoxically, behind these belief systems is a desire to get back to a more permanent reality. Gurus have often fallen because they have gone beyond accepted boundaries of reality, like drug taking. Jung asserted a particular foundation of reality drawing on Schopenhauer who interpreted Plato.[37] This is where his archetypes stem from, and a non-causal emphasis is zealously refuted within analytical psychology. An underlying connecting principle is asserted through synchronicity which is non-linear functioning as an unstated explanation for events and behaviour.

This non-linear performance equates with the transrational and Jung attempted to unite opposites to overcome binary oppositional paradigms at the heart of Western philosophy's origins. This was not just theoretical but had practical implications for wellbeing. For Jung the established Church had split off darkness, the deeper unknown, and it was his mission to unite this opposite with the whole, the Creator's consciousness coming through our consciousness.[38] Western culture, which increasingly suffers from mental health problems, unfortunately still operates via this splitting, by dividing up the inner and outer world for example. Without addressing this shadow, in Jungian terms, or the sinful self in Christian terms, we are doomed to ignorance, and history repeats itself but engaging with the transrationalism is a step out of this darkness.

A consideration of groups and corporate organisations illustrates this further. Through new technology corporate culture developed a zeal for unifying work and personal life, denying differences within these traditionally bifurcated realms. This blurring functions to create the insanity of the total institution where all is controlled and nothing remains unmonitored. The horrific implications of this are revealed by Dave Eggers in his 2013 dystopian novel *The Circle*, adapted for cinema by James Ponsoldt in 2017, where we learn about different styles of leadership within cult-like corporate culture. Despite a drive for diversity, in many organizations difference is discouraged, as it takes away power from the centralized agenda. This leads to a disincentive to originality and innovation that might challenge the status quo. Whether this is in religions, corporations, governments, or world organizations unable to change a fixed plan, this leads to corruption. Broken down in this fashion we see how groups can function through a collective 'madness', not based on any real assessment of endeavours. Time and again examples arise in the way institutions, such as the police, army, universities, church, and other organizations, have mismanaged people through denying real assessment of conduct, structures, objectives, and results.[39]

---

[37] Storr, op. cit., p. 99.

[38] Athony Stevens, *On Jung* (London: Penguin, 1991), p. 252.

[39] Despite overwhelming evidence, the head of London's Metropolitan Police refuses to admit the institutional racism of the police.

The trouble with Donald Trump and leaders like him with their acts of high drama that control the media narrative is that people sick with boring politicians are attracted by this 'mad' drama. This is an elusive 'madness' in the political and economic sphere, 'beyond the human pale: beyond full human comprehension and beyond effective human control'.[40] The leadership of Donald Trump can be interpreted as the id breaking free after the superego of former German leader Angela Merkel and others who for so long attempted to maintain global law and order. Russia's Vladimir Putin also appeals to his followers in this fashion and as a dictator like Trump he is a form of cult leader.

Entering directly into the unconscious and id, the savage 'madness' to paraphrase Foucault discussed previously, acting this out offers a form of pseudo-authentic freedom that on the surface seems refreshing but is regressive and atavistic. A surrender to the unconscious arising without being fettered by the super ego may appear falsely freeing, but this truth is a caged truth. In one reading, Jung never advocated a surrender to the unconscious, quite the reverse.[41] Donald Trump's over-inflated ego has dominated media discourse, but strictly speaking it is pre-ego as he works with the child-id of the nation.

From *Richard III* (1592 or 1594) to *Hamlet* (1600), from *Othello* (1604) to *King Lear* (1605 or 1606) and *Macbeth* (1606), Shakespeare reveals how at this level of leadership 'madness' and leaders are entwined. When we are no longer accountable to any other there is no one keeping our demons in check. The 'madness' of absolute power, of revenge, jealousy, and more, take over in Shakespeare, leading to a warning regarding the total loss of humanity. Without being held to account, the human becomes a primeval beast wrapped up in acting on a feeling which is often without base as in *Othello*.

Shakespeare is suggesting that the strongest are also the most gullible, most weak, most prone to be tricked because without equality there is no trust, there is no humanity. A general who is a Moor, Othello is an outsider highly acclaimed as a leader of men in battle. He does possess a high level of paranoia which may have helped him in battle, but in civilian life so much so he kills his innocent wife. In the 2001 television film version directed by Geoffrey Sax it is more noticeable how Othello's (Eamonn Walker) trust in others which helped him in battle is now his downfall. He seldom doubts Iago's lies, despite never actually having had 'the ocular proof' he asks for, other than seeing Cassio in possession of his handkerchief.

'Mad' by jealousy, Othello blindly believes erroneously that his wife Desdemona gave it to Cassio. This level of trust which is highly desirable on the battlefield can lead to gullibility and naivety in close relationships and politics with a natural leader in battle being easily led astray. Each leader has a flaw, such as Billy (Jaeden Martell) in the film version of the Stephen King novel *It* (Andy Muschietti, 2017). Like Othello, he just trusts too much. Because of this Billy remains the group's

---

[40] Brian Massumi, *The Principle of Unrest; Activist Philosophy in the Expanded Field* (Coventry: OHP, 2017), p. 9.

[41] R. Segal, *Jung* (Oxford: Oxford University Press, 1996).

leader confronting evil in their hometown. Psychiatrist Andrew Lobaczewski constructed the term 'pathocracy' after analysing psychological disorders and politics, recognising that psychopaths and narcissists are strongly attracted to power.[42] As noted, it would be wrong to demonize Donald Trump as 'mad' ignoring the system he inherited, and which created him.

Where selfish individualism becomes the mantra the sanity of believing in the human is challenged along with the definition of what it means to be human. If 'madness' is the inability to consider anything other than your own inner blinkered reality then this turbo-capitalism ideology is the ideology of 'madness', often accepted unquestionably as sanity and the nature of reality. Despite the inroads from the antipsychiatry movement and postcolonial theory and other progressive movements, the demonization of difference remains central to control in many organizations. To challenge anything seems 'mad' if this means the removal of our source of survival.[43] This bind keeps people in their place, accepting any horror and injustice; the mantra becomes: this is the way it is, only a fool (or a 'madman') would contest such behaviour.

7.2 Celebrity Culture and Group Psychosis

Celebrity culture is one of the most important mechanisms for mobilising abstract desire.[44] Hysteria surrounding celebrity culture can be termed mass hysteria and even group psychosis, turning the subject into an inanimate object for consumption, both the subject who worships the celebrity and the celebrity itself.[45] According to sociologist Max Weber the world is disenchanted; celebrity culture reinscribes the supernatural, re-enchanting the world offering an acceptable form of magic.[46] Diana, Princess of Wales, who instilled this form of magic was a global leader. The mass mourning following her death in 1995 produced a collective catharsis in Britain and the world. In one interpretation this mass grieving, what could be viewed as collective 'madness', was sane but group mourning broke out that was to some commentators disproportionate to the actual event, spurred on by the ever-present media that had been instrumental in her death. In his 2023 memoir *Spare* call the public grief hysterical, 'but the press's hysteria had veered into psychosis'.[47]

[42] S. Taylor, 'Pathological power: the danger of governments led by narcissists and psychopaths', *The Conversation*, September 19, 2019 https://theconversation.com/amp/pathological-power-the-danger-of-governments-led-by-narcissits-and-psychopaths-123118 (accessed 5 October, 2022).

[43] Never speak truth to power, as one conformist manager said to me.

[44] Chris Rojek, *Celebrity* (London: Reaktion, 2000).

[45] Jason Lee, *Celebrity, Pedophilia, and Ideology in American Culture* (New York: Cambria, 2010), p. 51.

[46] Ibid., p. 52.

[47] 39.

Psychosis is frequently found to be real 'madness', and it is interesting to observe here how from one bereaved son's perspective the press was 'madder' than the people.

The death of such a well-known figure might well have brought about unhappiness, but with the extent of severe mass grief so extraordinary this was a singular event. Not known for its outpouring of feeling, Britain was offered this opportunity to feel with the combination of early death, royalty, and injustice brewing a heady concoction with multiple archetypes at play. Diana embodied in her life, but primarily her death, an unconscious archetype resonating with what I have termed the 'death mother'.[48] This archetype is at the heart of many great religions. Despite this surprising level of grief, it is unsurprising then that her death caused such a collective depth of emotion to be unleashed with the sense of loss palpable.

We have repeatedly seen how loss and 'madness' are inseparable. The need for the transrational was at work in this instance and to brand this as total 'madness' is ignorant. Stiff upper-lip right-wing media commentators, like Christopher Hitchens, found this public grieving abhorrent. For them it was anathema to everything Britain stood for; indeed, it was anti-British, just as Diana had appeared to be threatening the heart of the British establishment in her moves against the royal family. Branding this outpouring and transrational behaviour offensive, 'madness', or sick, dismisses and ignores its central purpose. Of course, those who branded the mourning over Diana as offensive would have found the excessive mourning over Queen Elizabeth II's death in 2022 perfectly legitimate. The national press, especially the BBC, worked hard for 10 days of official mourning to maintain the myth of the cost-effective monarchy during a cost-of-living crisis. There were no dissenting voices; homogeneity was the rule, with the perfect combination of the magic of celebrity and royalty supposedly uniting the nation.[49]

The conclusions of Chap. 3 noted the complexities concerning gender, celebrity, and transgression, along with the politics of resistance. The 'mad' conspiracy theory culture that mushroomed around Diana's death fed into the collective belief that an evil power was at work.[50] Conspiracy theories offer believers an overarching metanarrative in a fragmenting world, an answer, when there is no one answer.[51] Like 'madness', we need to contest the practicality of the term 'conspiracy theory'. Interestingly, in 2022 Emma Young surveyed multiple studies on conspiracy theories and concluded that the label 'conspiracy theory' is unlikely to promote scepticism about an idea.[52]

---

[48] See CJP Lee, *The Metaphysics of Mass Art – Cultural Ontology, Vol. II* (New York: Mellen, 1999).

[49] The fact difference and dissent were eliminated implies authorities feared it.

[50] The most believable theory is that the car was at fault, having recently been used in a robbery.

[51] Knight, op. cit.

[52] Emma Young, "Conspiracy theory' label does little to stop people from believing', *The Psychologist*, May 2022, p. 19.

Numerous documentaries and fiction films followed about Diana whose myth is perpetually dissected at anniversaries of her death. People were seeking a secular tabloid saint, but the fact that they emotionally valued Diana should not cause us to condemn this outpouring of grief as essentially 'mad'. As well as being a tabloid dream, Diana took a political stance against landmines showing radical leadership. Her partisan political stance, including going against official etiquette, caused the establishment to condemn her further but raised her above normal royalty adding to her saint-like status which of course was and is a myth. This is perpetuated today by comparisons between the Duchess of Cambridge and Princess Diana in the tabloid press.

The often cult-like belief in the power of saints can be condemned as insanity, but in the Catholic tradition saints are perfectly normal, performing miracles remotely. Within this and related belief systems their heavenly position influences the earthly realm, sometimes economically.[53] This unification of heaven and earth is far from 'mad' in many religions and we have seen it is a core part of analytical psychology belief. Saint worship has parallels to how celebrities like Diana are venerated. St Ignatius of Loyola, the founder of the Jesuits who had a cult following, would have been classified as having a mental illness today. Many saints would. Psychiatrist and Jesuit W.W. Meisner, in his brilliant analysis *The Psychology of a Saint*, paints the picture of the founder and leader of the Jesuit religious order as having what verged on a personality disorder.[54] Contemporary Ignatian leadership has the following characteristics: humility, freedom, consolation, sense of direction, discernment.[55] A strong argument can be made that without his 'madness' St Ignatius would not have been able to lead and develop the largest religious order of its kind in the world.

By drawing together work on masochism and sadism, Meisner reveals how cult members sacrifice all signs of individuality.[56] This might be thought of as 'mad', but conversely this sacrifice can be viewed as the epitome of sanity if the self as currently known is a myth as we see in Chap. 8, or is damaging to true wellbeing given a focus on the other rather than the self is known medically to enhance wellbeing.[57] Here we approach the concepts of the False Self and True Self, the latter being at one with the God-head the former clinging to ego, separateness, and death.[58] There is a choice: slavishly follow the ideals of one's culture, such as celebrity worship and consumer culture, or resist. Female saints and celebrities can possess powerful transgressive powers with the magical martyrdom of saints cohering with the burning of the witches.[59]

---

[53] Lee 2015.

[54] Meisner, op. cit.

[55] S. Broscome, 'What is Ignatian leadership?' *Thinking Faith*, 1 September 2017, https://www.thinkingfaith.org/articles/what-ignatian-leadership (accessed 5 October 2022).

[56] Meisner, op. cit., p. 232.

[57] See Chap. 8 which contains this view from the NHS.

[58] Richard Rohr, *Immortal Diamond – the search for our true self* (London: SPCK, 2013), p. 62.

[59] G. Greer, The Change: Women, Aging, and Menopause (London: Bloomsbury, 2018), p. 404.

The social competence argument as proof of sanity is even harder to make with group psychosis. Social competence can mean acting in a 'mad' way to other 'mad' people which then in group terms is sanity. As noted, people have wrongly made this claim regarding Donald Trump. Cults have a central doctrine that condemns all those outside the cult as not knowing the one truth. The outsiders are 'mad', so it is easy to call belief within this framework collective group psychosis. Economics is often at the heart of a cult's ideology. Cults can be part of mainstream religion, as explained in Tara Westover's exquisite memoir *Educated*.[60]

Who has the truth exactly? This is a question Pontius Pilate puts to Jesus of Nazareth the day before his crucifixion and to Christians the irony is the truth is standing right in front of Pilate. Only a 'madman' might claim to have the whole truth, but there is a further deeper truth. 'Nothing is true which compels us to exclude'.[61] Camus goes on to claim for Marx nature is to be subjugated and for Nietzsche nature is to be obeyed to subjugate history. He notes what we desire is 'well-being', but this comes about through spiritual slavery. Within this logic much of mainstream Christianity, with its claims about who is in the right group or not (sheep and goats) and doing the right rituals or believing the right things, is untrue. We have also seen how 'madness' concerns itself with an exclusive truth, like visionary belief which is a trait of leadership. Frequently people who are 'mad' do not just know they are right—they KNOW. This inflexibility is sometimes thought to be evidence of strong leadership, such as George Osbourne 'madly' sticking to austerity as chancellor of the UK (2010 to 2016), against all the financial evidence.

Some thought Princess Diana was 'mad' because she spoke truth to power and dared voice her opinions against the British monarchy, an institution not without its own history of 'madness'. 'Madness' within the monarchy has been popularized by films such as *The Madness of King George* (Nicholas Hytner, 1995). Despite sometimes sensationalizing 'madness' these films can educate. Princess Diana's death in 1997 was a transrational mediated event that produced a grief that was atavistic filling a primal need, but personally she had been viewed as someone progressive and challenging the staid monarchy. This attitude can be viewed as sanity with this popular grief informed by a sane sense of mourning at the hope of change that was felt to be lost with her death. The attention given to Diana as a leader focused on her being a servant first, often a sign of a good leader. As with all great leaders, following Ghaemi's work discussed, she had several mental health problems including depression, anxiety, and bulimia. She was demonised as 'mad', as having 'advanced stages of paranoia' according to government minister Nicholas Soames.[62] Having a good level of paranoia is an essential trait in a good leader. We can compare Soames's attitude to those who condemned women for having a voice in other historical periods, including the Witch Craze.

[60] Tara Westover, *Educated* (New York: Windmill Books, 2018).

[61] A. Camus, *The Rebel* (London: Penguin, 1995), p. 68.

[62] Ibid.

This level of public grief can be called hysteria or psychosis, but it had a logic to it which breaking down false binary boundaries further. As noted, the rational is part of the transrational. Of course, we should be careful before calling any form of behaviour 'mad', insane, psychotic, or paranoid, especially in a group context; if it is normal within the group then it is not 'mad'. This moment of mourning was a liminal transrational time. Psychosis may be a clearer clinical definition than any other mental health term, but even here there is so much variation as to its causes, manifestations, and cure. When the majority act in an apparently irrational fashion this means group psychosis and seemingly 'mad' behaviour is sane. With the death of a globally renowned princess a timely and timeless myth was enacted in the media, involving the public in rituals providing a group transrational function. The barriers between sane and insane come down; as one of Britain's greatest psychiatrists and psychoanalysts put it the, 'sane are madder than we think; the mad are saner'.[63]

In the case of serial killers who have become cult figures and leaders in their field examples disprove that sanity is linked to functionality. Dennis Nielsen killed up to 15 young men over 4 years while Jeffrey Dahmer killed 17 people over approximately the length of time. In the 2020 ITV three-part drama *Des*, starring David Tenant as Nielsen, the defence barrister uses the legal term 'res ipsa loquitur', the thing speaks for itself, to make his point about diminished responsibility—if a man kills so many men, cuts them up, or puts them dead in a chair and chats to them when watching TV, is this 'mad'? His argument is hard to argue with. These are planned acts. This is not normal behaviour within 1980s Britain, but was Nielsen insane when he killed all these men and boys, the youngest known one being 14? His rational methodical approach suggests Nielsen was sane, although he was often blind drunk and in a 'mad' frenzy. Both Dahmer and Nielsen were declared sane at their trials because they were not manifesting any signs of known mental illness. Their behaviour could suggest otherwise. This confirms the point made continually about the blurring of the lines between 'madness' and sanity. The same is true of British doctor Harold Shipman who murdered as many as 700 of his patients.

Popular religious journalism dismisses followers of people like cult leader Charles Manson as insane.[64] This is an easy approach subverted skilfully by Quentin Tarantino in *Once Upon a Time in Hollywood* (2019). Experts agree that Manson may have had manipulative powers beyond the norm, just as any 'good' leaders do, but those who followed him and murdered at his request were acting out of their own personal choices. This needs to be remembered before we start believing in the dark arts, the powers of the occult, or brainwashing. Serial killers, 'constitute an extreme example of how grossly abnormal individuals can be considered sane by modern psychiatric taxonomy, and therefore responsible in law'.[65] There are many more

---

[63] Storr (1997), op. cit., p. 152.

[64] P. Berman, 'The Charles Manson Fallacy', *Tablet*, November 20, 2017.

[65] Storr, op. cit., p. 153.

schizophrenics in the general population than we realize.[66] Spree killer Michael Ryan was thought to be schizophrenic, but there was no evidence for this. Often people steer clear of asylums because deeper abnormality is covered up by a more socially acceptable neurosis, compulsion, phobia, or hysteria.[67]

Most guru-leader figures have gone through a period of mental illness and then return with a message, but it is difficult to explore these episodes in detail.[68] British arch-conspiracy theorist David Icke is a classic example. Icke went through a period of re-alignment of values, moving from being a footballer, television broadcaster and media figure, to a strong believer in a higher power. In religious terms this is the dark night of soul made popular by St John of the Cross where an individual realises fully their mortality and then deepens their perception of life's real purpose.[69] Religious texts in all cultures are full of these experiences: the call to wake up. Without going through this dark night, incorporating the shadow, people will continue to lead immature unconscious lives. We have seen how this relates to the immature narcissistic leader. Icke and those like him have projected this shadow onto all the usual suspects: high finance, governments, royalty, the Free Masons, and so on.

Using the ability to function as proof of sanity is unfortunate; in this definition someone is sane if they are a productive cog in the machinery of capitalism. This is an obvious definition, but weak if we look at the human overall. The opposite can be argued with the system being revealed as insane—the only way to sanity therefore is to resist the system's compulsion for production. We do not have to be Buddha, Jesus Christ, or even conspiracy theorist David Icke, to experience this wake-up call. This is played out in numerous cultural forms, such as the films *American Beauty* (Sam Mendes, 2000) and *Fight Club* (David Fincher, 1999).

A new belief system, whether it looks sane or not to others, is a way of attempting to solve a problem.[70] Over half the world's population are monotheistic believers from the same Abrahamic root. If we locked up everyone who had belief in the supernatural, such as UFOs, ghosts, or any invisible presence like a god, then it would be hard to find anyone deemed sane. Indeed, is it these 'mad' beliefs that keep people sane? From this it can be deduced that there are acceptable irrationalities or, to take this to an extreme, acceptable forms of 'madness' and there is one form that it is at the heart of society, literally. Religions promote, 'all you need is love'.[71] God is Love is a Christian mantra. Without it you are not fully human, fully alive, but what love might be is complex and has historically been linked to 'madness'. Lovers used to be denoted as 'moonstruck', like lunatics. As Philip Roth writes, one of his characters finds it impossible to not focus on a beautiful woman, and it is torment

[66] Ibid.

[67] Ibid.

[68] Ibid.

[69] Ibid.

[70] Ibid., p. 171.

[71] As does popular music, see The Beatles, 'All You Need Is Love', Lennon and McCartney, 1967.

to walk away from her; it was, 'an affront to common sese and a menace to his sanity .... He had not just to hide his hunger; so as to not go mad he had to annihilate it'.[72]

Freud referred to the state of being in love as a form of 'madness' and psychosis.[73] From this perspective 'madness' in this guise is essential for civilization to exist and grow, for happiness of the deepest kind. Religious and cult leaders are believed to be the experts in love. If society has normalized many traits of 'madness' and psychosis, this implies society is psychotic. Normal people, including leaders, have traits like schizophrenia, including 'telepathic' thoughts, auditory or visual hallucinations, and paranoid thinking, to name a few attributes of 'madness'.[74] These can have a positive element, but in the face of stress this schizotopy may manifest as schizophrenia.[75] The creative act brings order from the over stimulus of these states.[76] In Chap. 6 the value of hearing voices in all fields was explained; 'unexpected associations, the discovery of connections between concepts or phenomena hitherto unperceived, are essential elements of creative thinking in science'.[77]

'Mad' ways of being can lead to positive results in science and mental health, fantastic belief systems boost self-esteem.[78] Systems of belief offer a narrative that imbues lives with a higher meaning and purpose. It is not just the size of support that makes an idea 'mad' or otherwise, but the length of time for which ideas are held. The monotheistic religions of the world are given credibility due to their history, despite many of their ideas being farfetched. Christianity was once thought to be a Jewish cult. For Nietzsche, to be passionate about anything involves a form of 'madness' which is part of the artist's need for spiritual discipline.[79] 'When comparing the beliefs held by psychotics with religious beliefs it is impossible to say that one set of beliefs is delusional while the other is sane'.[80] Many people hold beliefs that cannot be proven rationally and often these are concerned with self-esteem.[81]

Chapter 1 addressed the happiness industry, including new age gurus, and the medical leaders and gurus in the happiness industry—the psychiatrists—who have a monopoly on pharmacotherapy. Faith has something the medical profession does not offer. Psychotherapy works better if both the therapist and client believe in the process possessing a form of faith. People of faith have higher levels of social

[72] P. Roth, *Everyman* (London: Vintage, 2007), p. 131.

[73] Storr, op. cit., p. 188.

[74] Ibid., p. 191.

[75] Ibid.

[76] Ibid.

[77] Ibid., p. 192.

[78] Ibid., p. 201.

[79] Ibid., p. 207.

[80] Ibid., p. 203.

[81] Ibid., p. 206.

interaction and lead healthier lifestyles, living on average 4 years longer.[82] Group beliefs, while looking psychotic and possibly 'mad' to outsiders, are often intrinsic for a society's wellbeing. This leads to wider questions which have political, biological, philosophical, and anthropological ramifications, such as: is 'madness' necessary for survival, or should we just reframe how we view group belief? On a personal and group level we must accept transrational knowledge, given we cannot fully function deeply and humanely otherwise. Bifurcation between sanity and insanity is unhelpful, as is the blind deification of data, the new God. Ignorantly, we might dismiss faith as the essence of ignorance and unreason, but when framed as Nietzsche's view on passion this is a paradigm for benign living and wellbeing, incorporating the transrational.

7.3 Conclusions: Witches Old and New

Contemporary authorities on the Witch Craze write of the 'holocaust' against women, and in England approximately 92% of those accused in the sixteenth and seventeenth centuries were women, but the reasons for this are manifold.[83] Women who were unable to take part equally within governing institutions took up other roles and professions, like prophetess or witch which challenged power and control. Entrenched misogyny was an important factor with women thought to be more likely to be corrupted by the Devil, but historical changes in social structures were also important. In this period 40% of women lived without the social protection of men, leaving them more open to accusations of witchcraft.[84] Women were 15 times more likely than men to give evidence in a witch trial than in other cases, the process giving the voiceless a sense of power.[85]

Despite this appearing like group psychosis, from our current perspective it would be wrong to condemn these people as lunatics.[86] Part of the stigma of mental illness comes from the need to view it as entirely other and expurgated from an agreed established normality re-asserting the status quo. This otherness is in all.[87] Humans never stop finding 'other others' to attack. As well as Jews, communists, and homosexuals, the Nazis murdered those considered disabled and 'mad'. From Jews to Muslims, women to homosexuals, groups have been demonized throughout

---

[82] Micaela Ricaforte, 'Why Do People of Faith Live Longer', Azusa Pacific University, 26 June 2018, https://www.apu.edu/articles/why-do-religious-people-live-longer/ (accessed 19 November 2020)

[83] Tracy Borman, *Witches. James I and the English Witch-Hunts* (London: Vintage, 2014), pp. 104–106.

[84] Ibid.

[85] Ibid.

[86] Keith Thomas, *Religion and the Decline of Magic* (London: Penguin, 1978), p. 173.

[87] Ghaemi, op. cit., p. 258.

recent history, and those termed 'mad' have been part of this. As we saw in Chap. 1, to those in the anti-psychiatry movement mental health patients are the new witches challenging the status quo's power.

This chapter explained how successful leaders enter periods of transnationality which enhances their abilities to lead and, as Ghaemi has revealed, in a time of crisis a truly great leader will be the one who has suffered from a mental illness. This transcends time, place, and culture, with empirical research and multiple historical case studies proving this.[88] Our 'mad' obsession with rationality is part of the problem. Simultaneously, a lust for the paranormal, and the cultural appetite for witchcraft, manifests itself in a wide range of media and cultural forms, including the acclaimed *Harry Potter* franchise.

In the history of Western thought as soon as reason was confirmed as the absolute truth there was a return of religious irrationality.[89] The Witch Craze was one of the widest and most significant forms of what could be called group psychosis and mass hysteria. The great Witch Craze of the sixteenth and seventeenth centuries that spread throughout Europe and America was part of this. There are overt parallels with other persecutions such as the American persecution of communists at home, where belief in a political system other than the American was believed to be a mental illness. Between 1400 and 1800 forty to fifty thousand people died from charges of witchcraft.[90] These killings began when large scale persecution of heretics by monarchs waned.[91] 'Fantasy', 'paranoia', and 'pathology' are all terms used to describe this activity by historians of the period.[92]

The DSM uses the term mass psychogenic illness for mass hysteria.[93] Since the Middle Ages there have been accounts of mass hysteria involving laughing, shaking, and even meowing.[94] What in the past was called possession is found in cases of extreme mass hysteria even today. Here the conscious mind and ordinary sense perception seem eclipsed. This is found in the frenzy of Balinese sword dancing which causes dancers to enter trances, sometimes even attacking themselves with swords.[95] When many rejected the more unconscious mystical practices of Catholicism, replacing them with Protestantism, the 'subconscious ran amok'.[96]

---

[88] Ibid.

[89] K. Armstrong, *The History of God* (New York: Alfred A. Knopf, 1993), p. 75.

[90] Diamaid MacCulloch, *Reformation – Europe's House Divided* (1490–1700) (London: Penguin, 2004), p. 563.

[91] Ibid.

[92] Ibid.

[93] DSM.

[94] Robert Youngson, *The Madness of Prince Hamlet and Other Delusions* (London: Robinson Publishing, 1999).

[95] C. G. Jung, M.-L. von Franz, J.L. Henderson, J. Jacobi, and A. Jaffé, *Man and his Symbols* (New York: Dell, 1968), p. 21.

[96] Armstrong, op. cit.

While those on either side of the religious and social conflict attempted to claim religious superiority through styles of worship, this binary approach was not the reality. 'Popery' was a general insult hurled in Protestant communities and did not necessarily relate to Rome.[97] The Protestant reformers saw necromancy at the heart of Catholicism, but by using petitionary prayer they too were performing a form of conjuring and magic.[98] For Jung the collective unconscious contained uncanny parallels across time and cultures with Joseph Campbell's examination of myth confirming this.[99] Interestingly, there is further evidence of this in the context of allegations of witchcraft. The same stories from the sixteenth century resurfaced in recent times, including implausible and delusional accusations of sexual practices with demons and ritual sacrifice.[100]

The fantasies of the unconscious have remained similar over hundreds of years, producing attractive clickbait on online news sites. Attributes of the Witch Craze returned in the twentieth and twenty first centuries in the form of mass allegations of satanic ritual abuse (SRA) whipped up by the media and linked to wider conspiracy theories.[101] When God became remote and alien s/he also became demonic; 'fear and desires were projected upon the imaginary figure of Satan, depicted as a monstrous version of humanity'.[102] 'The new scientific rationalism, which took no cognizance of these deeper levels of mind, was powerless to control this hysterical outburst'.[103] Paradoxically, this absurd unreason within the Witch Craze and related crazes was caused by an avoidance of a deeper religious transrationalism, especially a literalism and fundamentalism in Christian far-right America.

The stamping out of mysticism and an over-reliance on rationality had in part caused this great Witch Craze which can be framed as group psychosis. But behind this Witch Craze there was more than a psychotic belief in the dominance of Satan and witches; economics and finance were at its heart. Europe's witch trials concerned non-price competition between the Catholic and Protestant churches for the religious market share. By 'leveraging' the belief in witchcraft, these witch-prosecutors 'advertised their confessional brands' thus revealing, 'their commitment and power to protect citizens from worldly manifestations of Satan's evil'.[104] Keith Thomas argued that staging a trial could be expensive, but this does not include the long-term economic benefits.[105]

---

[97] Michael Braddick, *God's Fury, England's Fire – A New History of the English Civil Wars* (Allen Lane: London, 2008).

[98] Thomas, op. cit., p. 167.

[99] Joseph Campbell, *The Hero's Journey* (London: HarperCollins, 1990).

[100] Lee (2005), op. cit.

[101] Lee in Knight, op. cit., p. 642.

[102] Armstrong, op. cit.

[103] Ibid.

[104] P. Leeson and J. Russ, 'Witch Trials', *The Economic Journal*, Vol. 128, Issue 613, August 2018, pp. 2066–2105.

[105] Thomas, op cit.

From an analysis of 43,000 people across 21 countries between 1300 and 1850 it has been argued that before the Reformation, plus where Protestantism never gained ground after it, there was no need for witch trials, since religious market contestation was minimal.[106] Challengers of the Roman Church were dealt with through the application of a decisive competitive strategy—compelled conversion or annihilation, carried out through crusades and inquisitions.[107]

In the seventeenth century supernatural reasons were given for mental disorders and those trained in religious matters were the main psychotherapists.[108] Initially the establishment, including royalty and medical doctors, did not believe in medical treatment for curing mental disease. As explained in Chap. 1 once medical treatments were accepted improvements in mental conditions did not follow. In the main those who were seen as antisocial, and this would include those suffering from various types of 'madness', were viewed as having an allegiance to the devil.[109] These beliefs are held today; groups such as Breaking Free in America, a sexual ritual abuse (SRA) survivors' organisation, link SRA rings to the Jesuits and the Freemasons, seeing SRA as another way of bringing about the New World Order. To true believers 60,000 people a year are killed from SRA.[110] During the 1980s and early 1990s belief in Satanic movements molesting children became rampant, driven and normalized by the media. After the movement away from liberalism and the rise of the Christian right during the Regan era, there was a backlash in the 1990s against SRA belief. The public and juries became sceptical of accusations seeing them as the product of vivid imaginations imbued with stories from the Christianity right rather than reality.[111] These beliefs returned to the fore under Donald Trump.

Formed in 2016, QAnon believes Trump is the saviour-paedophile hunter who will rid the earth of SRA.[112] This is a form of group psychosis driven by social media with parallels to the earlier beliefs previously explained. Although recent cases have surfaced of child sexual abuse in England and Wales that include elements linked to aspects of pseudo-Satanism, we can position these claims in the wider contexts of conspiracy theories. Despite their horrific psychotic nature of these beliefs, they offer comfort. Their defined structure position fixed yet mysterious enemies, giving meaning and purpose in combatting them. US presidential candidate Hillary Clinton in 2016 was condemned for being 'pathological', due to her ambition as a woman and psychologist Rodolfo Mendoza-Denton explained this was due to voters experiencing her candidacy as a 'norm violation'.[113] The mob was incited, once

[106] Leeson and Russ, op. cit.

[107] Ibid.

[108] Thomas, op. cit., p. 16.

[109] R. Marshall, *Witchcraft: The History and Mythology* (New York: Crescent Books, 2009), p. 126.

[110] Lee in Knight, op. cit.

[111] Lee (2005), op. cit.

[112] Lee (2021), op. cit.

[113] See Caroline Criado Perez, *Invisible Women. Exposing women data bias in a world designed for men* (London: Chatto and Windus, 2019), p. 267.

more, to 'burn the witch'. Those who break norms are perceived as 'mad'. The large number of voters who went to the extremes of calling for her to be burnt as witch it can be argued were experiencing group psychosis as their belief in this was often literal.

Because witches had cures for 'madness' they were a threat to the established economic system. Scotland saw a much higher percentage of women charged with witchcraft including Janet Horne executed in 1727. In 1944 Scottish medium Helen Duncan was one of the last people to be prosecuted under the 1735 Witchcraft Act. Chapter 2 explained this belief lingered into contemporary Protestantism in Scotland as revealed in film by Lars von Trier. The Witch Craze and satanic child abuse craze are both related mass hysteria or, following the DSM, mass psychogenic illness.[114] New stories of apparent demonic creatures surface today, often as real 'others' in the form of immigrants entered European societies and asserted influence so, 'imaginary ones lost their existential menace' to a degree.[115] Those branded witches transgressed power and gender norms threatening the established hierarchy. The most vulnerable social scapegoats were accused of being 'handmaidens of the devil'.[116] The difference between legitimate church ministers and magicians and witches was not in what they claimed to achieve through supernatural activities, but in their social position.[117] Where the authority of their claims came from defined them; the pope, 'canonizeth the rich for saints and banneth the poor for witches'.[118] Those called witches were different to the social norms resisting the hierarchy. One way of controlling them was branding them insane.

The chapter has examined how gurus pass through a process of what could be termed mental illness where the illusions of society are stripped away. While certain behaviours of the mentally ill might be seen as social deviant, the treatment of the 'mad' can be directly compared to that of witches in the Middle Ages who threatened the status quo.[119] Like demonic possession and accusations of evil, concepts of mental illness and psychopathology are circular explanations for behaviour that is often otherwise unfathomable. One method is to compare two approaches; that which is personality-based and 'open' and that which is behaviour-based and 'closed'.[120] Diagnosis explains little and is tautological. Medical physical diagnosis and treatment can be objective and empirical, but all the sub-categories of 'madness' are subjective and inferential.

---

[114] Trevor A. Harley, *The Science of Consciousness. Waking, Sleeping and Dreaming* (Cambridge: Cambridge University Press, 2021), p. 150.

[115] R. Marshall, op. cit., p. 128.

[116] Van Arragon in Knight, op. cit., p. 740.

[117] Thomas, op. cit., p. 56.

[118] Elizabethan Reginal Scot in Thomas, ibid., p. 56.

[119] We noted this in Chap. 1 with reference to the so-called anti-psychiatric movement.

[120] S. Lilienfeld, 'Conceptual problems in the assessment of psychopathy', *Clinical Psychology Review*, Vol. 14, Issue 1, 1994, pp. 17–38.

If we brand someone a witch, possessed, evil, or 'mad', we remove from their actions a sense of responsibility. The Reformation called for the removal of magic in religion, but the rise of Calvinist belief in predetermination removed a sense of responsibility. Science-fictions, such as the BBC television series *Devs* (2020) and the HBO remake of *Westworld* (2016–2022), examine aspects of this further through analysing the relationships between science and ethics in terms of free-will and predetermination. If we could step back or forward in time would we change anything or can we change anything, if God has already decided everything? The questions these fictions address concern the ethics of humans playing God.

From ancient religious myths to contemporary films, the role of the guru and hero is to demonstrate that only by challenging the system can the protagonist break through to a new level of reality, including a new level of sanity which initially may look 'mad'. A group behaving collectively in one way will believe their behaviour is sane when it might be part of a mass psychogenic illness. This chapter commenced by relating this to gurus and cults, moving on to that of leaders, conspiracy theories, celebrities, and how people were demonized historically and today. If we fail as individuals or societies to incorporate our 'dark matter' we project this onto others with disastrous consequences; here it is clear the transrational should not be ignored. The ramifications of the early Witch Craze were examined, recognizing issues of gender, economics, and finance. Our final chapter examines these myths further, including the politics of self and authenticity, and the media and the law, furthering our understanding of 'madness' and the importance of the transrational.

Part IV
Philosophy and Law

Chapter 8
Conclusions: Transrational Hope

8.1 The Grand Transgressor

Known as the 'grand transgressor', 'madness' is the motive for transgression plus a justification for having transgressed.[1] The uses and meanings of 'madness' have been scrutinized and the importance of the transrational explained via film, media, and culture. We have examined how words can create illness and if the *Diagnostic and Statistical Manual of Mental Disorders* was applied literally everyone would have a mental health problem.[2] If everyone has a mental health problem then it might be argued no one does, but it could be the case that everyone does because, following Laing, your 'madness' keeps you safe.[3] This book has expounded on how positioning mental problems as medical was certainly not inevitable; when this happened the levels of mental illness did not decrease. Indeed, positioning mental wellbeing as a medical phenomenon within a scientific paradigm could be antithetical to its enhancement. Across the sciences research is not robust, two-thirds of experiments not replicable.[4] Mental health science is dominated by the drug industry, 70% of science papers untruthful, all major medical journals publishing drug treatment studies and drug sponsorship rules rather than health treatment.[5] As the band the Verve sang the 'drugs don't work'; neither does the science of 'madness'.

---

[1] Chris Jenks, *Transgression* (London: Routledge, 2003), p. 36.

[2] Darian Leader, *What is Madness?* (London: Penguin, 2011).

[3] R.D. Laing, *The Politics of Experience* and *The Bird of Paradise* (London: Penguin, 1967).

[4] Tom Feilden, 'Most scientists 'can't replicate studies by their peers', BBC News, 22 February, 2017, Most scientists 'can't replicate studies by their peers' - BBC News (accessed 26 January, 2023).

[5] Bessel van der Kolk, *The Body Keeps the Score: Mind, Brain and Body in the Transformation of Trauma* (London: Penguin, 2014), p. 38.

J. Lee, *Culture, Madness and Wellbeing*, https://doi.org/10.1007/978-3-031-37530-9_8

Media images define and are part of integral reality; they make the critical, aesthetic, and ethical gaze along with the political reality difficult to differentiate.[6] The media offers the framework for definitions of what is perceived appropriate, what is sane or insane, often in a mistaken binary fashion. That is exacerbated by the primal nature of online clickbait which is designed to appeal to the id. The transrational offers up a different and deeper form of knowledge moving beyond the biological approach. Virtuality, 'comes close to happiness only because it surreptitiously removes all reference from it'.[7] 'Madness' similarly offers meaning within the gap of socially defined meaning, freeing us from the original illusion. Often this is without an externalised understanding. The condemnatory phrase 'they are mad' refuses all comprehension as a way of denying understanding, positioning this other in a category outside the human, in the realms of the otherworldly. We have seen throughout how an understanding of 'madness' relates with that of the uncanny.

As Albert Camus put it, all greatness is rooted in risk.[8] Entrepreneur Elon Musk has a touch of 'madness' about him, enabling him to take risks. People who are creative need to branch out beyond what is considered normal and sane; what might be thought of initially as 'mad' can eventually be believed to be sane like going to moon or, in Musk's case, Mars. Each work of art, every utterance, comments on 'madness', as it negotiates signifiers of normality, or alternatives resisting or challenging the status quo. So, favouring the elite perpetuates the 'madness' of global destruction. Black Lives Matter and Black Marxist movements have pointed out turbo-capitalism, born out of slavery, creates slavery capturing people in its 'madness'. Capitalism is a form of legitimized 'madness'—a system that believes in no boundaries, no checks, and no balances. Unfettered, it is the ultimate transgressor and in this sense is the pure 'madness' that has been accepted as normal hiding its ideological origins by its ubiquity.

Chapter 3 explained how all aspects of being a woman have been psychopathologized. The category of woman as an object of study arose post-World War 2, along with those of 'youth' and 'race', and we noted how research on the older woman is still in its infancy.[9] For Germaine Greer once women were set free from bondage to fathers, husbands, and sons, from a lifetime of being told that they are 'irrational creatures', they would make a principle out of 'instability and unreason', using superstition to subvert religious and secular authority.[10] This has an important resonance concerning 'madness' and the significance of the transrational which incorporates the rational, including the economic. As Chap. 7 explained, those

[6]Jean Baudrillard, *The Intelligence of Evil – Or the Lucidity Pact*, trans. Chris Turner (London: Bloomsbury, 2013), p. 59.

[7]Ibid., p. 63.

[8]Albert Camus, *Create Dangerously* (London: Penguin, 2018), p. 31.

[9]Germaine Greer, *The Change: Woman, Ageing, and The Menopause* (London: Bloomsbury, 2019).

[10]Ibid., p. 400.

women who were unable to take part equally within the institutions that governed took up other roles, including those of prophetess and witch. From our current perspective it is wrong to condemn these people known as witches as lunatics.[11]

Part of the stigma of mental illness comes from the need to view it as entirely other, as a separate species. There is the desire to have 'madness' expurgated from an agreed normality which is time and location based. This is formulated through ideologies, including patriarchal power and racism, plus related bio-medical systems that ignore the social, but this otherness is in all.[12] Unfortunately, humans never stop finding other others to attack. As well as Jews, communists, and homosexuals, the Nazis murdered the differently abled, the neuro-diverse, and the 'mad'.[13] We have analysed how for those in the anti-psychiatry movement, including psychiatrists, psychologists, and service users, mental health patients are constructed as the new witches.[14] Fundamentally, we saw in Chap. 7 that the level of unreason within the Witch Craze was caused by the avoidance of a deeper transrationalism. This is a stark example of the relationship between the denial of the transrational and the increase in mental ill-health. Furthering ideas of feminism, it is useful to draw on other political traditions: 'black feminism', 'indigenous feminism', 'socialist feminism', 'communism', 'Third World feminism', and 'queer feminism'.[15]

'Madness' for those in the mental health industry and those impacted by that industry was examined in Chap. 5 through real-life accounts. Interview A.28 was a vivid account of what it is like to experience mental ill-health, and what happens when professionals deal with the end process. Medication was seen here as part of a solution, as is a clear diagnosis and in their words 'cracking your code'. Even here it was explained that all is a construction and a narrative with storytelling the key. According to Joan Didion we tell stories to live with life made up entirely by 'the impression of a narrative' full of disparate images' and 'shifting phantasmagoria which is our actual experience'.[16] Didion is only half right because she underestimates the nature of story. Conversely, we may force ourselves to believe in a non-narrative of incoherency that drives against narrative, just to keep sane, when an apparently insane event happens in our lives. We say it is 'mad' because it just does not fit the known story and, by doing, so we keep sane. Interview A.22 makes a similar point where the term 'mad' is used in the NHS when a patient manifests behaviours outside the normal framework. In this sense, 'madness' is the secret that is not revealed, and it is that which keeps us safe. The antithesis of the secret,

[11] Keith Thomas, *Religion and the Decline of Magic* (London: Penguin, 1978), p. 173.

[12] Nassir Ghaemi, *A First-Rate Madness: Uncovering the Links Between Leadership and Mental Illness* (London: Penguin, 2011), p. 258.

[13] Jason Lee, *Nazism and Neo-Nazism in Film and Media* (Amsterdam: Amsterdam University Press, 2018).

[14] See Chaps. 1 and 7.

[15] B. Bhandar and R. Ziadah, *Revolutionary Feminisms – Conversations on Collective Action and Radical Thought* (London: Verso, 2020).

[16] Joan Didion, *The White Album* (New York: Open Road, 1979), p. 1.

confessional culture, can be damaging as explained with reference to reality television.

Photography and film are, 'the mirror of imagination'.[17] We have examined narrative codes, such as the hermeneutic code following Barthes and how the enigma and secret.[18] For A.28 clients enter a mental health facility believing they are 'mad'.[19] They are then educated, and a specific diagnosis is found which optimistically leads to them feeling less desperate and alone. For A.6 reality is questioned via physics making our analysis all the harder when it comes to ascertaining what we are dealing with on a personal and social level. Labels may not always be helpful, but A.28 believes in their own diagnosis of anxiety, plus they also had mild psychosis so PTSD might be an appropriate diagnosis given some of their reactions. Real life and reality, if we believe in such a thing, is far wider than a single cause or a multitude of external causes; it includes the imagination and the mirror of imagination—culture.

In Chap. 1 it was perceived how disorders and diagnoses change over periods due to cultural changes. Chapter 4 elucidated how psychiatry developed during colonialization and how this impacted on racist dynamics of the discipline which had a global impact that still has impact. The culture examined in this book reveals a more progressive approach to 'madness' over time, especially concerning certain disorders such as PTSD as examined in Chap. 2. But there are discrepancies with reality. Those who attack postmodernism's relativism fail to grasp how it highlights inaccuracies of often simplistic positivist teleological metanarratives which dominate ideological belief systems. All ideologies that are accepted as normal need challenging and this unquestionably pertains to mental health ideologies. Once language was perceived as copying a ready-made order, but this was part of the damaging literalism of the Enlightenment.[20] As explained in Chap. 1, the belief in progress can be viewed as part of the cult of rationalism from the eighteenth century, although this does not have to lead to despair as our final conclusions on the hope of transrationalism reveal.

Globally we cannot divide the constructions and use of 'madness' from political repression. The number of cases of those incarcerated internationally in mental institutions for political reasons is on the increase.[21] This is especially the case in Russia where public dissent is outlawed. For example, Mikhail Kosenko was one of the accused in the May 2012 Bolotnaya Square protest against Vladimir Putin and was sentenced to forced psychiatric treatment.[22] Since the 1950s the Moscow School

[17] This point has been made by many critics and artists, including photographer Antonio Palmerini.

[18] Roland Barthes, *S/Z*, trans. Richard Miller (London: Blackwell, 1990).

[19] Despite one definition of 'madness' being you do not know you are 'mad'.

[20] Don Cupitt, *After God* (London: Weidenfeld & Nicolson, 1997), p. 112.

[21] Robert van Voren, 'Ending political abuse of psychiatry: where we are at and what needs to be done', *BJPsych Bull*, 40(1), February 2016, pp. 30–33.

[22] Shaun Walker, 'Bolotnaya trial: man sentence to indefinite psychiatric treatment', *The Guardian*, 8 October 2013, Bolotnaya trial: man sentenced to indefinite psychiatric treatment | Russia | The Guardian (accessed 22 February, 2021)

of Psychiatry monopolized treatment protocols in Russia. Political or religious dissenters and other 'bothersome citizens' are locked up in psychiatric hospitals due to ideology.[23] This treatment of dissidents is practical because hospitalisation has no end; unlike most prison sentences, people can be locked up indefinitely. These political dimensions to psychiatry have not disappeared, but there have been improvements.

Declaring someone mentally ill means there is no need to respond to them, but regimes employ lengthy trials to offer a veneer of transparency. In England and America, we saw that institutionalisation matched gendered and racial power dynamics which due to colonisation has had a global long-lasting impact. China has many cases where people are incarcerated in mental hospitals for political reasons and often these are petitioners, people who travel to Beijing from the rural provinces to issue a formal complaint and are then hospitalized for causing dissent.[24] International psychiatry has responded by adopting an ethical code, including the condemnation of psychiatry for non-medical purposes.[25] While this has not entirely stopped psychiatry being used for political repression, it has led to a worldwide committee on ethics and the review of abuses.

First published in 1949 in *Nineteen Eighty-Four* 'Reality Control' involves lying about the past so it becomes the truth. Any method, including rewriting external or personal internal history, is employed to avoid the horror of insanity. By avoiding the feared insanity, the 'madness' is unavoidably embedded as the system of reality. By 'lack of understanding they remained sane'.[26] But in Orwell's world which in many respects has come to fruition the question remains—what is sane? Here sanity relates to survival. Being sane could also involve taking responsibility for our actions, acknowledging free will and choice exist and being able to move forward. Unfortunately, due to predictions based on data and what I have explained elsewhere as mediated fate, where the media constructs a false level of predetermination in society, free will and responsibility are sacrificed leading to inaction.[27]

We have seen that since the 1950s literature and film have frequently advocated the view that to avoid 'madness' you need to avoid being dictated to by others. This is problematic when consumption is the defining action, reflecting the capitulation to the manipulation of desire. Some hoped the COVID-19 pandemic may have altered this, but it has just increased online demand for consumer goods, often as a solace in difficult times. This ideology replaces mental health with mental illness. From French director Claire Denis to African American Spike Lee, from Scottish director Lynne Ramsay discussed in Chap. 2, to American Richard Linklater, numerous filmmakers have explored these intricacies artistically. They do so by offering up an overt moral message and dissection of the damage done by the ideologically driven

[23] van Voren, op. cit.

[24] Ibid.

[25] Ibid.

[26] George Orwell, *1984* (London: Penguin, 1983), p. 138.

[27] Jason Lee, *The Psychology of Screenwriting* (London: Bloomsbury, 2014).

status quo. The Coen brothers do the same, using transgressive comedy for political purposes. Entertainment culture is often dismissed as ephemera, bubble gum for the eyes, and yet these important communications define what we think, feel, and who we are ontologically; we have also seen its therapeutic value.

'Mad' has meant many things, including annoyed, excited, enthusiastic, disturbed, wildly gay and extravagant, and much else, as previously explained. 'Madness' is a criterion often defined by a group of experts in collusion with the family and in Laing and Esterson's *Sanity, Madness and the Family* the 'mad' daughter Mary is found to be not suffering from any illness at all.[28] The authors contend that their work has, 'historical significance no less radical than the shift from a demonological to a clinical viewpoint three hundred years ago'.[29] Here the interviewed schizophrenics are not considered pathological in a biological sense, but in a familial sense. Even today this is still radical.

Belief in magical possession is still with us and increasing in belief. There are still 36 countries in the world where literal witch-hunts take place.[30] With reference to film, Catherine Malabou has shown how paranoia and schizophrenia coincide with two different ways of running away in the absence of 'elsewhere'.[31] In *Son of Saul* (László Nemes, 2016), where people are gassed on an industrial scale during the holocaust, this could be interpreted as group 'madness' and psychosis with one man's delusion his sanity. To stay alive the Jewish protagonist is helping Germans in their destruction of his fellow Jews and wrongly believes one victim his son. He wants a proper funeral for him and a frightened rabbi will not assist him. Saul's (Géza Röhrig) insanity in needing to provide some dignity in death for the boy reveals how hope can remain, even amongst such devastation and evil.[32]

Only a certain level of 'madness' can achieve this sanity, this being a paradox about what gives meaning in life inside and outside such a desperate situation. Whether Saul is psychotic or not, it does not matter. This confirms the work of Ghaemi discussed in Chap. 7 on leadership and 'madness'.[33] 'Madness' functions as resistance to a group psychosis that is beyond 'madness' with the group devoid of all humanity. What needs to be emphasised, particularly with reference to the holocaust, is that life does have meaning, despite some thinking such a view is complete 'madness'. The protagonist Saul creates sanity for himself by creating meaning, giving the plot a rescue narrative theme. Underlying the rescue of the boy's body is the rescuing of his own humanity and sanity. To attempt this here through insanity

[28] R.D. Laing and A. Esterson, *Sanity, Mandess, and the Family* (London: Pelican, 1964), p. 204.

[29] Ibid., p. 27.

[30] The campaigning work of Scottish QC Claire Mitchell details how the rights of women have been deleted through the lens of witch hunts.

[31] Catherine Malabou, 'Masks and Symbols: In Between Paranoia and Schizophrenia', in *Portable Gray*, 3:2, 2020, pp. 217–223.

[32] Jason Lee, *Nazism and Neo-Nazism in Film and Media* (Amsterdam: Amsterdam University Press, 2018).

[33] Nassir Ghaemi, *A First-Rate Madness. Uncovering the Links Between Leadership and Mental Illness* (London: Penguin, 2011).

enables us to see the necessity of 'madness' and the importance of transrationality for survival and a deeper wellbeing.

Can someone choose to go 'mad', or is this contradictory to the reality of 'madness' which comes upon the 'mad' possessing them without choice? As A.6 pointed out in Chap. 6, 'madness' is only known in retrospect after the event. In Chap. 1 we saw how people had entered mental hospitals and feigned 'madness' for research purposes and they succeeded in fooling the experts, meaning in this sense it is an act. People have pretended to be 'mad' for a variety of reasons, including famous legal cases, such as those with the Mafia.[34] Characters like R.P. McMurphy in *One Flew Over the Cuckoo's Nest* (Milos Forman, 1976) fake 'madness' to get out of what they, often mistakenly, think is a more stringent punishment in prison.

In the film *Midnight Express* (Alan Parker 1978), based on a true story, the American protagonist is placed in the mental hospital wing of a Turkish prison after trying to smuggle drugs. When confronted by one 'mad' man as to why he is walking the wrong way around a column, being informed by the inmate they will send him back to the factory, the protagonist screams, 'I'm from the factory, I make the machines!' This offers hope, suggesting the protagonist still has free will and has not sunken to the depths of his peers. Whether 'madness' is chosen or not, manifestations of 'madness' are a performative act. 'Madness' and theatre were explored in Chap. 2 where 'madness' is akin to obsession. By this we do not mean literally acting 'mad', like Brad Pitt (Jeffrey Goines) in *12 Monkeys* (Terry Gilliam, 1996). As Catherine Malabou explains this is not escaping closure, but escaping within closure and, in the absence of any outside; the only possible solution to the impossibility of fleeing consists in wearing a mask.[35]

8.2 The Monstrous and The Law

'Madness' takes on not merely an inevitability but a romantic cool tone, especially in certain forms of popular music such as Indie music. The romantic aspect of 'madness' was noted by interviewee A. 22. A definition of cool is you have seen it all before, nothing surprises you, but this is also akin to being a zombie. Indie bands like The Jesus and Mary Chain and Echo and the Bunnymen have atmospheric songs addressing 'cracking up' and having a 'breakdown'. With 'Cracking Up' by The Jesus and Mary Chain the rhythmic bass-tone of the song is demo-like adding to its apparent authenticity. 'Some said I was a freak', says one lyric. If you are a freak, which the next lyric concurs with, why not accept yourself, celebrate it? If you are 'incomplete', or 'mad'—rejoice! The song creates a trance-like experience, so when we get to the line, 'I'm cracking up, we're cracking up', this is shamanically ecstatic.

---

[34] John Dickie, *Cosa Nostra – A History of the Sicilian Mafia* (London: Hodder and Stoughton, 2007). One mafiaso pretended he was a bird in an ill-fated attempt to not go to prison.

[35] Malabou, op. cit.

'Madness' in can be beautiful, as in divine 'madness'. Through art, such as the films of Werner Herzog who has projects that appear 'mad' in their design and execution, a form of ecstasy can be achieved that is close to divine 'madness'.

We apprehended how Foucault's work on 'madness' and other subjects is ubiquitous, entering a multitude of disciplines, but the problem with Foucault's work on 'madness' is that he has a 'precomprehension of the concept'.[36] In Foucault's analysis the concept of 'madness' is the same as all that is under the rubric of negativity. This clearly needs challenging and leads also to further problems. 'Foucault, in rejecting the psychiatric and philosophical material that has always imprisoned the mad, winds up employing—inevitably—a popular and equivocal notion of madness, taken from an unverifiable source'.[37] This is a serious issue when it comes to unravelling the discourses of 'madness'. Any characterisation of insanity or 'madness' must be invested with caveats and this ambiguity is part of its beauty. Like Foucault, with a focus on the individual rather than the group, writer Virginia Woolf addressed questions of what wellbeing is.[38] This again could be a damaging trajectory given outside Western value systems social psychology challenges how individuality and autonomy are conducive to the optimal level of personality, cognitive, and moral development.[39]

An obsessive focus on individualism, which in reality is the dominance of the same, has led to mental illness and this was examined in Chap. 1 when we discovered the happiness industry is the unhappiness industry. Using his anthropological expertise, George Bataille tackles this problem with regards to the work of Jean-Paul Sartre, criticising Sartre's inability to move from a moral of liberty to a common morality, binding individuals in a system of obligations. 'Only a morality of communication—and loyalty based on communication—goes beyond utilitarian morality.'[40] Interdependence is a better way of putting it. Socialisation values and practices cannot be examined within individualistic ideology. Individual loyalties can co-exist with communal-familial loyalties with a new synthesis, rather than a mutual exclusivity.[41] This combines agency (autonomy, independence) with communion (relatedness, interdependence) in a positive way forward that requires emphasizing within social policy.

A simple way to avoid 'madness' is to keep away from extremes, but Chap. 1 explained that we are in an age where extremes have been normalized.[42] Shakespeare's use of 'madness' has been referred to throughout, 'his happy hunting

---

[36] Jacques Derrida, *Writing and Difference* (London: Routledge, 2001), p. 49.

[37] Ibid.

[38] See Woolf in Chap. 1.

[39] P. Smith and H. Bond, *Social Psychology Across Cultures: Analysis and Perspectives* (Hemel Hempstead: Harvester Wheatsheaf, 1993), p. 224.

[40] Georges Bataille, *Literature and Evil*, trans. Alastair Hamilton (London: Penguin, 2012), p. 178.

[41] Smith and Bond, op. cit., p. 224.

[42] Eric Hobsbawm, *Age of Extremes. The Short Twentieth Century 1914–1991* (London: Abacus, 1991).

ground of all minds that have lost their balance'.[43] While rooted in a time and place, his wok transcends East and West and his deep knowledge of psychopathology is clear. People go terribly 'mad' in tragic contexts (Titus, Ophelia, Lear), are comically 'mad' in error (Antipholus of Ephesus, Malvolio), and may pretend to be 'mad'; but there are those on the margins (Constance, Hamlet, Othello, plus Macbeth, and Leontes).[44] This final category makes us return to the liminal spaces in his work repeatedly, especially since these margins are paradoxically at the centre of culture. These categorisations help us to reframe the multiplicities of 'madness' and its nuances, with all categories being contestable, later cultural work drawn and drawing from these cultural and social paradigms. The relationship between 'madness' and evil has been analysed, especially in Chap. 2. Almost all staged 'madness' in Shakespeare's period had its moral dimension whereby error or evil is expressed and punished in affliction.[45] Excess of any passion is akin to 'madness', so it has a natural link to theatricality and performance.

As we observed in film, media, literature, theatre, and other culture analysed in Chap. 2, audiences in whatever format are 'mad' for 'madness', plus the process of spectatorship can be seen as 'madness' and has also driven people 'mad'. This could contradict an argument concerning 'madness' being taboo, but apart from the experimental mentioned in Chap. 2, 'madness' is still held at a distance. Using 'madness' in culture does not mean it is absorbed or accepted. This is especially true in the West where, like death, 'madness' informs entertainment and is still in many respects denied.[46] The mediated spectatorship of 'madness' can transfigure with more immersive media such as virtual reality, but the primacy of narrative and storytelling will always be maintained. This goes together with the argument that transrationality has been marginalised, exacerbating mental health problems. Only when we engage further with the transrational will wellbeing be achieved, and it was explained in Chap. 2 how media and culture can be a cure.

As Marshall McLuhan predicted, what was private is now public and what was public is now private with social media making this performativity central to normality. Those not on these platforms are the new freaks, considered deviant with something to hide. If you are not on Instagram, do you even exist given virtual existence is frequently prioritised and is the higher reality? For Baudrillard the world embodies 'madness' and signs are multiplying with a 'mad' over-determination, but this is nothing to be alarmed about because the world is saved by spectacle (evil), which is a deepening negative condition.[47] Here evil is a form of theatre and game.

---

[43] James Joyce, *Ulysses* (London: The Bodley Head, 1967), p. 320.

[44] I.I. Edgar, 'Shakespeare's Psychopathological Knowledge', *Journal of Abnormal and Social Psychology*, Issue 30, 1935, p. 71.

[45] Ibid., 18.

[46] See Jason Lee, *The Metaphysics of Mass Art – Cultural Ontology*, Vol. II (New York: Mellen, 1999b).

[47] J. Baudrillard, *Fatal Strategies,* trans. Philip Beitchman and W.G.J. Niesluchowski, ed. Jim Fleming (New York: Semiotext(e), 1990), p. 176.

There is no need for salvation without evil, so we can understand Baudrillard's position where the world in his sense is saved by evil. Derrida correctly found Foucault's work on 'madness' to be a discussion of blanket negativity but Baudrillard asserts negativity and appearance save us from chance in a Nietzschean sense.[48] Similar to Foucault's triumph of 'madness', Baudrillard is concerned with the triumph of the world as appearance and play.[49]

The mindfulness and back to nature part of the happiness industries are a realignment against a celebration of this 'mad' over-determination of signs. Ironically, this movement is counterproductive with the bombardment of messages about mental health and wellbeing, including Apps that help with mindfulness and the like, causing stress. This is part of the noise shouting for our attention ordering us to buy more. Concurrently the drive for emotional wellbeing for all masks the real need to address mental health problems. While it appears benign to observe many have mental health problems this removes the need to address specific needs and creates a victim culture where there is no scale of illness. At the other end of the spectrum are those who think Artificial Intelligence should dominate or currently is. This is akin to Baudrillard's view when he celebrates gaming as a theatrical form of immersive life that, like evil, should dominate. However, while calling the human a biological machine he asks: 'The creeping inhumanity coming out of artificial technicity—the most direct emanation of the reptilian brains of the species?'[50] We can see here the trajectory moving full-circle, where the machine that takes over is the primitive animal and the humane at the heart of humanity is eliminated.

In June 2020 British biotechnology company Puretech had the game EndeavorRx cleared by the US government as a prescription for children with attention deficit hyperactivity disorder (ADHD). This was the first game-based therapy to be granted authorisation for any condition. It was concerned with improving attention in children between eight and 12 with ADHD. The game does not function alone but is part of a package of clinician-directed therapy, medication, and education.[51] Video games have been considered with regards to therapeutic potential, including discussions in the 1990s on whether they might replace therapists.[52] There is the representation of heroic 'madness', especially in first-person-shooter games.[53] Rebutting the idea that games recreate an experience of 'madness' through linear representation two figures have been found within the genre: the 'monstrous double' and the

---

[48] Ibid.

[49] Ibid.

[50] Jean Baudrillard, *Fragments. Cool Memories III, 1990–1995*, trans. Emily Agar (London: Verso, 2007), p. 34.

[51] A. Ralph, 'Puretech EndeavourRx video game therapy wins US approval', *The Times*, 17 June 2020, p. 6.

[52] N. Wilkinson, R. Ang, D. Goh, 'Online Video Game Therapy for Mental Health Concerns: A Review', *International Journal of Social Psychiatry*, 54(4), 2008, pp. 370–382.

[53] Tom, Greenwood, 'Procedural Monsters: Rhetoric, Commonplace and 'Heroic Madness' in Video Games', *Journal for Cultural Research*, Vol. 22, No. 3, 2018, pp. 310–324.

'reaching tentacle'.[54] While these figures draw on existing tropes and processes associated with the cultural meanings of mental health, a rhetorical analysis of their use suggests that they are not simply recycling older clichés and they innovatively constitute a creative 'reobjectification' of 'madness'.[55]

Video games have often been vilified in the popular media for supposedly causing mental health problems, but there is a counter narrative worth considering which has a considerable history concerning social and psychological simulation. In 1986 the developer Activision developed a role-playing game *Alter Ego*, available for the Commodore 64 and Apple II, which concerned guiding a virtual personality through the seven stages of life. By doing so the aim was to achieve emotional, vocational, and physical balance; or, if you wanted to experiment, 'the most psychotic monster the process allows'.[56] The game is a form of, 'glorified Myers-Briggs psychometric questionnaire', having an ability to teach the player self-reflection.[57] If we consider how popular Myers-Briggs and related personality tests have become in human resources departments and educational settings, we can understand how such a game could have been valuable. In each stage of life, the player is confronted with moral conundrums with multiple choice scenarios to ascertain their moral development. These relate to whether, for example, as a baby you cry to get your mother's attention, or you keep calm, so she loves you, or as a teenager you join in getting drunk on a school night to be part of the gang. There is a score based on these behavioural choices, plus a commentary after each choice adding to personal insight. This was a precursor to the popular darker *Sim* series and while not commercially successful it was critically praised given it brought 'realism' to the 'text-based' adventure format.[58]

We detected how the contemporary world enforces synergy between surveillance, technology, and happiness. The risk of political solidarity in societies and cultures is viewed by governments and security forces as too high, and risk management is prioritised over freedom. A focus on a construct of wellbeing by employees and governments becomes a way to enact surveillance and control, rather than liberation. Chap. 2 illustrated how often good and evil are indistinguishable as are 'madness' and sanity. An absence of 'communication' is a greater evil; humans are driven to 'communication' (with both indefinite existence and themselves).[59] "Communication' cannot proceed from one full and intact individual to another. It requires individuals whose separate existence in themselves is *risked*'.[60]

---

[54] Ibid.

[55] Ibid.

[56] KS, *Alter Ego*, in *1001 Video Games You Must Play Before You Die*, ed. Tony Mott (London: Cassell, 2017), 110.

[57] Ibid.

[58] Ibid.

[59] Georges Bataille, *Bataille: Critical Reader*, ed. Fred Botting (Oxford: John Wiley & Sons, 1997), p. 93.

[60] Ibid.

Discrete individuals existing for this communication to take place are seen as a threat, but this de-individualisation needs resisting. Human activity is not reducible to production, morality, or utility, but the emphasis on the latter in the global economy is part of the subordination and rationalisation of all forms of human life to a, 'homogenized moral economy'.[61] Throughout this book an approach to being (ontology) that departs from defining the self through doing has been argued. The fallaciousness of the prioritisation of utility needs asserting in the context of 'madness'. As explained, definitions of 'madness' often correlate with definitions of what is thought to be a functional human being.

Those who were 'mentally incapacitated' and who committed crimes in mid-thirteenth century England became 'wards of the crown'.[62] During this period the 'mad' were not expelled from society but incorporated within it. Chapter 1 explained the historical rise and demise of the 'mad' house. The insanity defence legally was in place in the fourteenth century. Having to face the wrath of apparent unreason is at the heart of contemporary society with the punishment and threat of 'madness' not only at the heart of religious systems but framing political and social systems. In a secular age it is easy to forget that legal systems can include swearing an oath on the Bible, meaning perjury results in instigating the vengeance of the wrath of God in this world, or punishment in the next.[63] The belief is falsity and evil may result in 'madness' as a punishment. In the media age the media's influence is paramount in framing public debate on the sanity of perpetrators in high-profile cases which has led to significant legal ramifications.

John Hinckley Jr's shooting of American president Ronald Reagan in 1981 was one of the last high-profile cases in America where the insanity defence was accepted and 2% of homicide cases during this period used this defence.[64] The defence here claimed that their client had watched *Taxi Driver* (Martin Scorsese, 1976) 15 times, and that this is where they got the idea of attempting to kill a politician. Expert witnesses argued he was schizophrenic, had a personality disorder, and other mental problems, so he was legally insane. Here a court of law deemed it acceptable to blame media influence rather than the individual. The Hinckley case illustrates Foucault's point that psychiatry limits its domain by defining its discourse, giving it the status of an object, such as homicidal behaviour which is constructed as a deviance akin to 'madness'.[65] The outcry after this 'mad' verdict resulted in the 1984 Insanity Defence Reform Act.[66] Instead of the government having to prove a

---

[61] Ibid., p. 23.

[62] Aleksandra Pfau, *Medieval Communities and the Mad – Narratives of Crime and Mental Illness in Late Medieval France* (Amsterdam: Amsterdam University Press, 2020), p. 25.

[63] Keith Thomas, *Religion and the Decline of Magic* (London: Penguin, 1978), p. 49.

[64] Richard Henriques, *From Crime to Crime* (London: Hodder & Stoughton, 2020).

[65] Michel Foucault, *Madness and Civilisation. A History of Insanity in the Age of Reason*, trans. Richard Howard (London: Tavistock/Routledge, 1989).

[66] David Charter, 'Assassination attempt that gave flawed security the bullet', *The Times*, April 3, 2021, p. 45.

defendant's sanity 'beyond a reasonable doubt' they had to prove insanity. Expert witnesses were no longer permitted to testify whether a defendant was legally sane or not. Hinckley was eventually released from institutional psychiatric care in 2016.

If functionality defines 'madness' then this seems contradictory given many 'mad' people function very well. Dennis Nilsen held down a normal job while managing to kill over a dozen men between 1979 and 1983. Brian Masters compared him to the American serial killer Jeffrey Dahmer and called him 'morally mad'.[67] His murders were only discovered because he called someone to fix his drains which were blocked with his victims' remains. This can be read psychoanalytically, as in he wanted to get caught. The fact he managed to publicly maintain a normal life and was not discovered by the police indicates a very methodical mind, far from the stereotype of a 'mad' chaotic killer or non-functional 'madman'. His psychopathic rationality enabled his murderous capabilities, a portrayal Tennant encapsulates precisely in the ITV mini-series *Des* (2020).

Two of the most famous cases in British history are trial of the killers of James Bulger and that of Dr. Harold Shipman who murdered hundreds of his patients. In such cases the defence initially attempts to move to a dismissal by arguing that the media attention would prevent a fair trial. Claims of direct media influence was at the heart of the Bulger case. On February 12, 1993, 2-year-old James Bulger was taken when his mother was distracted at a butcher in Bootle by two 10-year-olds Robert Thompson and Jon Venable. He was tortured and murdered on a railway track two and half miles away. An initial question was, did the culprits know what they were doing? One of the two psychiatrists in the case, Dr. Eileen Vizard, stated that Thompson did know the difference between right and wrong.[68] She was not called by the defence as a witness. His schoolteachers testified that he knew the difference between right and wrong. One could argue if he did not then his teachers would be at fault. 'Whilst he was suffering some post-traumatic stress, there was no evidence of any abnormality of mind at the time of the killing'.[69] Claims of any previous 'madness' were not of value to the defence, but we should question what is meant by abnormality.

Driven by the media, satanic and child abuse panic swept America and the UK through the 1980s and up until the early 1990s.[70] The trial of Thompson and Venables took place at the end of this phenomenon. This was when it became more popular to blame criminal behaviour on film viewing and the media rather than the Devil, although the two were often entwined. Not only did the extraordinary media attention on the trial raise issues in court, but media texts and products, especially the influence of 'video nasties', were argued to be influential. For Richard Henriques legally, 'argument that the boys were re-enacting *Child's Play 3* was

---

[67] Brian Masters, *Killing for Company: The Case of Dennis Nilsen* (London: Arrow, 1985).

[68] Henriques, op. cit.

[69] Ibid., p. 54.

[70] Ibid.

clearly tenable'.[71] This might have been an argument, but this is highly questionable from a media influence and police perspective. The converse legal argument was the correct one: it had no influence, and this was the official conclusion.

Politicians of the period, such as the chairman of the Home Affairs Select Committee, Conservative MP Sir Ivan Lawrence QC, claimed an increase in viewing such films was obviously linked to the rise in juvenile crime. The irony was Britain already had the tightest European laws on videos. Ireland's largest outlet withdrew this video from its stores. The director of the murder investigation, Albert Kirby, stated at the trial that Venables was not living with his father at the time, making it highly unlikely he had even viewed the film. Senior detectives went through around 200 tiles rented by the Venables family and found no evidence that would suggest a boy would go out and commit murder relating to any scene. The media storm over the case was fuelled by the trial judge Mr. Justice Morland claiming exposure to violent movies might have encouraged both murderers.[72] This statement shocked the police investigating the case who concluded the theory of the film's influence was just a convenient way for people to attempt to, 'understand the absolutely incomprehensible actions; and it was wrong'.[73]

As in the Reagan case, a defence team might push this as a cause, but it is difficult to prove people were acting out a film, one connection here being paint was thrown in the victim's face which occurs in *Child's Play 3* (Jack Bender, 1991). One of the most esteemed legal professionals of our era argued that children as young as four know an exact difference between right and wrong.[74] This definitive view needs questioning. Some children do have a knowledge of right and wrong but those under 12 might not know the extent of their wrong, despite knowing they have done wrong; this is especially true concerning death.[75] Children have a limited understanding of death. There is synchronicity between this fallacious belief in direct film influence on behaviour and conspiracy theories. Both require the believer to accept the unproven as fact. It is far easier to believe in media influence or a hidden conspiracy as a singular cause, rather than the reality of a more complex world of influences, including biological, social, economic, and cultural.

In December 1999 the European Court of Human Rights ruled that the 1993 trial had been unfair, awarding Thompson and Venables costs and expenses. The court also ruled that the then Home Secretary, Michael Howard, had breached human rights by intervening to raise the sentences of the killers. In 1997 the House of Lords had already ruled Howard had been unlawful by setting an inflexible sentence given

---

[71] Ibid., p. 63.

[72] Terry Kirby, 'Video link to Bulger murder disputed', *The Independent*, November 26, 1993, Video link to Bulger murder disputed | The Independent | The Independent (accessed 9 April 2021).

[73] Nama Winston, 'Inside the theory that Child's Play 3 motivated the murder of James Bulger', *MamaMia*, June 23, 2019, Inside the theory Child's Play motivated the murder of James Bulger. (mamamia.com.au) (accessed 9 April, 2021).

[74] Ibid.

[75] Adam Morton, *On Evil* (London: Routledge, 2004), p. 76.

the killers were under 18. Arguments concerning the boys being too young to comprehend criminal responsibility were rejected.[76] Despite this, there is resonance with Aristotle's *Ethics* where he notes that dumb beasts have no use of reason, nor do children, or 'mad' people, with nothing done deliberately.[77] This view has filtered into theology, as discussed in Chap. 2, where evil acts are always conducted unconsciously and therefore unintentionally.[78]

Some doctors if they have spare time play golf; Harold Shipman murdered old ladies.[79] One explanation as to why Shipman murdered people is his enjoyment of, 'the thrill of killing'.[80] Inevitably psychoanalytical reasons related to Shipman's mother. 'The psychiatrists warned me that it is possible that, in Shipman's own mind, there was a conscious motivation', but this has been doubted.[81] As with Dennis Nielsen, serial killer Dr. Shipman gained purpose, meaning, control, and pleasure from his murders. There was no financial motive, not initially at least. Perhaps he only then took money to cover up his crime, or to normalize it. Hannah Arendt wrote famously of the banality of evil with regards to Nazism.[82] With Shipman we have a similar banality and rational ordinariness. Banal evil has been glamourized by films and the media, making killers celebrities, lending them some supernatural power when in Shipman's case it was planned, boring, and mundane power. When the police released some details of their investigation to the local paper many defended Shipman. They were unable to accept the accusations against who they perceived was a thoroughly 'nice' man. One other explanation for this denial is there was a refusal to conceive that serial killers could hit the same area twice with Myra Hindley having struck there. Britain's most prolific serial killer, Shipman's rational logical approach to his murders is as far away from the transrational as you can get. He typifies the monstrousness of normality.

We find, 'certain women are capable of actions which other, 'normal', women are not: the system of classification stays intact by resisting the 'defilement' of the abhorrent case'.[83] Framing such behaviour as evil and 'mad' may lend serial killing a passion that glamourizes. As interviewee A.22 pointed out, there is a romantic view of 'madness'. Similarly, using the word evil to describe behaviour can do the same, elevating actions beyond human responsibility. This is not to suggest that evil is not the right word to use in this instance. In some cases, celebrity, and fame drives killers

[76] Henriques, op. cit., p. 64.

[77] T. Pfau, 'The Letter of Judgement: Practical Reason in Aristotle, the Stoics, and Rousseau', *The Eighteenth Century*, vol. 51, no. 3, 2010, pp. 289–316.

[78] How Richard Rohr proposes this has been analysed alongside the counterarguments against this view.

[79] Henriques, op. cit.

[80] Ibid., p. 95.

[81] Ibid.

[82] See Jason Lee, *Nazism and Neo-Nazism in Film and Media* (Amsterdam: Amsterdam University Press, 2018).

[83] Henriques, op. cit.

with the media culpable by promoting this attention which sells papers and fosters clickbait. In Myra Hindley's 1966 case we have a notorious serial killer. With her partner Ian Brady, Hindley initially confessed to three murders in 1966, then two more bodies were discovered. Physical and sexual abuse took place, Lesley Anne Downey's suffering tape-recorded and labelled the primal 'snuff tape'.[84] Media was utilized, and the killers gained pleasure from this recording as a form of pornography, pushing this event to another level of horror, supplemented by the new media technology of the era. Was it any surprise that forever-more the wider public claimed Hindley was a monster and evil? Calling someone a monster denies their affinity with the species; 'then we are blocked from blaming them, any more than one could blame a crocodile, but we are also less compelled to attribute human rights to them.'[85]

As with child murderer Mary Bell, and Rosemary West who sexually and physically abused eight of her own children, assisting in the murder of one daughter, plus killing 12 known other young women in the early 1990s, these female figures are 'unbearable'.[86] Society must create these monsters to prevent society's 'madness' and the media plays a powerful part in this social process as these cases testify. For female serial killers this concerns the restoration of the, 'primary image of the innate maternal and caring dispositions of womankind'.[87] This was achieved primarily via the news media, and related spin-off products including documentaries and re-enactments continually broadcast on crime channels. Women who had performed atrocities were confined to another category, 'essentialised through images of evil or pathology'.[88] They became the total monstrous 'mad' (m)other by which we sanitize ourselves and is one of the primary social functions of 'madness', when equated with evil, where the media defines social reality.

8.3 Conclusions: No Time for Time

Despite its reliance on the study of humours and astrology, Robert Burton's *The Anatomy of Melancholy* (1621) is useful for our era. Depression doubled in the UK during the COVID-19 pandemic of 2020 to 2021 with all the activities the media repeated for wellbeing in this period in Burton's work. This included a focus on diet, exercise, and the need for friendship to help depression.[89] Often the state of the world is 'mad', so a reaction to the world that is not 'mad' would be 'madness'. As J.G. Ballard wrote, what had started as a response to, 'The subliminal living and the

[84] Ibid., p. 183.
[85] Morton, op. cit., p. 76.
[86] Ibid., p. 185.
[87] Ibid.
[88] Ibid.
[89] Robert Burton, *The Anatomy of Melancholy* (London: Penguin, 2003).

uncontrolled extension of techniques of mass manipulation for political and economic ends', developed into an attack on the psychological sciences.[90] In this Ballardian world helping anyone who has a mental disorder is a criminal offence the world being a 'madhouse'. People were, 'gloating over the torments of the other'.[91] Most were unaware which side they were on. After illegally treating Christian, who thinks he has an obligation to act rationally and murder the man responsible for his father's death, Dr. Gregory believes it is this rational logic that is insane. In this book we have seen Dr. Gregory is correct, if rationality is taken to the extreme of excluding the transrational. When preference is given exclusively for rational logic, without a consideration of the transrational, 'madness' and dehumanization prevail.

'Madness' is just as much a part of the social process as it is part of the individual psyche. We have examined its cultural mediation in film, art, media, theatre, and scripture, which informs and often creates its socially constructed and psychological meanings. The problems, inaccuracies, and dangers of splitting off the 'mad' into a different paradigm have been shown to be overt. Philosophically, Chap. 2 recognized how developments in film theory were tied to theories of 'madness' and film-philosophy. We never perceive anything in its wholeness, including the image, only what interests us; this is directed by our desires, economic benefits, ideological beliefs, and psychological demands. While this is true, according to Deleuze a break or jam can subvert clichéd perception.[92] If we once more consider Bess (Emily Watson) in *Breaking the Waves* (Lars Von Trier, 1996), discussed in Chap. 2, we can understand that her thinking lacks this semiological screen. Her love is, 'not the subjugation or consummation of the other, but a respect for its irreducibility', which is, 'rhizomatic relatedness'.[93]

This is another economy, part of the profounder transrational world of intimate exchange, articulated on differences where we find—'faith replaces thinking, belief surpasses logic, gift challenges isolation, intimacy overcomes community, rational acts give way to an activism'.[94] Activism is far more open than might be assumed and includes, 'praying, hoping, dreaming, imagining; a world where miracles become possible and the virtual becomes effectuated'.[95] This is a way of being that draws on transrationality for profounder wellbeing and confirms our overarching argument. There is an overcoming of the established order where the limited

[90] J.G. Ballard, *The Atrocity Exhibition* (London: Jonathan Cape: 1986), p. 117.

[91] Ibid., p. 120.

[92] G. Deleuze, *Cinema 2. The Time-Image*, trans. Hugh Tomlinson and Robert Galeta (London: Routledge, 2011), p. 20.

[93] C. Nigianni, 'Becoming-Woman by *Breaking the Waves*', *New Formations: A Journal of Culture, Theory, Politics*, 2010, No. 68, p. 120.

[94] Ibid., p. 118.

[95] Ibid.

economy of being is contained within a linear conception of time and the morality of utility.[96]

Through a multitude of examples drawn from film, media, theatre, and culture, including music and video games, creative practice, plus interviews with professionals and those impacted by 'madness', and cultural and social theory, this subversive position has been explicated throughout this book. This draws us on to the ultimate question—the final question of being. There is a parallel here with Deleuze's passive vitalism.[97] Difference goes beyond political processes, the 'will, intent and agency' of individuals or subjects; passive vitalism is 'micropolitical', concerning differences, 'we do not intend, perceive, or command'.[98] Accepting psychopathologizing as an inherent illness entails absorbing an essentialist ontology, diminishing and removing the human, but the human through transrational knowledge is deeper than this.

Chapter 1 explained that in true shamanism the shaman possesses the spirits, rather than the shaman being possessed by them. As we have seen, Carl Jung, Susan Sontag, and shamans argue symptom formation is a product of individuation with illness a creative act. Instead of seeing symptoms as pathological they can be approached, 'as symbolic communications from the unconscious, indicating where the patient has become embroiled in the fundamental problems of life'.[99] From this perspective we learn from 'madness' if it is not bracketed off as merely pathological and without meaning.

Chapter 2 illustrated how Kubrick is pre-eminent in films on 'madness'. *The Shining* (Stanley Kubrick, 1980) deduces the timelessness of 'madness', demonstrating this shamanistic take, along with illuminating hauntological components, traversing time. Jack Nicholson's abusively 'mad' caretaker Sam Torrance is possessed by the murders in the hotel built on a First Nation burial ground. Sam is jealous of his visionary son Danny (Danny Lloyd), who is a form of shaman with the gift of the shining. Timelessness and trauma are also at the core of Kubrick's *2001* (1968) where a machine goes 'mad'.[100] *The Shining* demonstrates that if transrational knowledge is not engaged with leading to wellbeing then possession and evil may result. Wellbeing through film and culture has been explained in the previous chapters and we identified the popularity of horror films that focus on 'madness'. Traditionally, horror films have been equated with mental disturbance, but exposure to horror films (prepper genres such as alien-invasion, apocalyptic, and

---

[96] Ibid., p. 122.

[97] Ibid.

[98] Claire Colbrook, *Deleuze and the Meaning of Life* (London: Bloomsbury, 2010), p. 80.

[99] Anthony Stevens, *Jung* (Oxford: Oxford University Press, 1994), p. 170.

[100] P. Kuberski, *Kubrick's Total Cinema. Philosophical Themes and Formal Qualities* (London: Bloomsbury, 2012), p. 143.

zombie films) offer viewers more resilience to real-life horror, so people become more psychologically resilient.[101]

Interactions between constructions of 'madness', possession, and evil have been scrutinized. The prevailing economic system involves the surrender to things (products and production) and turns people into things. This is a form of evil and 'madness' if this is dominating our becoming via things; as Bataille explains, 'this is in the way that Satan inhabits the soul of someone possessed, unbeknown to him, or that the possessed, without knowing it, is Satan himself'.[102] This behaviour is hellish somnambulism, part of the zombie political and economic culture identified in Chap. 1 which led to chaos through subservience to the dominance of the main activity in capitalism.[103] This book has argued against this process and against the transformation of the human into mere utility. Unfortunately, often humans select the unity of the 'undifferentiated aggregate' by consenting to be only a thing.[104] The imperative action is to move from a morality of utility which imprisons individuals under the conception of 'normality', 'sanity', 'rationality', utility, and 'reason'.[105]

If time is standing still, is it impossible to know what time is at all? 'Time which is unreal casts over all things including ourselves a veil of unreality'.[106] Cinema is time, bits of time; 'the longer you can extend it, the more truth there is in the piece.'[107] One way of viewing psychotic time is the denial of the past and future, so there is no absence; 'consciousness of time also includes the idea of eternity in the present, owing to the idea of infinity.'[108] 'Madness' can be viewed as being stuck in an eternal present (the 'mad' broken record), a nirvana of sorts as well as a nightmare. And yet through popular meditation techniques and mindfulness people attempt to reach this infinity for sanity and wellbeing. Paradoxically, this popular route to wellbeing can be conceived as a form of 'madness' and is problematic. But there is a difference between entering the infinity of the moment which is open to

[101] Colten Scrivener et al., 'Pandemic practice: Horror fans and morbidly curious individuals are more psychologically resilient during the COVID-19 pandemic', *Personality and Individual Differences*, Vol. 161, 1 January, 2021, 110,397, Pandemic practice: Horror fans and morbidly curious individuals are more psychologically resilient during the COVID-19 pandemic - ScienceDirect (accessed 30 January, 2023).

[102] George Bataille, *The Accursed* Share, Vol. 1, trans. Robert Hurley (New York: Zone Books, 1991), p. 136.

[103] Henry A. Giroux, *Zombie Politics and Culture in the Age of Casino Capitalism* (New York: Peter Lang, 2009).

[104] Ibid., p. 138.

[105] Nigianni, op. cit., p. 122.

[106] Simone Weil, *Gravity and Grace*, trans. Emma Crawford and Mario von der Ruhr (London: Routledge, 1992), pp. 45–46.

[107] Devika Girish, 'There's A Blind Spot About What America Was', *Sight and* Sound, May 2021, Vol. 31, Issue 4, p. 30. (26–33).

[108] Wouter Kusters, *A Philosophy of Madness – The Experience of Psychotic Thinking*, trans. Nancy Forest-Flier (Massachusetts: MIT, 2020), p. 105.

anything and being stuck in a 'madness' of a collapsed moment on a loop. Going beyond a fixed time is a path within this discourse to wellbeing.

There is a critical need for enhanced mental health care and more analysis of what mental health, 'madness', and wellbeing are and might be.[109] Optimistically, it can be more than an industry for social and political conformity and an acceptance of the status quo; a new path opens-up through transrationality. The concept of the self is a major part of the problem but is extremely difficult to overcome. According to Confucius to become good and therefore happy we must overcome the self by submitting to rituals.[110] In Chinese philosophy the self is not an entity that exists within which we must get in touch with for happiness, but an amalgamation of all our reactions that are learnt over a lifetime. If we can learn about these reactions and then unlearn them then we are free. We can understand that there is freedom in this philosophy from the concept of the self that has come to dominate in the West where the self is prioritised.

Playing itself is therapeutic and there is a direct continuity between the construction of reality through play in childhood with adult activities, including art, film, media, culture, and religion.[111] We all construct our make-believe, our individual myths functioning as a guide to the world which hopefully aids wellbeing.[112] One way of constructing these personal myths is online, the use of which has been demonized as detrimental to mental health. There is evidence online activity is no more damaging than watching television; one extensive longitudinal study published in 2021 in *Clinical Psychological Science*, involving data from over 430,000 people aged 10 to 15 in the UK and US, found no evidence of a link between mental ill health and screen use.[113] However, issues with this research were: it was self-reporting, and it is known that people tend to over and under report use; it did not say how people were using devices (whether talking to friends or looking at pro-anorexia sites for example); thirdly, it gathered data from 1991 to 2017, and its main finding was that mental health had not got worse over time; finally, participants graded their feelings according to set questions rather than describing their emotions and this has methodologically weaknesses when it comes to nuances.[114]

Alternatively, a report in 2019 found adolescents were more likely to be depressed, self-harm, and not sleep well if they over-used social media, and a study by the Education Policy Institute and Prince's Trust tied increase in mental

---

[109] See Bark in Chap. 3.

[110] R.D. Laing, 'The Obvious', in Stokely Carmichael, David Cooper, R.D. Laing, Herbert Marcuse, *The Dialectics of Liberation* (London: Verso, 2015), p. 19.

[111] M. Lenormand, 'Winnicott's theory of playing: a reconsideration, *The International Journal of Psychoanalysis*, Vol. 99, Issue 1, 2018, pp. 82–102.

[112] R. Segal, *Myth: A Very Short Introduction* (Oxford: Oxford University Press, 2004), p. 139.

[113] Tom Knowles, 'Social Media 'no worse than TV' for mental health of teenagers', *The Times*, May 5, 2021, p. 4.

[114] Ibid.

ill health with heavy social media use.[115] Concern was raised in October 2022 over the charity Mermaids promoting a youth forum and recommending children to use Discord, an instant messaging social media platform that started for gamers and claims 350 million subscribers. There are numerous accounts of children being sexually groomed on the platform and those with autism are noticeably vulnerable. Mermaids failed to clarify what training their moderators received, but claimed any discourse about this was a targeted smear campaign.[116] On its website, Mermaids had stated young people use, 'an email address their primary carers have no access to,' because LGBT children may live in 'hostile environments'.[117] While denying it gives medical advice, users may discuss experimental drug treatments and medical transitions, leading some to claim this environment is a lawless zone, like the wild west of the internet, with no age limits, making it a zone for paedophiles which is damaging.

Chapter 3 showed how an acceptance of the transrational is healthy, but a rejection leads to horror and insanity, revealing how past, present and future coalesce within transrational knowledge. Wellbeing has been defined as the state of being comfortable, healthy, or happy. We observed how for one of the most significant psychologists of our era happiness can be viewed as a mental illness.[118] The UK's National Health Service states these steps for mental wellbeing: good relationships; physical activity; learning new skills; giving to others; paying attention to the present moment (mindfulness).[119] As explained, the transrational supersedes the rational while including the rational. The transrational is larger than cause and effect, but since the Enlightenment the common modality is a cause-and-effect mindset. Mental unwellness is caused by a disengagement with the transrational. The transrational relates to the five steps for mental wellbeing, taking us beyond the fixity of the limited horizon of a mindset (the headset), moving us beyond the mind into the emotion and imagination. This informs current innovative practices, including storytelling that fuses with psychiatry in medical school training programmes.[120]

For the second century Roman emperor and Stoic philosopher Marcus Aurelius the object of life was not to be on the side of the majority, but to escape into finding oneself in the ranks of the insane.[121] The importance of engaging with 'madness' and the transrational in relation to contemporary media and culture has been explained. In the preface to Fanon's *The Wretched of the Earth*, Jean Paul Sartre

---

[115] Ibid.

[116] Lucy Bannerman, 'Trans charity's chatroom for children condemned as irresponsible free-for-all', *The Times*, Saturday October 1, 2022, p. 27.

[117] Ibid.

[118] See the work of Richard Bentall discussed in detail in Chap. 1.

[119] '5 steps to mental wellbeing', https://www.nhs.uk/mental-health/self-help/guides-tools-and-activities/five-steps-to-mental-wellbeing/ (accessed 4 October, 2022).

[120] Dr. Ahmed Hankir's work at the Maudsley Hospital UK is noteworthy here.

[121] Marcus Aurelius, *Meditations*, trans. Martin Hammond (London: Penguin, 2009).

wrote he believed we were living in a time which would see the end of fetishes.[122] Sartre did attempt to move away from the fetishism of dualism. This book has identified how rationalism is more deified than ever, especially inhuman data. A move away from the confines of such a system is essential for our survival. An absolute reliance on transrational knowledge may lead to 'madness', but we are living in a time when the prerational, the rational, and the transrational can unify.[123] This is possible by moving beyond the binary, beyond dualism. 'Doctors in all ages have made fortunes by killing their patients by means of their cures. The difference in psychiatry is that it is the death of the soul.'[124]

While being aware of a naive optimism, we must move beyond a didacticism in 'madness' studies which often fixates on the dangers of a neutralizing of the patient via the clinical gaze in Foucault's sense. This takes us in the direction of Deleuze and Guattari and their concepts of subjectivity and assemblage.[125] Media and culture can function in a transrational fashion, optimistically deepening our sense of the human, going beyond the view in the film *Ran* (Akira Kurosawa, 1986) that in a 'mad' world only the 'mad' are sane. Concurrently, media is 'madness' and this includes the human 'madness' of desire to be the image, and the dominance of celebrity culture which ultimately dehumanizes. As the universe fills with enhanced image spam that is too good to be true the 'profane rapture of consumption' is held up before people.[126] These are the new virtual demons and angels of mystic speculation, hegemonically infiltrating the everyday, creating: bulimia, steroid overdose, and personal bankruptcy.[127]

Empire of Light (Sam Mendes, 2023) offers a powerfully optimistic take on 'madness'. Olivia Coleman plays Hilary, a woman who has just spent time in the local mental institution and is on lithium but feels this deadens her. During the film she compliantly goes back to the same mental institution then returns to work and is accepted, her 'madness' in some sense overcome. Working as the duty manager in a cinema in Margate, Hilary learns about the healing power of film through its transrational knowledge, an area previously discussed here. The film reveals that art will not be thwarted by the exploitation of the vulnerable, be this through racism or those with mental health problems. This is an acknowledgement of transrational knowledge. For Kant there are universal laws that relate to a rational being with a being equalling an end-in-itself.[128] The other has been positioned as starkly alone and different including woman as other as argued by Simone de Beauvoir; the 'mad';

---

[122] See Chap. 4.

[123] Richard Rohr (2013), op. cit., p. 116.

[124] Ibid.

[125] Adam Szymanski, *Cinemas of Therapeutic Activism – Depression and the Politics of Experience* (Amsterdam: Amsterdam University Press, 2021), p. 17.

[126] Hito Steyerl, *The Wretched of the Screen* (Berlin: Sternberg Press, 2009), pp. 161–167.

[127] Ibid.

[128] Kant Immanuel, *Groundwork of the Metaphysics of Morals*, trans. and ed. Mary Gregor (Cambridge: Cambridge University Press, 1997), p. 43.

the racial other as discussed in Chap. 4; or God as the Other following Levinasian philosophy. Positively, Jean-Luc Nancy moves from this Levinas's position of absolute otherness, bringing together Heideggerian Being with Levinas's totally separate otherness, so they are then under a co-essentiality.[129] Here Being and Being-with co-exists at the heart of existence, fulfilling an aim of this book to move beyond the restrictive binary of the rational, moving us within the transrational.

One aspect of modern character that distinguishes us is that suffering is viewed as unusual.[130] This is of course a good thing. We live longer and have many more ways to alleviate our suffering, drugs being one of them. But an evasion of suffering through all manner of normalized and abnormal behaviour is neurotic; 'a desired state is one of "wellness", a perfect peace of mind and body that is supposed to be not only sublime but normal. Suffering represents a kind of failure.'[131] Grief is good an example. There is a medicalization of experiences that previously were known as, 'non-negotiable aspects of being human'; the fourth edition of *The Diagnostic and Statistical Manual of Mental Disorders* excluded grief, but the fifth includes it.[132] While there could be pathological grief, so an inclusion of this nature makes sense, the argument that today the belief, 'our bodies and our minds can be optimised for maximum efficiency, achievement, happiness and ideological purity', making us akin to a new MacBook, or perfectible machines, is a strong one.[133]

At the same time pain is worn as a badge in victim culture and this is often pain caused by others using the wrong words, but what pain is it in reality? This is exacerbated by culture wars on social media which over-emphasises an agreed normality that is part of purification process; you are correct, or otherwise, which is an oversimplification tied to the dualism that needs overcoming. Our obsession with this purity is our new 'madness'. The worship of robots encapsulates this.[134] The problem here though is again still how 'madness' is perceived and felt. Often 'madness', like grief, is viewed as disease which can be caught, and we have seen how 'madness' is seen as a threat to the group. It is something, 'safest to steer clear of, the enduring sort of grief that, like all forms of madness, feels threatening, possibly even contagious.'[135]

The current culture wars can be considered in the context of how 'madness' is perceived and dealt with. Those who condemn 'snowflakes' for jumping on a victimhood bandwagon are dualistically reacting against the Oprahfication of society which turned everything, especially the media, into a form of therapy. Publicly externalising our personal victimhood is very different to internally dealing with

---

[129] Daniel Rugo, *Jean-Luc Nancy and the Thinking of Otherness* (London: Bloomsbury, 2013).
[130] James Marriott, 'If we want to live we have to suffer and weep,' *The Times*, July 29, 2021, p. 24.
[131] Ibid.
[132] Ibid.
[133] Ibid.
[134] Jason Lee, *Sex Robots – The Future of Desire* (London: Palgrave, 2017).
[135] Jonathan Franzen, *Freedom* (London: Fourth Estate), p. 579.

areas such as grief and can be counterproductive; if we are all a victim, then no one is. Drawing on evolutionary psychology, we need to recognise that the heart has its reasons too, 'but these are not the reasons of means-ends *reasoning*', given emotions are not about how to achieve an end, but also concern what to pursue in the first place.[136] In this sense feeling, the transrational, comes before the rational and, as established in Chap. 1 with reference to Richard Rohr, it contains the rational but is more than the rational. This larger question is often overlooked but can be framed as 'ecological rationality' or 'evolutionary rationality', because our emotions are innately designed to help us thrive.[137] If only we could draw more on this transrational knowledge, rather than relegating it.

Researchers from the Finnish Institute for Health and Welfare, drawing on 16,000 randomly selected residents of three major Finnish cities, found a strong correlation between visits to green spaces and lower odds of using mental health drugs. Compared with less than one weekly visit, those who visited three to four times weekly were associated with 33% lower odds of using mental health drugs.[138] Ecological warnings have been presented in significant films such as *Soylent Green* (Richard Fleischer, 1973) and *China Town* (Roman Polanski, 1974).[139] As explained, moving beyond a Descartean binary logic that has facilitated planetary devastation and mass destruction is critical is achieved by further engagement with the transrational. Overall, this concerns creating a sustainable and meaningful life.[140] Call it the spirit, the divine, the still small voice, an inner 'madness', it does not matter what you call it, if this guides us in service to life.[141] Through film, media, and culture we have repeatedly found non-binary transrational knowledge central to wellbeing and this approach includes reconciling oppositions. 'The religious faculty is the art of taking the opposites and binding them back together again', enabling us to move away from contradiction where we are, 'able to entertain simultaneously two contradictory notions and give them dignity'.[142] This book has stressed the inaccuracy of a prevailing Hegelian hangover which blindly accepts the formula: 'All that exists is rational, all that is rational exists', which feeds scientific determinism, materialism, and the idea of historical progress'.[143]

---

[136] Dylan Evans, *Emotion* (Oxford: Oxford University Press, 2003), p. 124.

[137] Ibid.

[138] Damien Gayle, 'Visiting green spaces deters mental health drug use, researchers find', *The Guardian*, 17 January, 2023, p. 12.

[139] Jason Lee, *Pervasive Perversion. Paedophilia and Child Sexual Abuse in Media/Culture* (London: Free Association Books, 2005), pp. 117–123.

[140] Anon., *Why We Rebel* (Extinction Rebellion, 2019) p. 10.

[141] Ibid.

[142] Robert A. Johnson, *Romantic Love as Shadow, Owning Your Own Shadow: Understanding the Dark Side of the Psyche* (San Francisco: Harper, 1991), pp.84–85. Think not only of uniting dualism, but also the three in one of the Trinity.

[143] Ralph Matlaw, intro. and trans., Fyodor Dostoevsky, *Notes from Underground & The Grand Inquisitor* (New York: E. Dutton & Co., 1960), p. xiii.

With such an emphasis on gender in many of chapters in this book it is right to close on Virginia Woolf, a central transgressive writer we began with. Commentary on her *A Room of One's Own* reveals how radically different her style was, and how hard it was for some critics in the establishment to accept she was breaking new ground. An unsigned review in the *Times Literary Supplement*, 31 October 1929, was generous, but noted the main 'path' of the essay was the spiritual and material elements necessary for female writers.[144] Some, like Vita Sackville-West in the *Listener*, 6 November 1929, highlighted how the work was neither novel nor pure criticism.[145] We can see from this how it transgressed boundaries and while remaining political it included transrational knowledge. Arnold Bennett, dismissively calling her imagination her 'fancy', claimed this is what made it digress too much. Later female critics then linked its subject and style, among them Winifred Holtby, Alix Fox, Annabel Robinson, Jane Marcus, Julie Robin Solomon, Hermione Lee, and Marion Shaw.[146] The work engaged unorthodox methods and a complex 'compendium' of various disciplines, and has been compared to John Dryden's *Of Dramatick Poesie* and Sir Philip Sidney's *Defence of Poetry*.[147] While many have situated this and other work by Woolf as the commencing period of foundational Modernism, my central point of emphasising her at this final juncture is to reveal how we can see her work has powerful transrational merits that discombobulated critics, especially male critics. Within this discourse it embodies the power of the transrational.

This work has explained what makes us human has been maligned, as if only the deified data-field is legitimate knowledge. We have seen how this data-field is not objective but is driven primarily by patriarchal and racist paradigms. The dangers of a data-field approach have been exposed in this volume through reinvigorating the transrational. German philosophers and sociologists Theodor Adorno and Max Horkheimer traced the origin of reification and alienation back to instrumental reason, that is, the will to technological domination, 'a priori to the whole of human history, but no longer rooted in any concrete historical formations'.[148] The totality is not capitalism, or even commodity production, given capitalism is the manifestation of instrumental reason.[149] Through a refocus on transrationalism there is an alternative to this false totality of reason. We commenced this analysis through an explanation of how the happiness industry has become the unhappiness industry and how false science and profit have driven this. We witnessed how imagination restores the balancthrough emotions which are part of the transrational and this has

[144]Christiane Bimberg, 'The Poetics of Conversation in Virginia Woolf's *A Room of One's Own:* Constructed Arbitrariness and Thoughtful Impressionism', *Connotations – A Journal of Critical Debate*, Vol. 11.1 (2001/2002), p. 24.

[145]Ibid.

[146]Ibid.

[147]Ibid.

[148]Slavoj Žižek, *Living in the End Times* (London: Verso, 2011), p. 205.

[149]Ibid.

been confirmed, ironically, through empirical psychological experiments. This moves us beyond the sociology of insanity, reinscribing the importance of narrative. Once this realm of the transrational is engaged with the endemic 'madness' due to blind rationalism is overcome. Through the unprescribed non a priori openness of transrational knowledge a deeper wellbeing is enabled.

References

Adler, Alfred. 2009. *Understanding Life. An Introduction to the Psychology of Alfred Adler*. London: Oneworld.

Adorno, Theodor. 2002. In *Aesthetic Theory*, eds. Gretel Adorno and Rolf Tiedemann, trans. Robert Hullot-Kentor. London: Continuum.

Al-Krenawi, A. 2005. Mental health practice in Arab countries. *Current Opinion in Psychiatry* 18 (5): 560–564.

Andrews, Kehinde. 2016. The psychosis of whiteness: The celluloid hallucinations of *Amazing Grace* and *Belle*. *Journal of Black Studies* 47 (5): 435–445.

Andrews, Sarah. 2019. *Creativity and Mental Health*, Media Discourse Centre seminar presentation, De Montfort University, March 10.

Anonymous. 1977. *The Bible*, Revised Standard Version. London: Collins.

———. 1990. *The New Jerusalem Bible*. London, Darton: Longman & Todd.

———. 2004. *BBC News Channel, Theatre attacks Sikh play protest*, 19 December, BBC NEWS | England | West Midlands | Theatre attacks Sikh play protest (accessed 26 January, 2023).

———. 2007. *The Bible*, New Living Translation. London: Tyndale House.

———. 2018. *NHS workforce statistics*, 28 October, NHS Workforce Statistics - July 2021 (Including selected provisional statistics for August 2021) - NHS Digital (accessed 26 January, 2023).

———. 2019a. *Why We Rebel. Extinction Rebellion*.

———. 2019b. Support for Central Americans. *Monitor on Psychology* 50 (9): 46–52.

———. 2021. BibleHub, https://biblehub.com (accessed 26 January, 2023).

———. 2022a. *Discrimination in mental health services*, 23 June, Discrimination in mental health services | Mind, the mental health charity - help for mental health problems (accessed 23 June, 2022).

———. 2022b. Woeful scarcity: NHS psychiatrist decries lack of mental health beds. *The Guardian*, April 24, 'Woeful scarcity': NHS psychiatrist decries lack of mental health beds | Mental health | The Guardian (accessed 26 January, 2023).

———. 2022c. Confessions of a junior doctor. *The Times Magazine*, August 13.

———. 2022d. *5 steps to mental wellbeing*, https://www.nhs.uk/mental-health/self-help/guides-tools-and-activities/five-steps-to-mental-wellbeing/ (accessed 26 January, 2023).

Armstrong, K. 1993. *The History of God*. New York: Alfred A. Knopf.

———. 2000. *Islam: A Short History*. London: Penguin.

———. 2001. *The Battle for God*. London: Ballantine Books.

———. 2009. *The Case for God*. New York: Knopf.

J. Lee, *Culture, Madness and Wellbeing*, https://doi.org/10.1007/978-3-031-37530-9

Aroyewun-Adekomaiya, K. 2017. *Representation of Mental Illness: An Examination of Movies and Professional Perspectives in Nigeria*, unpublished PhD, De Montfort University.
Attwood, Feona. 2021. *Sex on Stage: Rethinking the Sexual Vocabularies of Objectification*, Research Seminar, University of Northumbria, 5 May.
Aurelius, Marcus. 2009. *Meditations*, trans. Martin Hammond. London: Penguin.
Badious, Alain. 2012. *Ethics. An Essay on the Understanding of Evil*, trans. Peter Hallward. London: Verso.
Badley, Linda. 2022. *Lars von Trier Beyond Depression*. New York: Columbia University Press.
Bakhtin, M.M. 1982. *The Dialogic Imagination: Four Essays*, ed. Michael Holquist, trans. Caryl Emerson and Michael Holquist. Texas: University of Texas Press.
Ballard, J.G. 1986. *The Atrocity Exhibition*. London: Jonathan Cape.
Bannerman, Lucy. 2022. Trans charity's chatroom for children condemned as irresponsible free-for-all. *The Times*, 1 October, p. 5.
Barnes, Julian. 2012. *The Sense of an Ending*. London: Vintage.
Barthes, Roland. 1973. *Le Plaisir du Texte*. Paris: Éditions du Seuil.
———. 1990. S/Z. Trans. Richard Miller. London: Blackwell.
Bataille, Georges. 1991. *The Accursed Share*, Vol. 1. Trans. Robert Hurley. New York: Zone Books.
———. 1997. *Bataille: Critical Reader*, ed. Fred Botting. Oxford: Wiley.
———. 2012. *Literature and Evil*. Trans. Alastair Hamilton. London: Penguin.
Bateman, A. and Fonagy, P. 2019. *Mentalisation-treatment Training*. NHS training the Anna Freud Centre, July/October.
Baudrillard, J. 1990. *Fatal Strategies*. Trans. Philip Beitchman and W.G.J. Niesluchowski, ed. Jim Fleming. New York: Semiotext€.
———. 2005/2013. *The Intelligence of Evil – Or the Lucidity Pact*. Trans. Chris Turner. London: Bloomsbury.
Baudrillard, J. 2007. *Fragments. Cool Memories III, 1990–1995*. Trans. Emily Agar. London: Verso.
Baudrillard, J. 2013. *The Spirit of Terrorism*. New York: Verso.
Becker, Ernest. 1973. *The Denial of Death*. New York: Free Press.
Beddard, Ryne. 2017. 'Anselm's atonement theory – "Unmaking" The indebted man', *Religious Theory*, 3 January. Rethinking Anselm's Atonement Theory – "Unmaking" The Indebted Man (Ryne Beddard) – RELIGIOUS THEORY (jcrt.org) (accessed 22 March, 2021).
Bentall, Richard. 1992. A proposal to classify happiness as a mental disorder. *Journal of Medical Ethics* 18 (2): 94–98.
———. 2004. *Madness Explained – Psychosis and Human Nature*. London: Penguin.
Bergson, Henri. 1998. *The Creative Mind: An Introduction to Metaphysics*. London: Kensington Publishing Corps.
Berman, P. 2017. The Charles Manson Fallacy. *Tablet*, 20 November, p. 12.
Bernstein, Jerome. 2000. Listening in the borderlines. *The Salt Journal* 2 (2): 13–21.
Bhabha, Homi. 2009. *The Location of Culture*. London: Routledge.
Bhandar, Brenna, and Rafeef Ziadhah, eds. 2020. *Revolutionary Feminisms – Conversations on Collective Action and Radical Thought*. London: Verso.
Bimberg, Christiane. 2001/2002. The poetics of conversation in Virginia Woolf's *a room of one's own:* Constructed arbitrariness and thoughtful impressionism. *Connotations – A Journal of Critical Debate* 11(1):24.
Bishop, Claire. 2012. *Artificial Hells. Participatory Art and the Politics of Spectatorship*. London: Verso.
Blakely, Rhys. 2020. Why the path to enlightenment is an ego trip. *The Times*, 29 December, p. 1.
———. 2021. Ketamine on prescription at first psychedelic psychotherapy clinic. *The Times*, 27 February, p. 7.
———. 2022. Journals run fake Chinese science papers. *The Times*, 1 October, p. 5.

Blakemore, Sarah-Jayne. 2018. *Inventing Ourselves: The Secret Life of the Teenage Brain*. London: Doubleday.
Blatty, William. 1971. *The Exorcist*. New York: Harper & Row.
Bloom, Ursula. 1970. *Rosemary for Frinton*. London: Robert Hale.
Bly, Robert. 1997. *The Sibling Society*. London: Penguin.
Boddy, C., R. Ladyshewsky, and P. Galvin. 2010. Leaders without ethics in global business: Corporate psychopaths. *Journal of Public Affairs* 10 (3): 121–138.
Borman, Tracy. 2014. *Witches. James I and the English Witch-Hunts*. London: Vintage.
Boulter, A. 2007. *Writing Fiction: Creative and Critical Approaches*. London: Palgrave.
Bourdieu, Pierre, ed. 1999. *The Weight of the World: Social Suffering in Contemporary Society*. Stanford: Stanford University Press.
Braddick, Michael. 2008. *God's Fury, England's Fire – A New History of the English Civil Wars*. London: Allen Lane.
Bradshaw, P. 2008. *W* review – Dubya presidential biopic without dramatic fizz. *The Guardian* 7 November: 7.
Brand, Russell. 2007. *My Booky Wook*. London: Hodder & Stoughton.
Breggin, Peter. 1994. *Toxic Psychiatry: Why Therapy, Empathy and Love Must Replace the Drugs, Electroshock, and Biochemical Theories of the "New Psychiatry"*. New York: St. Martin's.
Brewster, Scott. 2018. Access denied: Memory and resistance in the contemporary ghost film. In *Uncanny Modernity – Cultural Theories, Modern Anxieties*, ed. Jo Collins and John Jervis, 112–127. New York: Palgrave.
Brindle, James. 2019. *New Dark Age: Technology and the End of the Future*. London: Verso.
Bronfen, E. 2008. Night and the uncanny. In *Uncanny Modernity – Cultural Theories, Modern Anxieties*, ed. Jo Collins and John Jervis. New York: Palgrave.
Brooke, Roger. 2015. *Jung and Phenomenology*. London: Routledge.
Brooks, Peter. 1991. The body in the field of vision. *Paragraph – A Journal of Modern Critical Theory* 14 (1): 46–67.
Broscome, S. 2017. What is Ignatian leadership? *Thinking Faith*, September 1. https://www.thinkingfaith.org/articles/what-ignatian-leadership (accessed 27January, 2023).
Bukowski, Charles. 2009. *Tales of Ordinary Madness*. London: Virgin.
Burke, Seán. 2008. *The Death and Return of the Author. Criticism and Subjectivity in Barthes, Foucault and Derrida*. Edinburgh: Edinburgh University Press.
Burston, Daniel. 1996. *The Wing of Madness. The Life and Work of R.D. Laing*. London: Harvard University Press.
Burton, Robert. 2003. *The Anatomy of Melancholy*. London: Penguin.
Butler, Judith. 1992. *Gender Trouble: Feminism and the Subversion of Identity*. London: Routledge.
Calkwell, T. 2004. Interview. In *Schrader on Schrader*, ed. K. Jackson, 71. London: Faber & Faber.
Campbell, Joseph. 1990. *The Hero's Journey*. London: HarperCollins.
———. 1993. *The Hero with a Thousand Faces*. London: Fontana.
Campbell, Gordon. 2021. The World's Favourite Bible – The remarkable story of the King James Version. *St Mary Magdalen Church research presentation*, Leicester, 25 October.
Camus, A. 1995a. *The Rebel*. London: Penguin.
———. 1995b. *Summer*. London: Penguin.
Camus, Albert. 2018. *Create Dangerously*. London: Penguin.
Caplan, Paula. 1996. *They Say You're Crazy – How the World's Most Powerful Psychiatrists Decide Who Is Normal*. London: Hachette Books.
Carbado, D.W. 2013. Colorblind intersectionality. *Signs* 38 (4): 811–845.
Carey, John. 2020. Review of Tom Stoppard by Hermione Lee. *The Times*, 4 October, p. 7.
Carmichael, S., D. Cooper, R.D. Laing, and H. Marcuse. 2015. *The Dialectics of Liberation*. London: Verso.
Carney, Ray, and Leonard Quart. 2000. *The Films of Mike Leigh – Embracing the World*. Cambridge: Cambridge University Press.

Cerny, C., S. Friedman, and D. Smith. 2014. Television's "crazy lady" trope: Female psychopathic traits, teaching and influence of popular culture. *Academic Psychiatry* 38 (2): 233–241.

Chambers-Cooper, B. 2022. *British Television Drama and Caribbean Families*, unpublished PhD, De Montfort University.

Charter, David. 2021. Assassination attempt that gave flawed security the bullet. *The Times*, 3 April, p. 12.

Chesterton, G.K. 2001. In *The Penguin Dictionary of Epigrams*, ed. M.J. Cohen. London: Penguin.

Chilcott, Rob. 2021. *Peter Whitehead Interview, Incomplete and Unpublished PhD*. De Montfort University.

Christie, I., and D. Thompson. 2003. *Scorsese on Scorsese*. London: Faber & Faber.

Clare, Anthony. 1989. *Psychiatry in Dissent – Controversial Issues in Thought and Practice*. London: Routledge.

Clay, R. 2019. Psychotherapy in China. *Monitor on Psychology* 50 (9): 27.

Cockerham, William. 2017. *Medical Sociology*. London: Routledge.

Cohen, J., J. Johnson, and P. Orr, eds. 2015. *Video and Filmmaking as Psychotherapy: Research and Practice*. London: Routledge.

Cohn, Norman. 1993. *The Pursuit of the Millennium: Revolutionary Millenarians and Mystical Anarchists of the Middle Ages*. London: Pimlico.

———. 2001. *Cosmos, Chaos, and the World to Come: The Ancient Roots of Apocalyptic Faith*. London: Yale University Press.

Colbrook, Claire. 2010. *Deleuze and the Meaning of Life*. London: Bloomsbury.

Conlin, J. 2019. The $10 billion business of self care. *LA Times*. 19 May. The $10-billion business of self-care - Los Angeles Times (latimes.com) (accessed 25 January, 2023).

Connolly, Angela M. 2009, review of Greg Singh's *Film after Jung: Post-Jungian approaches to film theory*. London: Routledge in *Journal of Analytical Psychology*, 2011, 56, 134–147.

Creed, B. 1998. *The Monstrous-Feminine: Film, Feminism, Psychoanalysis*. London: Routledge.

———. 2000. Kristeva, femininity, abjection. In *The Horror Reader*, ed. Ken Gelder, 64–70. London: Routledge.

Criado Perez, Caroline. 2019. *Invisible Women. Exposing Women Data Bias in a World Designed for Men*. London: Chatto & Windis.

Crowcroft, Andrew. 1977. *The Psychotic. Understanding Madness*. New York: Penguin.

Crystal, S., et al. 2016. Rapid growth of antipsychotic prescriptions for children who are publicly insured has ceased but concerns remain. *Health Affairs* 35 (6): 974–982.

Cupitt, Don. 1997. *After God*. London: Weidenfeld & Nicolson.

Curtis, Adam. 2002. The century of the self. *Episodes* 2: BBC 2.

De Luca, R. 2019. Dermatology as screenology: The films of Lynne Ramsay. *Film Criticism* 43: 1.

de Maupassant, Guy. 1973. *Pierre and Jean*. London: Penguin.

DeGruy Leary, J. 2005. *Post Traumatic Slave Syndrome. America's Legacy of Enduring Injury and Healing*. New York: Uptone Press.

Dein, S., and A.S. Illaiee. 2013. Jinn and mental health: Looking at jinn possession in modern psychiatric practice. *The Psychiatrist* 9: 290–293.

Deleuze, Gilles. 1989. *Cinema 2: The Time-Image*. Trans. Hugh Tomlinson and Robert Galeta. London: Continuum.

Deleuze, Gilles and Guattari, Félix. 2011. *A Thousand Plateaus – Capitalism and Schizophrenia*. Trans. Brian Massumi. London: Continuum.

Delgado, R., and J. Stefancic. 2017. *Critical Race Theory: An Introduction*. New York: New York University Press.

Derrida, J. 2001. *Writing and Difference*. London: Routledge.

———. 2009. *Specters of Marx*. London: Routledge.

Dickie, John. 2007. *Cosa Nostra: A History of the Sicilian Mafia*. London: Hodder & Stoughton.

———. 2020. *The Craft: How the Freemasons Made the Modern World*. London: Hodder & Stoughton.

Didion, Joan. 1979. *The White Album*. New York: Open Road.

Dostoevsky, Fyodor. 1960. *Notes from Underground & the Grand Inquisitor.* Trans. And Intro Ralph Matlaw. New York: E. Dutton & Co.
Droit-Volet, S., Fayolle, L. and Gil, S. 2011. Emotion and time perception: Effects of film-induced mood. *Frontiers in Integrative Neuroscience.* 9 August, Vol. 5, https://doi.org/10.3389/fnint.2011.00033 (accessed 27 January, 2023).
Dryden, Windy, and Rhena Branch, eds. 2011. *The CBT Handbook.* London: Sage.
du Maurier, Daphne. 1981. *Rebecca.* London: Pan.
Dunst, Alexander. 2016. *Madness in Cold War America.* London: Routledge.
Durek, Shaman. 2019. *Spirit Hacking: Shamanic Keys to Reclaim Your Personal Power, Transform Yourself and Light up the World.* California: Hay House.
Dyer, Wayne. 2006. *The Power of Intention,* 121. California: Hay House.
Eagleton, Terry. 2007. *The Meaning of Life.* Oxford: Oxford University Press.
———. 2009. *Trouble with Strangers: A Study of Ethics.* Oxford: Wiley-Blackwell.
Edgar, I.I. 1935. Shakespeare's psychopathological knowledge. *Journal of Abnormal and Social Psychology* 30: 71.
Egeci, I., and F. Gençöz. 2017. The use of cinematherapy in dealing with relationship problems. *The Arts in Psychotherapy* 53: 64–71.
Elliott, R., D. Shapiro, J. Firth-Cozens, W. Stiles, G. Hardy, S. Llewelyn, and F. Margison. 1994. Comprehensive process analysis of insight events in cognitive-behavioral and psychodynamic-interpersonal therapies. *Journal of Counseling Psychology* 41: 449–463.
Engdahl, F. W. 2016. *Shocking report from medical insiders.* NEO: New Eastern Outlook, 18 June, Shocking Report from Medical Insiders | New Eastern Outlook (journal-neo.org) (accessed 4 January 2022).
Engdahl, Jesse and Hosney, Jim. 1995/6. Review of kids. *Film Quarterly* 49(2):39–42.
Epicurus. 1996. *Being Happy.* London: Penguin.
Evanier, M., Patton C. and Blyberg, W. 1985. *The new DNAAgents.* California: Eclipse Comics, 4; 28: 11.
Evans, Dylan. 2001. *Emotion.* Oxford: Oxford University Press.
Fanon, Frantz. 1973. *Black Skin, White Mask.* London: Penguin.
Feilden, Tom. 2017. Most scientists 'can't replicate studies by their peers, *BBC News,* 22 February, Most scientists 'can't replicate studies by their peers' - BBC News (accessed 26 January, 2023).
Fenton, Natalie, et al. 2020. *The Media Manifesto.* Cambridge: Polity Press.
Feuerstein, Georg. 2006. *Holy Madness: The Shock Tactics and Radical Teachings of Crazy-Wise Adepts, Holy Fools, and Rascal Gurus.* London: Penguin.
Fleming, Michael, and Roger Manvell. 1986. *Images of Madness: Portrayal of Insanity in the Feature Film.* Vancouver: Fairleigh Dickinson University Press.
Fortier, Mark. 2004. *Theory/Theatre: An Introduction.* London: Routledge.
Foucault, Michel. 1978. *The History of Sexuality.* Trans. Robert Hurley. Paris: Gallimard.
———. 1989a. *The Archaeology of Knowledge.* London: Routledge.
———. 1989b. *Madness and Civilisation. A History of Insanity in the Age of Reason.* Trans. Richard Howard. London: Tavistock/Routledge.
Franzen, Jonathan. 2011. *Freedom.* London: Fourth Estate.
Freshwater, Helen. 2009. *Theatre and Audience.* London: Macmillan.
Freud, S. 1996. *New Introductory Lectures on Psychoanalysis.* Trans. James Strachey. London: Penguin.
Fromm, E. 1976. *To Have or To Be?* London: Routledge.
———. 1989. *The Fear of Freedom.* London: Routledge.
Furedi, F. 2001. How sociology imagined 'mixed race'. In *Rethinking 'Mixed Race',* ed. David Parker and Miri Song. London: Pluto.
———. 2004. *Therapy Culture: Cultivating Vulnerability in an Uncertain Age.* London: Routledge.
Gago, Verónica. 2020. *Feminist International – How to Change Everything,* trans. Liz Mason-Deese. London: Verso.

Garber, Marjorie. 2013. *Dream in Shakespeare. From Metaphor to Metamorphosis*. New Haven: Yale University Press.
Gask, L., M. Evans, and D. Kessler. 2013. Personality disorder. *British Medical Journal* 34 (7924): 28–32.
Gayle, Damien. 2023. Visiting green spaces deters mental health drug use, researchers find. *The Guardian* 17 January: 12.
Geddes, L. (2020). 'Psychedelic drug DMT to be trialled in UK to treat depression', *The Guardian*, 9 December, Psychedelic drug DMT to be trialled in UK to treat depression | Drugs | The Guardian (accessed 24 January, 2022).
Gendzier, I. 1979. *Frantz Fanon: A Critical Study*. New York: Pantheon.
Georges, Bataille. 2008. *The Accursed Share*. Vol. 1, trans. Robert Hurley. New York: Zone Books.
Ghaemi, Nassir. 2011. *A First-Rate Madness: Uncovering the Links Between Leadership and Mental Illness*. London: Penguin.
Gibson, Mel. 2010. 'Sick fictions: Contamination, disease, and addiction in accounts of young people's reading of comics. In *Cultures of Addiction*, ed. Jason Lee. New York: Cambria.
Gilroy, Paul. 2002. *There Ain't No Black in the Union Jack*. London: Routledge.
Ginsberg, Allen. 1955. *Howl and Other Poems*. San Francisco: City Lights.
———. 2001. *Spontaneous Mind. Selected Interviews 1958–1996*. ed. David Carter. New York: Perennial.
Girish, Devika. 2021. There's a blind spot about what America was. *Sight and Sound* 31 (4): 26–33.
Giroux, Henry A. 2009. *Zombie Politics and Culture in the Age of Casino Capitalism*. New York: Peter Lang.
Glasser, David, and S. Frosh. 1988. *Child Sexual Abuse*. London: Macmillan.
Goffman, Erving. 1991. *Asylums – Essays on the Social Situation of Mental Patients and Other Inmates*. London: Routledge.
González, J., and J. Torres. 2012. *News for All the People. The Epic Story of Race and the American Media*. London: Verso.
Gray, John. 2007. *Black Mass – Apocalyptic Religion and the Death of Utopia*. London: Farrar, Straus, and Giroux.
Greenberg, D.M., S. Baron-Cohen, N. Rosenberg, P. Fonagy, and P.J. Rentfrow. 2018. Elevated empathy in adults following childhood trauma. *PLoS One* 13: 10.
Greenwood, Tom. 2018. Procedural monsters: Rhetoric, commonplace and 'heroic madness' in Video Games. *Journal for Cultural Research* 22 (3): 310–324.
Greer, G. 1970. *The Female Eunuch*. London: MacGibbon & Kee.
———. 1986. *The Madwoman's Underclothes: Selected Journalism 1963–1985*. New York: Atlantic Grove.
———. 2019. *The Change: Woman, Ageing, and the Menopause*. London: Bloomsbury.
Grim, B., and M. Grim. 2016. The socio-economic contribution of religion to American society: An empirical analysis. *Interdisciplinary Journal of Research on Religion* 12: 1–31.
Hall, Martin, ed. 2022. *The Women of Woody Allen*. Amsterdam: Amsterdam University Press.
Hand, Sean. 2009. *Emmanuel Levinas*. London: Routledge.
Harewood, D. 2021. I came close to death. David Harewood on racism and psychosis. *The Guardian*, August 21. 'I came close to death': David Harewood on racism and psychosis | David Harewood | The Guardian.
Harley, Trevor A. 2021. *The Science of Consciousness. Waking, Sleeping and Dreaming*. Cambridge: Cambridge University Press.
Hart, David Bentley. 2021. *That All Shall Be Saved: Heaven, Hell, and Universal Salvation*. New Haven: Yale University Press.
Hassan, Stephen. 2019. *The Cult of Trump*. New York: Free Press.
Heidegger, Martin. 1977. *The Question Concerning Technology and Other Essays*, Trans. William Lovitt. New York: Harper and Row.
Hellman, M., and V. Rantala. 2012. Codependence, madness, and glamour. In *Cultures of Addiction*, ed. J. Lee. New York: Cambria.
Henriques, Richard. 2020. *From Crime to Crime. From Harold Shipman to Operation Midland. 17 Cases that Shocked the World*. London: Hodder & Stoughton.

High, M. 2014. *Taxi Driver* and veteran trauma. In *A Companion to Martin Scorsese*, ed. A. Baker. Oxford: Wiley.

Hoad, Phil. 2020. Madness in the movie: in defence of going gothic. *The Guardian*, 24 January, Madness in the movie: in defence of going gothic | Film | The Guardian (accessed 26 January, 2023).

Hobsbawm, Eric. 1991. *Age of Extremes. The Short Twentieth Century 1914–1991*. London: Abacus.

Homes, A.M. 1999. *Music for Torching*. London: Granta.

hooks, bell. 1996. *Reel to Real. Race, Sex and Class at the Movies*. London: Routledge.

Huggan, Graham. 2000. Ghost stories, bone flutes, cannibal countermemory. In *The Horror Reader*, ed. Ken Gelder. London: Routledge.

Hunter, E. 1997. Evan Hunter (Ed McBain) remembers with Hitchcock on *The Birds* and *Marnie* – the complete journal. *Sight and Sound* 7 (6): 26.

Huskinson, Lucy. 2021. Uncanny places. *The Psychologist*, Dec:40.

Immanuel, Kant. 1997. *Groundwork of the Metaphysics of Morals*, Trans. and ed. Mary Gregor. Cambridge: Cambridge University Press.

Irigaray, Luce. 2002. *The Way of Love*, Trans. Heidi Bostic and Stephen Pluháek. London: Continuum.

———. 2004. *Key Writings*. London and New York: Continuum.

———. 2007. *Je, Tu, Nous – Toward a Culture of Difference*. Trans. Alison Martin. London: Routledge.

Jackson, Joe. 2021. *Call for Submissions, ScreenWorlds*, April 26.

James, William. 1982. *The Varieties of Religious Experience: A Study in Human Nature*. London: Penguin.

James, E.L., A. Lau-Zhu, I.A. Clark, R.M. Visser, M.A. Hagenaars, and E.A. Holmes. 2016. The trauma film paradigm as an experimental psychopathology model of psychological trauma: Intrusive memories and beyond. *Clinical Psychology Review* 47: 106–142.

Jason, Lee. 1999. *The Metaphysics of Mass Art - Cultural Ontology*. Vol. II. New York: Mellen.

Jason, Lee. 2021. Facebook, paedophile hunters, and surveillance - mediated transnational abuse. *The Journal of New Media and Culture* 1 (1) http://ibiblio.org/nmediac/2021/facebook_Paedophile_Hunters.html. Accessed 17 July 2023.

Jay, Martin. 1994. *Downcast Eyes: The Denigration of Vision in Twentieth-Century French Thought*. Berkley: University of California Press.

———. 2017. *Reason After Its Eclipse. On Late Critical Theory*. Madison: University of Wisconsin.

Jenks, Chris. 1996. *Childhood*. London: Routledge.

———. 2003. *Transgression*. London: Routledge.

Jernigan, A. 2014. Paraliterary labors in Sylvia Plath's *The Bell Jar*. *Modern Fiction Studies* 60 (1): 1–27.

Johnson, R.A. 1991. *Romantic Love as Shadow, Owning Your Own Shadow: Understanding the Dark Side of the Psyche*. San Francisco: Harper.

Johnson, Malynnda, and Chris Olson, eds. 2021. *Normalizing Mental Illness and Neurodiversity in Entertainment Media: Quieting Madness*. New York: Routledge.

Jones, Amy. 2018. *Gender Differences in the Experience of Psychosis*, unpublished PhD, University of East London.

Josselson, R. 2020. *Narrative and Cultural Humility: Reflections from "The Good Witch" Teaching Psychotherapy in China*. Oxford: Oxford Scholarship Online.

Joyce, James. 1967. *Ulysses*. London: The Bodley Head.

Jung, C.G. 1932. *The Psychology of Kundalini Yoga: Notes of the Seminar Given in 1932 by C.G. Jung*. Princeton, NJ: Princeton University Press.

———. 1966. *The Practice of Psychotherapy*. Princeton, NJ: Princeton University Press.

———. 1970. *Mysterium Conjunctionis: An Inquiry into the Separation and Synthesis of Psychic Opposite in Alchemy*. Princeton: Princeton University Press.

———. 1971. *Psychological Reflections: A New Anthology of his Writings, 1905–1961*. London: Routledge and Keegan Paul.

———. 1977. *Psychology and the Occult*. London: Routledge.
———. 1986. Psychological reflections. In *An Anthology of the Writings of C.G. Jung*, ed. Jolande Jacobi. London: Routledge & Kegan Paul Ltd.
———. 1995. *Memories, Dreams, Reflections: An Autobiography*. London: Fontana.
———. 1998. *The Essential Jung*. London: Fontana.
———. 2006. *Psychological Types*. London: Routledge.
———. 2008. *Children's Dreams: Notes from the Seminar Given in 1936–1940*. Princeton, NJ: Princeton University Press.
Jung, C.G., M.-L. von Franz, J.L. Henderson, J. Jacobi, and A. Jaffé. 1968. *Man and his Symbols*. New York: Dell.
Kael, P. 1976. Underground man. *The New Yorker*, February 9, https://newyorker.com/magazine/1976/02/09/underground-man (accessed 06 January, 2022).
Karpf, A. 1988. *Doctoring the Media: The Reporting of Health and Medicine*. London: Routledge.
Keesler, M., and D. DeMatteo. 2017. How media exposure relates to laypersons' understanding of psychopathy. *Journal of Forensic Sciences* 62 (6): 1522–1533.
Kempley, Rita. 1995. "Review of kids". *The Washington Post*, August 25, available online, http://www.washingtonpost.com/wpsrv/style/longterm/movies/videos/kidsnrkempley_c029f5.htm (accessed 23 March, 2018).
Kendi, I.X. 2017. *Stamped from the Beginning. The Definitive History of Racist Ideas in America*. London: Bodley Head.
King, John. 2000. *Magical Reels. A History of Cinema in Latin America*. London: Verso.
Kirby, Terr. 2021. Video link to Bulger murder disputed. *The Independent*, November 26, 1993, Video link to Bulger murder disputed | The Independent | The Independent (accessed 9 April, 2021).
Knight, P. 2003. *Conspiracy Theories in American History*. New York: ABC Clio.
Knight, C. 2018. Review of *kids, National post.*
Knowles, Tom. 2021. Social media 'no worse than TV' for mental health of teenagers. *The Times*, May 5.
Koutsourakis, Angelos. 2011. *A Film Should Be Like a Stone in Your Shoe': A Brechtian Reading of Lars von Trier*, unpublished PhD, University of Sussex.
KS. 2017. Alter ego. In *1001 Video Games You Must Play Before You Die*, ed. Tony Mott. London: Cassell.
Kuberski, P. 2012. *Kubrick's Total Cinema. Philosophical Themes and Formal Qualities*. London: Bloomsbury.
Kubrick, Stanley. 2022. Words and movies. *Sight and sound 90 years anniversary special*, Summer, 32;6:67.
Kuhn, Annette, ed. 2013. *Little Madnesses: Winnicott, Transitional Phenomena, and Cultural Experience*. London: I.B. Tauris.
Kusters, Wouter. 2020. *A Philosophy of Madness – The Experience of Psychotic Thinking*. Trans. N. Forest-Flier. Cambridge, MA: Massachusetts Institute of Technology.
Laing, R.D. 1967. *The Politics of Experience and the Bird of Paradise*. London: Penguin.
———. 2015. The obvious. In *The Dialectics of Liberation*, ed. S. Carmichael, D. Cooper, R.D. Laing, and H. Marcuse, 19. London: Verson.
Laing, R.D., and A. Esterson. 1964. *Sanity, Madness, and the Family*. London: Pelican.
Laing, R.D., and Aaron Esterson. 1970. *Sanity, Madness and the Family: Families of Schizophrenics*. London: Pelican.
Laouar, N. 2019. *Ghosts Within Us: A Study of Women of Gothic Modernism*, unpublished PhD, Canterbury Christ Church University.
Lawrence, B. 1998. *Social Work and Mental Health*, Unpublished PhD, University of York.
Lay, Kat. 2022. Antidepressant use rises by a fifth. *The Times*, July 8.
Leader, Darian. 2011. *What is Madness?* London: Penguin.
Leary, Timothy. 1968. *The Politics of Ecstasy*. Berkeley: Ronin Publishing.

Lee, Jason. 2005. *Pervasive Perversions: Paedophile and Child Sexual Abuse in Media/Culture*. London: Free Association Books.
———. 2010a. *Dr Cipriano's Cell*. London: Chipmunka.
———. 2010b. *Celebrity, Pedophilia, and Ideology in American Culture*. New York: Cambria.
———, ed. 2010c. *Cultures of Addiction*. New York: Cambria.
———. 2011. *Unholy Days*. London: Roman.
———. 2012. The Zoo Keeper's strife: Will self's psychiatric fictions. *Philosophy and Literature* 36 (1): 196–208.
———. 2014. *The Psychology of Screenwriting*. London: Bloomsbury.
———. 2018a. *Sex Robots – The Future of Desire*. London: Palgrave.
———. 2018b. *Nazism and Neo-Nazism in Film and Media*. Amsterdam: Amsterdam University Press.
———. 2018c. Smile, Hitler? Nazism and Comedy in Popular Culture. In *Comedy and the Politics of Representation – Mocking the Weak*, ed. Helen Davies and Sarah Illott, 223–240. London: Palgrave.
———. 2018d. Are you kidding? Reassessing morality, sexuality and desire in *kids*. *Film International* 16 (3): 16–26.
Lee, Jason, and A.K.A.C.J.P. Lee. 1999a. *The Metaphysics of Mass Art – Cultural Ontology*. Vol. I. New York: Mellen.
———. 1999b. *The Metaphysics of Mass Art – Cultural Ontology*. Vol. II. New York: Mellen.
Leeson, P., and J. Russ. 2018. Witch trials. *The Economic Journal* 128 (613): 2066–2105.
Lehrer, Jonah. 2009. *The Decisive moment. How the Brain Makes Up Its Mind*. Edinburgh: Canongate.
Leiba, Patrick Anthony. 1997. *Caretakers and the Rights of the Insane: An Historical Sociology*, unpublished PhD, University of London.
Leistedt, S., and P. Linkowski. 2014. Psychopathy and the cinema: Fact or fiction? *Journal of Forensic Sciences* 59 (1): 167–174.
Lenormand, M. 2018. Winnicott's theory of playing: A reconsideration. *The International Journal of Psychoanalysis* 99 (1): 82–102.
Levinas, Emmanuel. 1991. *Totality and Infinity*. Trans. Alphonso Lingis. London: Kluwer Academic Publishers.
———. 1996. In *Basic Philosophical Writings*, ed. A.T. Peperzak, S. Critchley, and R. Bernasconi. Bloomington: Indiana University Press.
Lewis, H. 2020. *Difficult Women. A History of Feminism in 11 Fights*. London: Vintage.
Lewis, G. (2021). Interview. Dr Natalie Ashburner interviews Professor Glyn Lewis: Antidepressants (rcpsych.ac.uk) (accessed 22 December, 2021).
Lilienfeld, S. 1994. Conceptual problems in the assessment of psychopathy. *Clinical Psychology Review* 14 (1): 17–38.
Lloyd, Genevieve. 1995. *The Man of Reason. 'Male' & 'Female' in Western Philosophy*. London: Routledge.
Long, Camilla. 2021. It's not just rich for Samantha Cameron to claim she's a victim – it's genuinely harmful. *The Sunday Times*, May 9.
Macalister, Todd. 2008. *Einstein's God – A Way of Being Spiritual Without the Supernatural*. Berkeley: Apocryphile Press.
MacCulloch, Diamaid. 2004. *Reformation – Europe's House Divided (1490–1700)*. London: Penguin.
Macey, David. 2000. *Frantz Fanon: A Life*. London: Granta.
Macnab, G. 2006. *The Making of Taxi Driver*. New York: Unanimous.
Maitland, Sara. 2008. *A Book of Silence*. London: Granta.
Malabou, Catherine. 2020. Masks and symbols: In between paranoia and schizophrenia. *Portable Gray* 3 (2): 217–223.
Manning, C. 2020. Researching autism. *The Psychologist*, March 17.
Mantel, Hilary. 2005. *Beyond Black*. London: Fourth Estate.

Marcuse, Herbert. 1973. *Eros and Civilization*. London: Abacus.

Marriott, J. 2020. Why a closed mind is key to a happy life. *The Times*, September 3.

———. 2021. If we want to live we have to suffer and weep. *The Times*, July 29.

Marshall, R. 2009. *Witchcraft: The History and Mythology*. New York: Crescent Books.

Martin, Ian. 2020. Algorithmic decision making. *The Times*, 5 November.

Massumi, Brian. 2017. *The Principle of Unrest; Activist Philosophy in the Expanded Field*. Coventry: OHP.

Masters, Anthony. 1977. *Bedlam*. New York: Michael Joseph.

Masters, Brian. 1985. *Killing for Company: The Case of Dennis Nilsen*. London: Arrow.

McCollum, V. 2016. *Post-9/11 Heartland Horror: Rural Horror Films in an Error of Urban Terrorism*. London: Routledge.

McDonnell, John J. and Silver, Jon. 2009. 'Hollywood dominance: will it continue?' In *What is film? Change and Continuity in the 21st Century*, November 6–7, Turnbull Center, Portland, Oregon (Unpublished).

McEwan, Ian. 1997. *Enduring Love*. London: Jonathan Cape.

Meissner, W.W. 2009. *Ignatius of Loyola: The Psychology of a Saint*. New Haven: Yale University Press.

Mental Health Foundation. 2023. *Good mental health for all*, https://www.mentalhealth.org.uk (accessed 27 January, 2023).

Merleau-Ponty, M. 2004. *Phenomenology of Perception*. Trans. Chris Smith. London: Routledge.

Metz, Christian. 1977. *The Imaginary Signifier, Psychoanalysis and the Cinema*. Trans. Celia Britton et al. Bloomington: Indiana University Press.

Metzl, J. 2009. *The Protest Psychosis: How Schizophrenia Became a Black Disease*. Boston: Beacon Press.

Michael, Fleming, and Manvell Roger. 1985. *Images of Madness: Portrayal of Insanity in the Feature Film*. London and Toronto: Fairleigh Dickinson University Press.

Micks, David. 2020. *Stanley Kubrick – American Filmmaker*. New Haven: Yale University Press.

Mills, Tom. 2018. *The BBC: The Myth of a Public Service*. London: Verso.

Milton, John. 1989. *Paradise Lost*. London: Penguin.

Moi, Toril. 1989. Patriarchal thought and the drive for knowledge. In *New Directions in Psychoanalysis and Feminism*, ed. Teresa Brennan, 189–205. London: Routledge.

Moncrieff, J., Cooper, R.E., Stockmann, T. et al. 2002. The serotonin theory of depression: A systematic umbrella review of the evidence. *Molecular Psychiatry*, June, https://doi.org/10.1038/s41380-022-01661-0

Moriarty, Liane. 2016. *Truly Madly Guilty*. London: Penguin.

Morrison, Toni. 1987. *Beloved*. New York: Alfred A. Knopf.

Mortimer, B. 1997. Portraits of the postmodern person in *Taxi Driver*, *Raging Bull*, and *The King of Comedy*. *Journal of Film and Video* 49 (1–2): 29.

Morton, Adam. 2004. *On Evil*. London: Routledge.

Moss, Robert. 2012. *Dreaming the Soul Back Home: Shamanic Dreaming for Healing and Becoming Whole*. New York: New World.

Muldoon, Paul. 2001. *Poems 1968–1998*. London: Faber & Faber.

Mulkerrins, J. 2021. The extraordinary life of Senator Tammy Duckworth. *The Times Magazine*, April 14.

Mulvey, Laura. 1975. Visual pleasure and narrative cinema. *Screen* 6 (3): 6–18.

Murakami, Haruki. 2002. *Sputnik Sweetheart*. Trans. Philip Gabriel. London: Vintage.

Murch, Walter. 2021. *In the Blink Of An Eye – A Perspective on Film Editing*. Los Angeles: Silman-James Press.

Murphy, L. 2020. *Writers & Lovers* by Lily King review – A novel about writing a novel, *The Times*, May 29, 15.

Muteanu, A. 2016. The aesthetics of depression in the work of Lars von Trier. *Ethical Considerations on "Depression Trilogy"*, unpublished dissertation, University of Bergen.

Myles, P., and R. Shafran. 2015. *The CBT Handbook: A Comprehensive Guide*. London: Constable & Robinson.

Nancy, Jean-Luc. 1999. *The Gravity of Thought*. Trans. François Raffoul and Gregory Rocco. New York: Humanity Books.

Neil, William. 1996. *One Volume Bible Commentary*. London: Hodder & Stoughton.

Nigianni, C. 2010. Becoming-woman by *Breaking the Waves*. *New Formations: A Journal of Culture, Theory, Politics* 68: 120.

Noll, Richard. 1994. *The Jung Cult: Origins of a Charismatic Movement*. London: Touchstone.

O'Brien, Edna. 2012. *Country Girl*. London: Faber and Faber.

O'Brien, Maeve. 2017. *The Courage of Shutting-up: Decisions of Silence in the Work of Sylvia Plath*, unpublished PhD, University of Ulster.

Obama, Michelle. 2022. *The Light We Carry – Overcoming in Uncertain Times*. New York: Viking.

Olsen, Mark. 2019. *Midsommar* explained: The filmmakers unpack the sex, rituals and shocking ending, *Los Angeles Times*, July 3, 'Midsommar' explained: The filmmakers unpack the sex, rituals and shocking ending - Los Angeles Times (latimes.com) (accessed 25 January, 2023).

Ondaatje, Michael. 2008. *The Conversations: Walter Murch and the Art of Editing Film*. London: Bloomsbury.

Orwell, George. 1983. *Nineteen Eighty-four*. London: Penguin.

Owen, Alex. 2004. *The Place of Enchantment: British Occultism of the Modern*. Chicago: University of Chicago Press.

Pappacostas, Savvas. 2015. *Madness and Leadership: From Antiquity to the New Common Era*. Cheltenham: Edward Elgar Publishing.

———. 2017. *A bit of madness is good for leadership potential, Business Review*, London School of Economics. https://blogs.lse.ac.uk/businessreview/2017/09/04/a-bit-of-madness-is-good-for-leadership-potential (accessed 25 January, 2023).

Patton, Paul. 1996. *Deleuze: A Critical Reader*. London: Routledge.

Pfau, T. 2010. The letter of judgement: Practical reason in Aristotle, the Stoics, and Rousseau. *The Eighteenth Century* 51 (3): 289–316.

Pfau, Aleksandra. 2020. *Medieval Communities and the Mad – Narratives of Crime and Mental Illness in Late Medieval France*. Amsterdam: Amsterdam University Press.

Pfohl, Stephen. 1992. *Death at the Parasite Café. Social Science (Fictions) and the Postmodern*. London: Palgrave Macmillan.

Phelan, J.C., B.G. Link, A. Stueve, and B.A. Pescosolido. 2000. Public conceptions of mental illness 1950 to 1956: What is mental illness and is it to be feared? *Journal of Health and Social Behaviour* 41 (2): 188–207.

Phillips, J., and R. Potter. 2006. "Black skins and white masks": Postcolonial reflections on 'race', gender and second generation migration to the Caribbean. *Singapore Journal of Tropical Geography* 27 (3): 309–325.

Pick, Daniel. 1993. *War Machine: The Rationalisation of Slaughter in the Modern Age*. London: Yale University Press.

Pickens, Therí Alyce. 2019. *Black Madness :: Mad Blackness*. Durham, NC: Duke University Press.

Pinker, Stephen. 1995. *The Language Instinct: How the Mind Creates Language*. London: Penguin.

Plath, Sylvia. 2010. *The Bell Jar*. London: Faber & Faber.

Poidevin, Le, and Roboert. 2003. *Travels in Four Dimensions: The Enigmas of Space and Time*. Oxford: Oxford University Pres.

Porter, R. 1987/1996. *A Social History of Madness; Stories of the Insane*. London: Weidenfeld and Nicolson.

Powell, John. 2017. *Happiness is an Inside Job*. London: Kendall.

Price, S. 2013. *Worst-case Scenario? Governance, Mediation, and the Security Regime*. London: Bloomsbury.

Prince, Ron. 2018. OUT OF CONTROL Tom Townend/You were never really here. *British Cinematographer*, 7 May, *https://britishcinematographer.co.uk/tom-townend-you-were-never-really-here/* (accessed 15 July, 2022).
Prince Harry. 2023. *Spare*. New York: Random House.
Radeska, Tijana. 2019. "The Horror": A look inside the grueling madness of making apocalypse now, *Vintage News*, February 16.
Ralph, A. 2020. Puretech EndeavourRx video game therapy wins US approval. *The Times*, June 17.
Rancière, Jacques. 2011. *Mute Speech*. Trans. James Swenson. New York: Columbia University Press.
Regan, Jenny. 2018. *Improving representations of mental health on TV*, 19 January, Improving representations of mental health on TV | Mind, the mental health charity - help for mental health problems (accessed 26 January, 2023).
Ricaforte, Micaela. 2018. *Why do people of faith live longer*, Azusa Pacific University, June 26, https://www.apu.edu/articles/why-do-religious-people-live-longer/ (accessed 25 January, 2023).
Ridley, Matt. 2003. *Nature via Nurture: Genes, Experience, and What Makes us Human*. London: HarperCollins.
Roberts, R. and Itten, Theodor. 2021. Francis Huxley and the human condition. *The Psychologist*, May: 69.
Robinson, Paul. 1969. *The Freudian Left*. Wilhelm Reich, Gerza Roheim, Herbert Marcuse. New York: Harper and Row.
Rogers, A., and D. Pilgrim. 2010. *A Sociology of Mental Health and Illness*. Maidenhead: Open University Press.
Rohr, Richard. 2011. *Falling Upward: A Spirituality of the Two Halves of Life*. London: SPCK.
———. 2013. *Immortal Diamond – The Search for Our True Self*. London: SPCK.
———. 2019. *The University Christ*. London: SPCK.
Rojek, Chris. 2000. *Celebrity*. London: Reaktion.
Rosanoff, A., L. Handy, I. Plesset, and S. Brush. 1934. The etiology of so-called schizophrenic psychoses, with special reference to their occurrence in twins. *The American Journal of Psychiatry* 91: 247–286.
Rose, Jacqueline. 2013. *The Haunting of Sylvia Plath*. London: Virago.
Roth, P. 2007. *Everyman*. London: Vintage.
Roth, Martin, and Jerome Kroll. 1986. *The Reality of Mental Illness*. Cambridge: Cambridge University Press.
Rousselle, Duane. 2022. *Call for papers – Negative psychoanalysis: Nurturing negativity, death, and trauma*, ed. Julie Reshe & Duane Rousselle, January 21.
Rovito, Maria. 2020. Toward a new madwoman theory – Reckoning the pathologization of Sylvia Plath. *Journal of Literary and Cultural Disabilities Studies* 143 (3): 317–332.
Rugo, Daniel. 2013. *Jean-Luc Nancy and the Thinking of Otherness*. London: Bloomsbury.
Russ, S. 2015. In eds. A. Kaufman and J. Kaufman, *Animal Creativity and Innovation*. New York: Academic Press.
Said, Edward. 1994. *Culture and Imperialism*. London: Routledge.
Samaritans. 2021. *Latest Suicide Data*. Latest suicide data | Suicide facts and figures | Samaritans (accessed 30 January, 2023).
Sanghera, Sathnam. 2021. My relatives, the slave owners. *The Times Magazine*, May 1.
Schneider, Pat. 2003. *Writing Alone and with Others*. Oxford: Oxford University Press.
Scott Peck, M. 1990. *The Road Less Travelled: A New Psychology of Love, Traditional Values and Spiritual Growth*. London: Arrow Books.
Scott, Michael, and Stephen Stradling. 1992. *Counselling for Post-traumatic Stress Disorder*. London: Sage.
Scott, M., and S. Stradling. 1994. *Counselling for Post-traumatic Stress Disorder*. London: Sage.
Scrivener, C., et al (2021). Pandemic practice: Horror fans and morbidly curious individuals are more psychologically resilient during the COVID-19 pandemic, *Personality and Individual*

Differences, 161, 110397. Pandemic practice: Horror fans and morbidly curious individuals are more psychologically resilient during the COVID-19 pandemic - ScienceDirect (accessed 30 January, 2023).
Scull, Andrew. 1979. *Museums of Madness: The Social Organization of Insanity in Nineteen-century England*. London: Allen Lane.
Segal, R. 1996. *Jung*. Oxford: Oxford University Press.
———. 2004. *Myth: A Very Short Introduction*. Oxford: Oxford University Press.
Selden, R., P. Widdowson, and P. Brooker. 2013. *A Reader's Guide to Contemporary Literary Theory*. Harlow: Pearson Longman.
Self, Will. 1991. *The Quantity Theory of Insanity*. London: Penguin.
Sergeant, Jason. 1999. *Deathtripping. An illustrated history of the cinema of transgression.*
Shaviro, S. 1993. *The Cinematic Body*. Minneapolis: University of Minnesota Press.
Showalter, Elaine. 1985. *The Female Malady: Women, Madness and English Culture, 1830–1980*. London: Virago.
Sifferlin, Alexandra. 2018. Fewer high school students are having sex, *Time*, January 4, https://yahoo.com/news/fewer-high-school-students-having-180241040.html (accessed 26 January, 2023).
Simpson, Joe. 1998. *Touching the Void*. London: Vintage.
Smith, Andrew. 2009. Moon dust. In *Search of the Men Who Fell to Earth*. London: Bloomsbury.
Smith, P., and H. Bond. 1993. *Social Psychology Across Cultures: Analysis and Perspectives*. Hemel Hempstead: Harvester Wheatsheaf.
Snelson, T. 2021. From *In Two Minds* to MIND: The circulation of 'anti-psychiatry' in British film and television during the long 1960s. *History of the Human Sciences* 34 (5): 53–81.
Sobchack, V. 1991. Postmodern modes of ethnicity. In *Unspeakable Images: Ethnicity in American Cinema*, ed. Lester Friedman, 329–352. Urbana: University of Illinois Press.
Sontag, Susan. 1978. *Illness as Metaphor*. London: Penguin.
Spitzer, Jennifer. 2012. *Article Abstract*, unpublished, Transgressive Culture.
Stajic, Malden. 2015. *The best movies about INSANITY*, The best movies about INSANITY - IMDb (accessed 24 January, 2023).
Stam, Robert. 2000. *Film Theory: An Introduction*, 2000. Oxford: Blackwell.
Sterling, Bruce. 2016. *Preface to William Gibson, Burning Chrome*. London: Gollancz.
Stevens, Anthony. 1991. *On Jung*. London: Penguin.
———. 1994. *Jung*. Oxford: Oxford University Press.
———. 1996. *Private Myths: Dreams and Dreaming*. London: Penguin.
Steyerl, Hito. 2012. *The Wretched of the Screen*. Berlin: Sternberg.
Stock, Kathleen. 2021. *Material Girls – Why Reality Matters for Feminism*. London: Fleet.
Storr, Anthony. 1970. *Human Aggression*. London: Penguin.
———. 1991. *The Dynamics of Creation*. London: Penguin.
———. 1996. *Feet of Clay – Saints, Sinners, and Madmen: A Study of Gurus*. London: HarperCollins.
Strinati, Dominic. 1995. *An Introduction to Theories of Popular Culture*. London: Routledge.
Summers, M. 2010. 'Suitable care of the African when inflicted with insanity': Race, madness, and social order in comparative perspective. *Bulletin of the History of Medicine* 84 (1): 59.
Swain, Kelley. 2016. *The Naked Muse*. Scarborough: Valley Press.
Swallow, Michael. 1999. French cinema, audiences, and madness. *Essex Research Seminars*, September.
Sweet, Mathew. 2022. Thomas Newman in conversation. *BBC Radio 3*, Sound of Cinema, 16 April.
Szasz, Thomas. 1970. *Ideology and Insanity – Essays on the Psychiatric Dehumanization of Man*. New York Syracuse: University Press.
Szymanski, Adam. 2021. *Cinemas of Therapeutic Activism – Depression and the Politics of Experience*. Amsterdam: Amsterdam University Press.
Taylor, Elayne. 2000. Script comments. *Creative Screenwriting* 7 (1): 14–15.

Taylor, S. 2019. Pathological power: The danger of governments led by narcissists and psychopaths, *The Conversation*, September 19, https://theconversation.com/amp/pathological-power-the-danger-of-governments-led-by-narcissits-and-psychopaths-123118 (accessed January 25, 2023).

Thomas, Keith. 1978. *Religion and the Decline of Magic*. London: Penguin.

Thompson, Guy M. 1993. *The Death of Desire. An Existential Study of Sanity and Madness*. London: Routledge.

Titley, Gavin. 2019. *Racism and Media*. London: Sage.

Tolle, Ekchart. 2003. *Stillness Speaks. A Guide to Spiritual Enlightenment*. London: New World.

Townend, Tow. 2022 *New shoots: Visual storytelling masterclass* with Tom Townend, Shooting People.

Trotter, W. 1917. *Instincts of the Herd at Peace and War*. London: T. Fisher Unwin.

Trueth, M.J. 1994. Revisiting fluoxetine (Prozac) and suicidal preoccupations, *The Journal of Emergency Medicine*, September–October, 12;5:685–687.

Turda, Marius. 2007. Review of Harriet A. Washington, *Medical Apartheid: The Dark History of Medical Experimentation on Black Americans from Colonial Times to the Present* (New York: Doubleday, 2006), in *Social history of medicine*, October: 620–621.

Tuval-Mashiach, R., B.W. Patton, and C. Drebing. 2018. "When you make a movie, and you see your story there, you can hold it": Qualitative exploration of collaborative filmmaking a therapeutic tool for veterans. *Frontiers in Psychology* 9: 1954.

Twenge, Jean. 2015. Are mental health issues on the rise?. *Psychology Today*, October 12, Are Mental Health Issues On the Rise? | Psychology Today (accessed January 25, 2023).

van der Kolk, Bessel. 2014. *The Body Keeps the Score: Mind, Brain and Body in the Transformation of Trauma*. London: Penguin.

van Voren, Robert. 2016. Ending political abuse of psychiatry: Where we are at and what needs to be done. *British Journal of Psychology Bulletin* 40 (1): 30–33.

Vannoy Adams, Michael. 2004. *The Fantasy Principle. Psychoanalysis of the Imagination*. New York: Brunner-Routledge.

Vargas, R. A. 2022. Mother of Dahmer victim condemns Netflix series: 'I don't see how they can do that, *The Guardian*, October 10, Mother of Dahmer victim condemns Netflix series: 'I don't see how they can do that' | US news | The Guardian (accessed 11 October, 2022).

Walker, Shaun. 2013. Bolotnaya trial: Man sentenced to indefinite psychiatric treatment, *The Guardian*, October 8. Bolotnaya trial: man sentenced to indefinite psychiatric treatment | Russia | The Guardian (accessed 22 February, 2021).

Wark, McKenzie. 2019. *Capital is Dead: Is this Something Worse?* London: Verso.

Waugh, Evelyn. 1945. *Brideshead Revisited – The Sacred and Profane Memories of Captain Charles Ryder*. London: Penguin.

Wear, D. 2010. Review of *the protest psychosis: How schizophrenia became a black disease. The Journal of the American Medical Association* 303 (19): 1984.

Weaver, L. 2009. *Theatre and Audience*. London: Bloomsbury.

Webb, Jen. 2015. *Researching Creative Writing*. Suffolk: Creative Writing Studies.

Weber, Max. 2012. *The Protestant Ethic and the Spirit of Capitalism*. New York, NY: Start Publishing LLC.

Weil, Simone. 1992. *Gravity and Grace*. Trans. Emma Crawford and Mario von der Ruhr. London: Routledge.

Westover, Tara. 2018. *Educated*. New York: Windmill Books.

Wig, N. 1999. Mental health and spiritual values. A view from the East. *International Review of Psychiatry* 11 (2–3): 92–96.

Wilbur, Ken. 1995. *Sex, Ecology, Spirituality – The Spirit of Evolution*. Boulder, CO: Shambhala.

Wiley, Norbert. 2003. Emotion and film theory. *Studies in Symbolic Interaction* 26: 169–187.

Wilkinson, N., R. Ang, and D. Goh. 2008. Online video game therapy for mental health concerns: A review. *International Journal of Social Psychiatry* 54 (4): 370–382.

Williams, Melanie. 2017. *Female Stars of British Cinema. The Women in Question*. Edinburgh: Edinburgh University Press.

Winston, Nama. 2019. Inside the theory that Child's Play 3 motivated the murder of James Bulger, *MamaMia*, June 23, Inside the theory Child's Play motivated the murder of James Bulger. (mamamia.com.au) (accessed 9 April, 2021).

Wooden, I. M. 2019. *Review of Wayways Lives, Beautiful Experiments: Intimate Histories of Social Upheaval.* by Saidiya Hartman. New York: W. W. Norton. *Theatre Journal*, 71(4):537–538.

Woolley, B. 2002. *The Queen's Conjuror: The Life and Magic of Dr Dee*. London: HarperCollins.

Wurtzel, Elizabeth. 1994. *Prozac Nation*. New York: Riverhead.

Wyatt, S. Aldridge, S. Callaghan, D. Dyke, A. Moulin, L. 2019. Exploring mental health inpatient capacity across sustainability and transformation partnerships in England, *NHS Midlands and Lancashire*, Midlands and Lancashire Commissioning Support Unit: The Strategy Unit, November.

Young, Neil. 1975. *World on a String*. Reprise Records.

Young, Emma. 2022. Conspiracy theory' label does little to stop people from believing. *The Psychologist*, May:19.

Youngson, Robert. 1999. *The Madness of Prince Hamlet and Other Delusions*. London: Robinson Publishing.

Žižek, Slavoj. 2006. *How to Read Lacan*. London: Granta Books.

———. 2011. *Living in the End Times*. London: Verso.

Index

J. Lee, *Culture, Madness and Wellbeing*, https://doi.org/10.1007/978-3-031-37530-9

SPRINGER NATURE

GPSR Compliance

The European Union's (EU) General Product Safety Regulation (GPSR) is a set of rules that requires consumer products to be safe and our obligations to ensure this.

If you have any concerns about our products, you can contact us on ProductSafety@springernature.com

In case Publisher is established outside the EU, the EU authorized representative is:

Springer Nature Customer Service Center GmbH
Europaplatz 3
69115 Heidelberg, Germany

The manufacturer's authorised representative in the EU is Springer Nature Customer Service Centre GmbH, Europaplatz 3, 69115 Heidelberg, Germany. If you have any concerns regarding our products, please contact ProductSafety@springernature.com

Printed and bound by CPI Group (UK) Ltd, Croydon, CR0 4YY
28/09/2026
02224070-0007